VARCAROLIS'
Clinical Companion for Psychiatric Nursing
An Interprofessional Approach

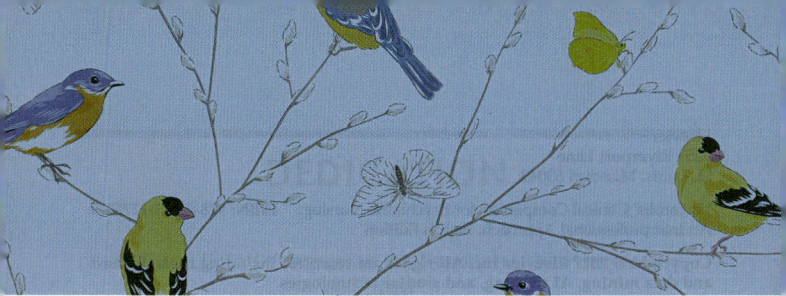

VARCAROLIS'
Clinical Companion for Psychiatric Nursing
An Interprofessional Approach

8TH EDITION

Margaret Jordan Halter, PhD, APRN
Editor, Foundations of Psychiatric–Mental Health Nursing,
    Essentials of Psychiatric-Mental Health Nursing
Former Clinical Nurse Specialist, Cleveland Clinic Akron
    General, Akron, Ohio
Former Faculty, Malone College, Canton, Ohio
University of Akron, Akron, Ohio
State University, Columbus, Ohio
Former Associate Dean, Ashland University, Mansfield,
    Ohio

**Christina A. Fratena, MSN, APRN, CNS-BC,
    PMHCNS-BC**
Clinical Nurse Specialist, SpringHaven Counseling
    Center, Dundee, Ohio
Faculty, Malone University, Canton, Ohio
University of Akron, Akron, Ohio
Former Clinical Nurse Specialist, Aultman Hospital,
    Canton, Ohio

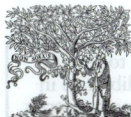

ELSEVIER

3251 Riverport Lane
St. Louis, Missouri 63043

DEDICATION

Varcarolis' Clinical Companion for Psychiatric Nursing: ISBN: 978-0-443-12759-5
An Interprofessional Approach, Eighth Edition

This Clinical Companion for Psychiatric Nursing is
dedicated to:

Those on the hard journey toward recovery.

The compassionate nursing students and dedicated
nurses who walk beside them.

Previous editions copyrighted 2023, 2019, 2015, 2011, 2006, 2004, and 2000.

Executive Content Strategist: Sonya Seigafuse
Senior Content Development Manager: Lisa P. Newton
Publishing Services Manager: Deepthi Unni
Senior Project Manager: Nayagi Anandan
Design Direction: Brian Salisbury

Printed in India

Last digit is the print number: 9   8   7   6   5   4   3   2   1

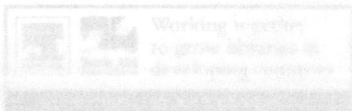

REVIEWERS

J'Andra Antisdel, MSN, RN-BC
Visiting Clinical Assistant Professor
Indiana University South Bend
South Bend, Indiana

Josephine M. Britanico, MSN, RN, PNP
Assistant Professor of Nursing
Borough of Manhattan Community College/
    City University of New York
New York City, New York

Debra Forbes, MSN, RN
Associate Professor of Nursing
Kirkwood Community College
Cedar Rapids, Iowa

Chris Paxos, PharmD, BCPP, BCPS, BCGP
Director of Pharmacotherapy
Professor of Pharmacy Practice
College of Pharmacy, Northeast Ohio Medical University
Rootstown, Ohio;
Associate Professor of Psychiatry
College of Medicine, Northeast Ohio Medical University
Rootstown, Ohio

PREFACE

As with previous editions, the eighth edition of the *Varcarolis' Clinical Companion for Psychiatric Nursing* supports students and practitioners in planning realistic, evidence-based, and individualized nursing care for their patients. This thoroughly updated edition of the *Clinical Companion* provides readers with a foundation for clinical work in contemporary psychiatric settings. The chapters are logically and intuitively arranged in five parts:

- Part I lays the foundation for care with essential psychiatric nursing concepts and tools, focusing on the nursing process, therapeutic relationships, and therapeutic communication.
- Part II delves into specific diagnostic groups, offering an overview of major disorders within these groups and providing guidelines for developing effective psychiatric nursing care.
- Part III addresses psychiatric crises, such as suicide and family violence, outlining the nursing process specific to managing these urgent situations.
- Part IV is devoted to pharmacological treatment modalities for psychiatric disorders, typically administered by advanced practice professionals such as psychiatric nurse practitioners and psychiatrists. This section covers pharmacotherapy with a focus on drug classifications, including antipsychotics and antidepressants.
- Part V explores nonpharmacological approaches to psychiatric care. This part includes a summary of psychological therapies, such as cognitive-behavioral therapy. The final chapter is devoted to other somatic approaches to psychiatric care that fall under the umbrella of neuromodulation. They include older treatments such as electroconvulsive therapy and new treatments such as vagus nerve stimulation.

The organization of the clinical chapters reflects the order of chapters in the *Diagnostic and Statistical Manual of Mental Disorders*, fifth edition, text revision (*DSM-5-TR*). Descriptions of the disorders are also aligned with *DSM-5-TR* criteria to ensure consistency in understanding and assessing symptoms of psychiatric conditions.

Classical references have been retained to provide foundational knowledge. Additionally, all citations have been updated throughout to reflect current research and best practices in psychiatric care.

The International Council of Nurses' nursing diagnosis classification system is the foundation for nursing diagnoses and outcomes. The *International Classification for Nursing Practice (ICNP)* uses logical, understandable, and interprofessional terminology to describe responses to psychiatric disorders.

ACKNOWLEDGMENTS

Thanks to our Elsevier colleagues for coordinating and completing another successful project! Kudos to Yvonne Alexopoulos, our former senior content strategist, for getting the ball rolling with this eighth edition. Sonya Seigafuse recently assumed the role of senior content strategist and has been a welcome addition. As always, cheers go out to Lisa Newton, our senior content development manager, who keeps us on track, responds to emails promptly, and sends positive greetings. A big thanks to Nayagi Anandan, our senior project manager, for meticulously pulling all the details together, ensuring consistency, and producing a reader-friendly edition.

In this eighth edition of the manual, we continue to incorporate standardized nursing diagnoses from the International Classification for Nursing Practice (ICNP). Developed and published by the International Council of Nurses (2019), an affiliate of the World Health Organization, the ICNP offers a comprehensive set of standardized terms that are logical, relevant, and align with terminology in other healthcare disciplines.

We are thrilled to welcome Chrissy Fratena back as a collaborator for this edition. Chrissy, a former student of Margaret Halter, approached her own psychiatric nursing rotation with remarkable enthusiasm and professionalism. Over the years, she gained graduate education in psychiatric nursing and extensive experience in both clinical practice and nursing education. Her expertise and unwavering passion for psychiatric nursing have added great depth and value to this edition.

This clinical companion is designed to be a valuable resource as you embark on the transformative journey of learning in the psychiatric setting. As you develop and apply your knowledge, compassion, and dedication, you will have a profound impact on the lives of your patients. In turn, the experience of helping others will enrich and shape your own path as a nursing professional.

Best wishes,
Margaret Jordan Halter
Christina A. Fratena

CONTENTS

CONTENTS

CHAPTER 1

The Nursing Process

The nursing process serves as a fundamental problem-solving process. It is the basic framework for nursing practice with patients who are experiencing psychiatric disorders or conditions. According to the National Council of State Boards of Nursing (NCSBN, 2023), it is characterized as both a scientific and clinical reasoning approach to patient care. It encompasses the following key stages:

- Assessment
- Analysis (diagnosis)
- Planning
- Implementation
- Evaluation

It is important to highlight that the NCSBN refers to the second step of the nursing process as "analysis" instead of the conventional term "diagnosis." This adjustment stems from the fact that standardized nursing diagnoses, as outlined by such groups as NANDA-I (Herdman et al., 2021), are not commonly used in clinical care. In this book, we will be using diagnosis based on a global standardized classification system.

In 2023 the NCSBN test plan, which is known as the National Council Licensure Examination for Registered Nurses (NCLEX-RN®), underwent an expansion of the nursing process. They did so by incorporating a model of clinical judgment officially called the NCSBN Clinical Judgment Measurement Model. The framework, developed by researchers, aims to assess clinical judgment and decision-making skills through standardized examination items/questions. Clinical judgment, defined as a multistep process involving observation, assessment, prioritization of concerns, and the generation of evidenced-based solutions for safe patient care, is integral to this model (NCSBN, 2023).

Psychiatric nursing care involves supporting individuals who are experiencing psychiatric disorders, commonly known as mental illness or mental disorders. The *Diagnostic and Statistical Manual of Mental Disorders* (DSM), published by the American Psychiatric Association (APA), serves as the official guide for categorizing psychiatric disorders in the United States. Offering standardized criteria, the DSM is a valuable resource for clinicians, researchers, insurance companies, pharmaceutical firms, and policymakers. Clinicians rely on this publication as a guide for planning care and assessing the effectiveness of patients' treatments.

Originally published in 1952, the present manual represents the fifth edition of the DSM, commonly referred to as the *DSM-5-TR* (APA, 2022). This book adopts the *DSM-5* framework for organizing clinical chapters and detailing information on psychiatric disorders.

Terms Used to Describe Care Recipients

You may notice variations in the terminology utilized by textbooks, instructors, and clinical staff when referring to individuals receiving nursing care. These differences arise from organizational preferences, professional beliefs, and even personal choices. "Client" is a common term often used in community-based or private practice settings, while "consumer of mental healthcare" is another frequently employed phrase in similar contexts.

Among healthcare professionals, "patient" is one of the most widely used terms. This noun typically denotes an individual requiring a higher level of care and undergoing treatment in an acute care setting. Although not all readers of this manual may have clinical experiences centered in acute care settings, for the sake of simplicity and uniformity, the term "patient" will be consistently used to denote the recipient of nursing care in this manual.

ASSESSMENT

The psychiatric–mental health registered nurse provides a unique and comprehensive assessment of the patient's health status that guides the plan of care. Assessment is both an essential initial activity and one that is ongoing throughout the course of care. The focus and type of information that is gathered are based on the patient's specific condition and by anticipating future needs.

Individuals with psychiatric disorders are encountered by nurses working in psychiatric units. However, symptoms such as depression, suicidal thoughts, anger, disorientation, delusions, and hallucinations are experienced by patients in all settings. These settings include medical-surgical, obstetrical, and intensive care units; outpatient care; extended-care facilities; emergency departments; and community centers. Psychiatric symptoms are not always the result of psychiatric disorders, and they may stem from chemical imbalances, substance use, and other disease processes.

The assessment phase of the nursing process has several primary goals. They are to:

- Establish rapport by creating a supportive and non-judgmental environment that fosters trust, open communication, and a sense of safety for the patient.
- Determine the chief complaint (i.e., the perception of the problem in the patient's own words).
- Review physical status and obtain baseline vital signs.
- Identify the impact of symptoms on the patient's life (e.g., self-esteem, loss of intimacy, role functioning, change in family dynamics, lifestyle change, and employment).
- Identify risk factors that may affect safety (e.g., confusion, suicidal ideation, or homicidal thoughts).
- Gather information related to previous illnesses, treatment, and hospitalizations.
- Identify psychosocial (i.e., psychological and social) aspects of the patient's life (e.g., family relationships, social patterns, interests and abilities, stress factors, substance use, social supports).

It may be helpful if the patient's support system (e.g., family members, friends, and relatives) participates during the data collection if possible and desirable to provide additional information. If law enforcement was involved in the admission, the nurse should gather details about the circumstances leading to police intervention to ensure a comprehensive understanding of the situation.

Past medical and psychiatric history can also supply valuable information. This is particularly important if the patient is experiencing psychosis, is withdrawn and mute, or is too agitated to provide an accurate history. Charts from previous hospitalizations or electronic medical records are extremely helpful. Laboratory reports also provide important information.

While not always practical from a time perspective or for brief encounters, a complete mental status examination may be conducted during the assessment phase of the nursing process. A patient-centered assessment is provided in Appendix A. This assessment not only provides a framework for a thorough mental status examination but also reinforces key terms and essential concepts.

Most healthcare facilities provide patient assessments in either paper or electronic format. While these tools are integral for gathering essential data, they can feel impersonal as question after question is asked. With practice, nurses may become proficient with a less formal approach to assessment by clarifying, focusing, and exploring information with the patient. This method allows patients to use their own words to express themselves and enables the nurse to observe a wide range of nonverbal behaviors. A unique style of interviewing congruent with the nurse's personality develops as comfort and experience increase. Box 1.1 presents areas that are typically evaluated during the assessment phase.

Issues for Which Referral May Be Indicated

Patients may be referred to other disciplines within the healthcare team, such as social services or occupational therapy, and might need further investigation when planning long-term care. This is especially important in the case of serious mental illness and if any of the following problems are present:

- Inadequacy of primary support (e.g., due to death, illness, divorce, sexual or physical abuse, neglect of a child, discord with siblings, birth of a sibling).
- Problems related to the social environment (e.g., death or loss of friends, inadequate social support, living alone, difficulty with acculturation, discrimination, life cycle transition such as retirement).
- Educational problems (e.g., illiteracy, academic concerns, conflict with teachers or classmates, inadequate school environment).
- Occupational problems (e.g., unemployment, job insecurity, stressful work schedule, difficult work conditions, job dissatisfaction, job change, conflict with boss or coworkers).
- Economic problems (e.g., poverty, inadequate finances, insufficient welfare support).

Box 1.1 **Common Assessment Areas**

Previous psychiatric treatment
Educational background
Occupational background
    Employed? Where? How long?
    Special skills?
Social patterns
    Describe family
    Describe friends
    With whom does the patient live?
    Describe a typical day
Sexual patterns
    Sexually active? Practices safe sex? Practices birth
      control?
    Sexual orientation
    Sexual difficulties
Interests and abilities
    What do you enjoy doing?
    What sport, hobby, or leisure activity does the patient
      enjoy?
Medications/substances
    What medication(s) does the patient take? How often?
      How much?
    What herbal or over-the-counter drug(s) does the
      patient take? How often? How much?
    Describe alcohol use: How often? How much? Last use?
    What recreational drugs does the patient take or use?
      How often? How much? Last use?
    Does the patient identify the use of drugs as a problem?
Coping abilities
    What does the patient do when upset?
    To whom can the patient talk?
    What usually helps to relieve stress?

- Barriers to healthcare access (e.g., inadequate services, lack of available transportation to healthcare facilities, inadequate health insurance).
- Interaction with the legal system or crime (e.g., arrest, incarceration, litigation, victim of crime).

Cultural and Social Assessment

Healthcare providers in the United States engage with an ever-growing culturally diverse population. Providing effective care necessitates an awareness of and appreciation for an individual's cultural background. All healthcare professionals, especially mental health professionals, need to continually expand their knowledge and understanding of the complexity of the cultural and social factors that influence health and illness. It is especially important to broaden one's understanding of how health and illness are influenced by cultural and social factors.

Spiritual and Religious Assessment

The importance of spirituality and religious beliefs is an often-overlooked element of patient care. Spirituality and religious beliefs have the potential to exert an influence on how people understand meaning and purpose in their lives and how they use critical judgment to solve problems. Box 1.2 offers suggestions for gathering information to better adapt a plan of care to an individual patient's needs.

After the Assessment

Following the initial assessment, it proves beneficial to recap and discuss the gathered data with the patient. This summary not only assures patients that their concerns have been heard but also provides an opportunity for them to correct any potential misunderstandings.

It is crucial to inform the patient about the next steps. For instance, in a hospital setting, the nurse should outline upcoming meetings with other clinicians.

After conducting the initial assessment, the nurse informs the patient when and how often they will meet. If the nurse thinks a referral is necessary (e.g., a psychiatrist or advanced practice nurse, social worker, or medical personnel), this is also discussed with the patient.

Non–English-Speaking Patients

In 2019 nearly 22% of the US population did not speak English at home (US Census Bureau, 2022). The most frequently spoken languages other than English are:

- Spanish (61.6%)
- Chinese (5.2%)
- Tagalog (2.1%)
- Vietnamese (2.3%)
- Arabic (1.9%)

Box 1.2 Brief Cultural, Social, and Spiritual and Religious Assessment

Cultural Assessment

Language

What is your primary spoken language?

How would you rate your ability to speak and understand English?

Would you like an interpreter?

Communication style

Observe nonverbal communication (e.g., gestures, posture, eye movement)

What are your feelings about touch?

Observe how much eye contact the patient is comfortable with.

How much or little do people make eye contact in your culture?

Family unit

Describe the members of your family.

Who makes the decisions in your family?

Which family members can you confide in?

Health and illness beliefs

When you become ill, what is the first thing you do to take care of the illness?

How is this illness viewed by your culture?

Are there special practices within your culture that address your healthcare problem?

Are there any restrictions on diet or medical interventions within your cultural beliefs?

What are the attitudes of mental illness in your culture?

Who do you go to when you are medically ill?

Are there special practices within your culture that address psychiatric conditions?

Social Supports

Are there people outside the family, such as friends and neighbors, that you are close to and feel comfortable confiding in?

Is there a place where you can go for support (e.g., church, school, work, club)?

Spirituality and Religion

What importance does spirituality or religion have in your life?

Do your spiritual or religious beliefs relate to your healthcare? How?

Does your faith help in stressful situations? How?

Would you like to have a spiritual advisor or religious leader visit?

Who or what supplies you with strength and hope?

If a nurse does not speak the patient's language, data gathering may be inaccurate and incomplete, not to mention impossible. The Americans with Disabilities Act of 1990 has established federal standards to ensure that communication barriers do not impede equal access to healthcare for everyone.

All healthcare organizations must provide language interpreters, interpreters trained in sign language, telecommunication relay services for the deaf, closed-caption decoders for televisions, and amplifiers on phones. Translators are made available to provide written information in the patient's language.

Family members, friends, or neighbors are often used to communicate in emergency medical situations. However, using nonprofessional interpreters may have significant drawbacks. For example, a family interpreter might want to protect the patient and filter out information given to the patient. Conversely, the family member might want to filter out information to the healthcare provider. Using a professional interpreter reduces the risk of wrong procedures, medication errors, and other adverse events.

The following guidelines are recommended when working with an interpreter:
- Address the patient directly rather than speaking to the interpreter.
- Maintain eye contact with the patient to ensure patient involvement and strengthen personal connection.
- Avoid interrupting the patient and interpreter.
- Ask the interpreter to give you verbatim translations.
- Avoid using technical medical terms the interpreter or the patient might not understand.
- Avoid talking or commenting to the interpreter at length. The patient might feel left out and distrustful.
- Ask for permission to discuss intimate or emotionally charged topics first and prepare the interpreter for the content of the interview.
- Arrange for the interpreter and the patient to meet each other ahead of time, if possible, to establish some rapport.
- Aim for consistency by using the same interpreter for subsequent interactions.

There are occasions when an interpreter may not be readily available. In such situations, auxiliary tools such as picture charts or flash cards can prove valuable in facilitating communication between the nurse and the patient. These aids are particularly helpful in conveying essential basic information about the patient's immediate needs, such as indicating the degree of pain or addressing toileting needs.

Occasionally, patients with limited English proficiency may appear agreeable or nod affirmatively, either influenced by cultural norms or a desire to be helpful, even when they may not fully comprehend. To ensure accurate communication, it is beneficial to pose questions that require more than a simple "yes" or "no" response. This approach allows for a more comprehensive understanding of the patient's level of comprehension and ensures clarity in communication.

DIAGNOSIS

After conducting a thorough assessment, psychiatric-mental health registered nurses carefully analyze the gathered data to identify patient problems and potential concerns. It is noteworthy that the term "patient" in this context can be substituted with the words "family," "group," or "community," broadening the scope of analysis beyond the individual patient.

Nursing diagnoses identify unmet needs that are within the nurse's domain to treat. In this book, we use the diagnoses provided by the *International Classification for Nursing Practice* developed by the International Council of Nurses (2019). This classification system is a part of the World Health Organization family of classifications. It offers a standardized set of terms that are logical, useful, and consistent with other healthcare disciplines.

A well-chosen and well-stated nursing diagnosis is the basis for selecting therapeutic goals and interventions. A nursing diagnosis is usually composed of the problem, probable cause, and supporting evidence.

An example of a nursing diagnosis is the *risk for self-mutilation*. In this case, the nurse identified several characteristics during the assessment that indicate that the patient is at increased risk for this behavior.

Related Factors (Probable Cause)

The probable cause is linked to the nursing diagnosis with the term *related to*. This term identifies factors that contribute to or are related to the development or maintenance of a patient problem. The probable cause tells us what needs to be addressed to bring about change and identifies what needs to be targeted through nursing interventions. In the case of potential for self-mutilation, the addition of a second part of the patient problem results in:

Risk for self-mutilation related to anxiety.

This statement indicates that the nurse and healthcare team will initiate interventions that reduce the patient's anxiety. Anxiety can also be improved by increasing the patient's ability to express tensions verbally rather than act them out physically.

Consider the difference in a plan of care for someone with the same nursing diagnosis but with a different probable cause. For example, *risk for self-mutilation related to command hallucinations* indicates that the individual is experiencing auditory hallucinations instructing them to engage in self-harm. In this case, the self-mutilation (e.g., cutting) may relieve the anxiety brought on by the voices. Interventions will again be aimed at decreasing the patient's anxiety by finding a calmer environment or offering an as-needed medication. Teaching distraction techniques such as reading out loud, talking with others, engaging in an activity, and singing lightly may also be useful.

Defining Characteristics (Supporting Evidence)

Nursing diagnoses draw support from two fundamental types of data—signs and symptoms. Signs encompass objective and observable information, including manifestations like a rash, slumped posture, or hyperactivity. On the other hand, symptoms involve subjective reports provided by the patient, such as expressions like "I'm tired" or "I feel nervous."

Both types of data become the defining characteristics that are linked to the diagnosis and probable cause by the words *as evidenced by*. Supporting data that validate the diagnosis of *risk for self-mutilation related to anxiety* include:

- *Fresh cuts on forearms*
- *Scars on forearms*
- *"I cut myself to calm down."*

Types of Nursing Diagnoses

Problem-Focused Statements

For problem-focused statements, the nurse makes a judgment about a human response to a health condition or life process. An example of a problem-focused statement is:

Anxiety related to losing employment and financial burdens.

Risk Statements

Statements identifying potential problems highlight vulnerabilities that bear a heightened likelihood of leading to negative outcomes. Nursing diagnoses falling into this category encompass preventable occurrences like falls, self-injury, pressure ulcers, and infections.

This type of nursing diagnosis always begins with the phrase "risk for" followed by supporting evidence. Because the problem has not yet occurred, there is no probable cause (i.e., related to). An example of a potential problem statement is:

Risk for injury as evidenced by extreme agitation, hyperactivity, less than 2 hours rest at night, poor skin turgor, and abrasions on hands and arms.

Health Promotion Diagnosis

A health promotion diagnosis facilitates the progression of an individual, family, or community from a particular level of wellness to a higher state of well-being. Similar to risk statements, health promotion diagnoses do not necessitate a related factor. Instead, the defining characteristics serve as indicators of the individual's motivation to enhance their current state of health. For instance, "Readiness for effective coping" is evident when a person expresses sentiments like "Alcohol is ruining my life" and declares a willingness to explore alternative strategies for managing anxiety.

OUTCOMES

Outcomes are patient centered (e.g., "the patient will") and are written in positive terms. As a basis for evaluation, overall outcomes are formulated to reverse the problem stated in the nursing diagnosis. In the case of a patient with impaired coping, an overall outcome would be for the patient to demonstrate improved coping.

Outcome criteria are ideal outcomes that reflect the maximum level of health that the patient can realistically achieve through nursing interventions. In this clinical companion, overall desired outcome criteria are provided.

Short-term and long-term goals are steps toward the overall outcome(s). These goals are stated in behavioral and measurable terms and might have time factors such as "in 1 week," "by discharge," or "within 2 days." The goals are evaluated and revised as the patient progresses or does not progress. The amount of time needed to attain some of these goals will vary.

A patient with bipolar disorder in a manic phase may be extremely agitated. In this case, the nursing diagnosis may be:

Risk for injury as evidenced by hyperactivity, less than 2 hours rest at night, and poor skin turgor.

The overall outcome of this diagnosis is a reversal of the problem, that is, the patient will be free from injury.

Possible long-term goals and associated short-term goals might include the following:
1. The patient will return to pre-mania level of activity.
   a. The patient will spend 10 minutes in a quiet, non-stimulating area with a nurse each hour during the day (by time/date).
   b. The patient will engage in short 1:1 exchanges with the nurse while walking (by time/date).
2. The patient will sleep 6 to 8 hours per night within 1 week.
   a. The patient will sleep 3 to 4 hours per night with the aid of medication (by time/date).
   b. The patient will identify the connection between sleep loss and mania (by date).
3. The patient will maintain a sufficient daily fluid intake by (date).
   a. The patient will drink a total of 9 cups (females) or 12 cups (males) of liquids (e.g., water, juice, milk, or milkshakes) a day (by date).
   b. The patient's skin turgor will be within normal limits within 24 hours, as evidenced by the raised area disappearing in less than 4 seconds when the skin over the sternum is pinched and released.

PLANNING

On concluding an assessment and formulating nursing diagnoses, the next step involves prioritizing the identified problems. Maslow's hierarchy of needs serves as a valuable framework for this process (Fig. 1.1). Prioritization begins with addressing four deficiency needs required for basic survival. They include physiological needs, safety needs, love/belonging, and self-esteem. Four additional higher-order needs are referred to as growth needs. They are cognitive, esthetic, self-actualization, and transcendence (i.e., spiritual needs).

For each problem statement, the formulation of desired outcomes is followed by the selection of interventions aimed at achieving these outcomes. The nurse considers

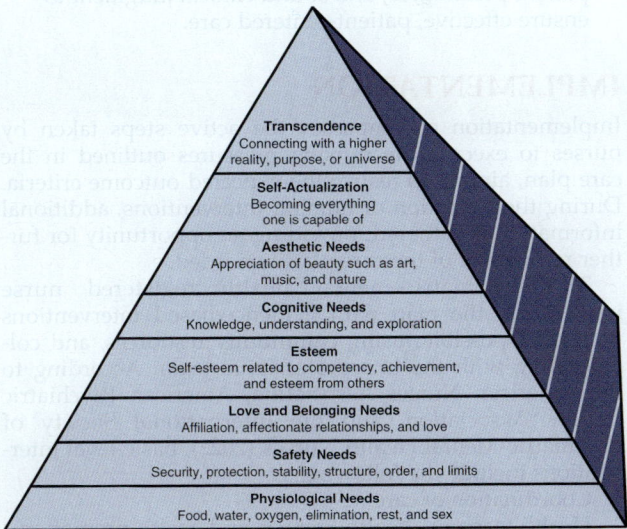

Transcendence
Connecting with a higher reality, purpose, or universe

Self-Actualization
Becoming everything one is capable of

Aesthetic Needs
Appreciation of beauty such as art, music, and nature

Cognitive Needs
Knowledge, understanding, and exploration

Esteem
Self-esteem related to competency, achievement, and esteem from others

Love and Belonging Needs
Affiliation, affectionate relationships, and love

Safety Needs
Security, protection, stability, structure, order, and limits

Physiological Needs
Food, water, oxygen, elimination, rest, and sex

Fig. 1.1 Maslow's hierarchy of needs. (Adapted from Maslow, A. H. [1954]. *Motivation and personality*, Harper and Row; Maslow, A. H. [1970]. *Motivation and personality*. Harper & Row; and Maslow, A. H. [1970]. *Religions, values, and peak experiences*. Penguin. https://www.worldcat.org/title/farther-reaches-of-human-nature/oclc/205658.)

the following specific principles when planning interventions:

- *Safe:* Interventions promote safety for the patient, as well as for other patients, staff, and family.
- *Compatible and appropriate:* Interventions are compatible with other therapies and with the patient's personal goals and cultural values, as well as with institutional rules.
- *Realistic and individualized:* Interventions are (1) within the patient's capabilities, given the patient's age, physical strength, condition, and willingness to change, (2) based on the availability of support staff, (3) reflective of the actual available community resources, and (4) within the student's or nurse's capabilities.
- *Evidence based:* Interventions should be grounded in the best available scientific evidence and clinical expertise. Evidence-based practice integrates research findings, patient preferences, and sound clinical judgment to ensure effective, patient-centered care.

IMPLEMENTATION

Implementation encompasses the active steps taken by nurses to execute the nursing measures outlined in the care plan, aiming to realize the expected outcome criteria. During the execution of nursing interventions, additional information is gathered, providing an opportunity for further refinement of the care plan as needed.

The psychiatric–mental health registered nurse implements the plan with evidence-based interventions whenever possible, using community resources, and collaborating with the interprofessional team. According to the American Nurses Association, American Psychiatric Nurses Association, and the International Society of Psychiatric-Mental Health Nurses (2022), basic-level interventions include the following:

1. Coordination of care
2. Health teaching, health literacy, and health promotion
3. Pharmacological/biological therapies
4. Complementary/integrative therapies
5. Milieu therapy
6. Therapeutic relationship

In addition to these six interventions, psychiatric–mental health advanced practice registered nurses are qualified to provide three higher-level interventions:

1. Consultation
2. Pharmacological/biological therapies and prescriptive authority
3. Psychotherapy

EVALUATION

Evaluation is an ongoing process that includes evaluating the effectiveness of plans and strategies and documenting the results. Desired outcome evaluation occurs in the context of the entire plan of care and represents a comprehensive approach to determining the success of the plan.

In addition to addressing the success of desired outcomes, nursing students may evaluate long-term and short-term goals. These goals can have three possible outcomes: The goal is met, not met, or partially met. Consider a previous example of a nursing diagnosis:

Risk for injury as evidenced by hyperactivity, less than 2 hours rest at night, poor skin turgor, and abrasions on hands and arms.

Evaluation of short-term goals might be documented as follows:

1. The patient will spend 10 minutes in a quiet, nonstimulating area with a nurse each hour during the day.

   Goal partially met: After 2 days, the patient continues restless and purposeless pacing and is only able to stay quiet with the nurse for 4 to 6 minutes per hour.

2. The patient will sleep 3 to 4 hours at night with the aid of medication (by time/date).

   Goal met: Within three nights, the patient was able to sleep 4.5 hours with the aid of a short-term benzodiazepine.

3. The patient will drink 8 oz of fluid (e.g., juice, milk, milkshake) every hour.

   Goal met: Patient takes frequent sips of fluid provided in cups with lids equaling 8 oz an hour during the hours of 9:00 a.m. to 4:00 p.m., with reminders from nursing staff.

4. The patient's skin turgor will be within normal limits within 24 hours, as evidenced by the raised area disappearing in less than 4 seconds when the skin over the sternum is gathered and released.

   Goal not met: At 8:00 a.m., the patient's skin turgor is still poor. The raised area from gathered skin over the sternum disappeared 4 seconds after release.

Evaluate the need for increasing daytime fluids from 9:00 a.m. to 9:00 p.m.

IN THE CHAPTERS THAT FOLLOW

This clinical reference guide is designed to assist nursing students in crafting a patient-centered plan of care. Parts II and III delve into specific *DSM-5* (APA, 2022) psychiatric disorders and psychiatric crises that may necessitate nursing interventions. Each disorder or phenomenon is accompanied by the presentation of common plans of care. For every nursing diagnosis, suggested outcomes are provided, along with specific nursing assessments and actions, supported by detailed rationales. Students have the flexibility to choose interventions suitable for their patients and make modifications as needed to address the unique needs of each individual.

The remaining chapters provide information to support nursing care through an overview of medical treatment modalities. Part IV is devoted to pharmacotherapy such as antidepressants and antianxiety agents. Part V focuses on nonpharmacological approaches such as psychotherapy (i.e., talk therapy) and neuromodulation.

CHAPTER 2

Therapeutic Relationships

Psychiatric–mental health nursing is based on principles of *science*. Knowledge of anatomy, physiology, and chemistry is the basis for providing safe and effective biological treatments. Knowledge of pharmacotherapy—a medication's mechanism of action, indications for use, and adverse effects based on evidence-based studies and trials—is vital to nursing practice. However, the caring relationship and the development of the interpersonal skills needed to enhance and maintain such a relationship make up the *art* of psychiatric nursing. This art comes to life through the therapeutic relationship where caring and healing can occur.

NURSE-PATIENT RELATIONSHIP

The nurse-patient relationship is the basis of all psychiatric–mental health nursing treatment approaches, regardless of the specific goals. We all have distinct gifts—unique personality traits and talents—that we can learn to use creatively to form positive bonds with others. The use of these gifts to promote healing in others is referred to as the *therapeutic use of self*. A positive therapeutic alliance, which is collaborative and respectful, is one of the best predictors of positive outcomes in therapy (Gordon & Beresin, 2016).

Talk Therapy

Basic-level psychiatric–mental health nurses use counseling techniques in the context of the therapeutic relationship. Counseling is a supportive face-to-face process that helps individuals to problem solve, resolve personal conflicts, and feel supported. Education and learning are also included under the counseling umbrella.

A formalized approach to talk therapy that is based on theoretical models is called *psychotherapy*. Healthcare providers with advanced training, such as psychiatric–mental health advanced practice registered nurses, psychiatrists, social workers, counselors, and psychologists, are licensed to practice psychotherapy. Evidence suggests that psychotherapy within a therapeutic partnership actually changes brain chemistry in much the same way as medication. Thus the best treatment for most psychiatric disorders is a combination of medication and psychotherapy.

Goals and Functions

A therapeutic nurse-patient relationship has specific goals and functions, including the following:
- Facilitating communication of thoughts and feelings.
- Assisting with problem-solving to help facilitate activities of daily living.
- Exploring self-defeating behaviors and testing alternative behaviors.
- Promoting self-care and independence.
- Providing education about medications and symptom management.
- Promoting recovery.

PERSONAL VERSUS THERAPEUTIC RELATIONSHIPS

Throughout life, we meet people in a variety of settings and share a variety of experiences. With some individuals, we develop long-term relationships. With others, the relationship lasts only a short time. Naturally, the kinds of relationships we develop vary from person to person and from situation to situation.

Personal Relationships

A personal or social relationship is an association that is initiated for the purpose of friendship, socialization, enjoyment, or accomplishment of a task. Mutual needs are met during social interaction. People may give advice and sometimes help meet basic needs such as lending money. During social interactions, roles may shift. For example, one day you may be the listener, and one day you may be listened to. Within a personal relationship, there is little emphasis on the evaluation of the interaction, although we sometimes reflect on what we have said or done. In the following example, notice the casual friend–like tone of the nurse:

Patient: "Oh, I just hate to be alone. It's getting me down, and sometimes it hurts so much."

Nurse: "I know how you feel. I don't like being alone either. Getting on Instagram might help you feel less alone, it does me." (In this nontherapeutic response, the nurse is minimizing the patient's feelings and giving advice prematurely.)

Therapeutic Relationships

In a therapeutic relationship, the nurse uses effective communication skills, knowledge of human behavior, and personal strengths to support and foster the patient's growth. Patients more easily engage in the relationship when the clinicians address their concerns, respect patients as partners in decision-making, and use straightforward language. The focus of the relationship is on the patient's ideas, experiences, and feelings. Together, the nurse and the patient identify areas that need exploration and periodically evaluate the degree of the patient's progress.

Although the nurse may take on a variety of roles (e.g., educator, counselor, socializing agent), the relationship is consistently focused on the patient's problem and needs. The nurse's needs are met outside the relationship.

Nursing students have the opportunity to develop therapeutic nurse-patient relationships with the support of both clinical faculty and nursing staff. This clinical supervision is a mentoring relationship characterized by feedback and evaluation. Typically, students experience a gradual increase in autonomy and responsibility.

Like staff nurses, nursing students may struggle with the boundaries between personal and therapeutic relationships because there is a fine line between the two. Students often feel more comfortable being a friend because it is a more familiar role, especially with patients close to their age. When this occurs, students need to make it clear to themselves and the patient that the relationship is a therapeutic one.

A therapeutic relationship does not require that the nurse is unfriendly. Talking about everyday topics such as television, weather, and children's photos is acceptable. Additionally, a small amount of self-disclosure on the

Professional Sexual Misconduct

The least common and most extreme form of boundary violation is professional sexual misconduct, which can be physical or verbal. It may include sexual gestures, physical contact, and expressions of feelings or thoughts that a patient could reasonably interpret as sexual. This breach of trust often leads to malpractice claims, loss of licensure, and reputational harm. Sexual misconduct must be reported to both the institution and the board of nursing.

Transference and Countertransference

Roles may be blurred in the nurse-patient relationship due to unrecognized transference or countertransference. These concepts originated from Sigmund Freud who believed that patients unconsciously displace (transfer) feelings and behaviors related to significant others in the patient's past. The individual from the past is usually an authority figure since healthcare providers are also in a position of authority. Transference may be positive or negative. If the patient is motivated to work with you, then the transference may be positive. Negative transference may result in intense feelings that impede the nurse-patient relationship.

Countertransference occurs when the nurse consciously or unconsciously allows personal experiences, feelings, or personal issues to interfere with a therapeutic relationship. For example, a nurse whose childhood was damaged by her father's alcohol use disorder may transfer those negative feelings toward a patient with the same disorder. Self-awareness is crucial in addressing these feelings.

When Values and Beliefs Do Not Match

Nurses must recognize that personal values and beliefs are not universal. It is essential to understand that:
1. Our values and beliefs stem from our own culture or subculture.
2. They are shaped by a range of choices.
3. We adopt them based on a variety of influences and role models.

Our values and beliefs guide us in making decisions and taking actions that we hope will make our lives meaningful, rewarding, and fulfilled.

Working with other people whose values and beliefs are different can be a challenge. Topics that cause controversy in society in general—including political ideology, religion, gender roles, abortion, war, drugs, alcohol, and sex—also can cause conflict between nurses and patients. What happens when the nurse's values and beliefs are different from those of a patient? Consider the following examples of possible conflicts:

- A patient plans to have an abortion, conflicting with the nurse's belief that life begins at conception.
- A nurse values cleanliness, while the patient believes that showering more than once a week wastes water and harms the environment.
- A nurse, who strongly supports feminism and women's rights, feels frustrated when a female patient defers to her husband's judgment.

Self-awareness supports patient-centered care and requires that we understand what we value and the beliefs that guide our behavior. Being self-aware helps us to accept the uniqueness and differences of others.

PEPLAU'S NURSE-PATIENT RELATIONSHIP

Hildegard Peplau introduced the concept of the nurse-patient relationship in 1952 in her groundbreaking book *Interpersonal Relations in Nursing*. This model of nurse-patient relationship is well-accepted as an important tool for all nursing practice. A professional nurse-patient relationship consists of a nurse who has skills and expertise and a patient who wants to feel better again, understands the illness and its treatment alternatives, alleviates suffering, finds solutions to problems, and improves the quality of life.

Peplau (1999) described the nurse-patient relationship as evolving through three distinct and overlapping phases. An additional preorientation phase, during which the nurse prepares for the orientation phase, is also included:

1. Preorientation phase
2. Orientation phase
3. Working phase
4. Termination phase

Most likely, you will not have time to experience all the phases of the nurse-patient relationship in your often brief psychiatric–mental health nursing rotation. However, it is important to be aware of these phases to recognize, practice, and use them later.

Preorientation Phase

The preorientation phase begins with preparing for your assignment. The patient chart is a rich source of information, including mental and physical evaluations, progress notes, and patient orders. You will probably be required to research your patient's condition, learn about prescribed medications, and understand laboratory results. Staff may be available to share more anecdotal information or provide tips on how to best interact with your patient.

Before meeting the patient, it is essential to recognize your thoughts and feelings. Self-awareness helps ensure that personal beliefs do not interfere with providing unbiased, patient-centered care.

Nursing students usually have many concerns and experience anxiety, especially on their first clinical day. These concerns include being afraid of those with psychiatric problems, of saying the wrong thing, and of not knowing what to do in response to certain patient behaviors. Table 2.1 identifies patient behaviors and gives examples of possible reactions and suggested responses.

Experienced faculty and staff monitor the unit atmosphere and have a sense of behaviors that indicate escalating tension. They are trained in crisis interventions, and formal security is often available on-site to support the staff. Your instructor will set the ground rules for safety during the first clinical day. These rules may include not going into a patient's room alone, staying where others are around in an open area, and reporting signs (i.e., what you observe) and symptoms (i.e., what a patient says) of escalating anxiety.

Orientation Phase

The orientation phase is the first time the nurse and the patient meet. Specific tasks of the orientation phase follow.

Introductions

The first task of the orientation phase is introductions. The patient needs to know about the nurse (i.e., who the nurse

Table 2.1 **Patient Behaviors, Possible Reactions, and Useful Responses**

If the patient threatens suicide

The nurse assesses whether the patient has a plan and the lethality of the plan. The nurse tells the patient that this is serious, that the nurse does not want harm to come to the patient, and that this information needs to be shared with other staff.

The nurse and patient can then discuss the thoughts, feelings, and circumstances that led up to suicidal thoughts.

If the patient asks the nurse to keep a secret

The nurse cannot make this promise. The information may be important to the health or safety of the patient or others:

"I cannot make that promise. It might be important for me to share it with other staff."

If the patient asks the nurse personal questions

The nurse may or may not answer the patient's query. The nurse may choose to answer a simple question with a brief response and then refocus on the patient. For example, "Yes, I have been enjoying nursing school. Let's talk about what is happening with your housing situation."

If the patient makes sexual advances

The nurse sets clear limits and boundaries: "I'm not comfortable with [name the behavior]. This is a professional relationship. We will focus on your problems and concerns."

The nurse might leave to give the patient time to reflect and gain control, saying: say: "I am going to leave for a bit. I'll be back at [time] to check on how you're doing."

If the patient cries

The nurse should stay with the patient and let the patient know that it is all right to cry.

"You are upset about your brother's death."

"What are you thinking right now?"

If the patient does not want to talk

The nurse might spend short, frequent periods (e.g., 5 minutes) with the patient throughout the day: "Our 5 minutes is up. I'll be back at 10 a.m. and stay with you 5 more minutes."

This approach helps the patient recognize the nurse as reliable and consistent while also providing time for the patient to feel less threatened and more comfortable.

If the patient gives the nurse a gift

Many organizations have guidelines regarding gift acceptance. In general

- If the gift is expensive or involves money, the only response is to graciously refuse.
- If the gift is inexpensive, it may be appropriate to graciously accept, particularly toward the end of the treatment period.
- If you are in doubt, consult a supervisor or ethics committee for guidance.

(Continued)

Table 2.1 Patient Behaviors, Possible Reactions, and Useful Responses–cont'd

If a patient interrupts a conversation with another patient
Maintain a focus on the original patient. This demonstrates that the session is important: "I am with Mr. Duff for the next 20 minutes. At 10 a.m. we can talk."

is and the nurse's background) and the purpose of the meetings. For example, a student might supply the following information:

Student: "Hello, Ms. Chang. My name is Ethan Jacobs, and I am a registered nursing student from Fairlawn University. I am currently in my psychiatric rotation and I will be here for the next six Thursdays. I would like to spend time with you during your stay. I'm here as a support person for you as you work toward your treatment goals."

Knowing what the patient would like to be called is also essential—names and titles are meaningful to most people. In the previous example, the student begins with a formal greeting of Ms. Chang. After reading the patient's identification band out loud, "Dorothy Chang," the student should ask, "What would you like to be called?" This approach demonstrates respect, promotes rapport, and ensures the patient feels acknowledged in a way that is comfortable for them.

Establishing Rapport

A major emphasis during the first few encounters with the patient is on providing an atmosphere in which trust and understanding, or rapport, can grow. As in any relationship, you can nurture rapport by demonstrating genuineness, empathy, and unconditional positive regard. Being consistent, helping in problem-solving, and providing support are also essential aspects of establishing and maintaining rapport.

Specifying a Contract

A contract, either stated, written, or both, contains the place, time, date, and duration of the meetings. Termination of the relationship is also discussed during the orientation phase.

Confidentiality

The patient has a right to know (1) who else will be given shared information and (2) that the information may be shared with specific people such as a clinical supervisor, the healthcare provider, the staff, or students in clinical conferences. The patient also needs to know that the information will not be shared with relatives, friends, or others outside the treatment team, except in extreme situations. Extreme situations include child or elder abuse and threats of self-harm or harm to others.

Working Phase

A strong working relationship allows the patient to safely experience increased levels of anxiety and recognize dysfunctional responses. New and more adaptive coping behaviors can be practiced within the context of the working phase.

A major focus of the working phase is on recognizing ineffective ways of coping and replacing them with healthier methods of coping. Sometimes the patient's coping methods were developed to survive in a chaotic and dysfunctional family environment. Although coping methods may have worked for the patient at an earlier age, they may now interfere with the patient's healthy functioning and interpersonal relationships.

Another important aspect of this working relationship is patient education. To facilitate this education, become familiar with biological factors (e.g., genetic, biochemical) and psychological factors (e.g., cognitive distortions, learned helplessness) that contribute to psychiatric disorders. Understanding medications, laboratory work and results, and other treatments is also essential. This knowledge enables nurses to educate patients effectively, empowering them to an active role in their own care and recovery.

Termination Phase

The termination phase is the final phase of the nurse-patient relationship. Termination may occur when the patient is discharged, when the student's clinical rotation ends, or another time based on the student's learning needs and the patient's wishes to continue meeting. The tasks of termination include the following:

- Summarizing the goals and objectives achieved.
- Reviewing education and providing written material.
- Discussing ways for the patient to incorporate new coping strategies into daily life.
- Identifying follow-up after discharge.

If a nurse senses that the patient is reluctant to be discharged, it is important to address this reluctance. A general question—such as "How do you feel about being discharged?"—may provide the opening necessary for the patient to describe feelings and fears.

Part of the termination process is to discuss the patient's plans for the future. If the termination is the result of a discharge, part of these plans has usually been discussed by the psychiatrist or advanced practice provider, including follow-up care and referrals. Registered nurses generally reinforce those plans and emphasize understanding of medications and recognizing when symptoms are increasing. Self-help groups can also be encouraged.

FACTORS THAT PROMOTE A PATIENT'S GROWTH

Personal characteristics of the nurse that promote change and growth in patients are (1) genuineness, (2) empathy, and (3) positive regard. These are some of the intangibles that are at the heart of the art of nursing and patient-centered care.

Genuineness

Genuineness refers to the nurse's ability to be open, honest, and authentic in interactions with patients. Being genuine is a key ingredient in building trust. When a person is genuine, others get the sense that what is displayed on the outside of the person is congruent with who the person is on the inside. Nurses convey genuineness by listening to and communicating clearly with patients.

Empathy

Empathy occurs when the helping person attempts to understand the world from the patient's perspective. This understanding is in contrast to sympathy, which involves feeling pity or sorrow for others. Although these are considered nurturing human traits, they may not be particularly useful in a therapeutic relationship.

The following examples clarify the distinction between empathy and sympathy. A friend tells you that her mother was just diagnosed with inoperable cancer. Your friend then begins to cry and pounds the table with her fist.

Sympathetic response: "I feel so bad for you *(tearing up)*. I know how close you are to your mom. She is such an amazing person. Oh, I am so sorry." (You hug your friend.)

Empathetic response: "This must be devastating for you *(silence)*. It must seem so unfair. What thoughts and feelings are you having?" (You stay with your friend and listen.)

Empathy is not a technique but rather an attitude that conveys respect, acceptance, and validation of the patient's strengths. Empathy may be one of the most important qualities that a psychiatric–mental health nurse can possess.

Positive Regard

Positive regard is the ability to view another person as inherently worthy of care and respect, recognizing their strengths and potential for growth. It is primarily conveyed through attitudes and actions rather than words alone.

Attitudes

One way to convey positive regard, or respect, is having a positive attitude about working with the patient. The nurse takes the patient and the relationship seriously. The experience is viewed not as "a job," or "part of a course," but as an opportunity to work with patients to help them develop personal resources and actualize more of their potential in living.

Actions

Some actions that manifest positive regard are attending, suspending value judgments, and helping patients develop resources.

Attending. Attending is a special kind of listening that refers to an intensity of presence or being with the patient. At times, simply being with another person during a painful time can make a difference.

Suspending Value Judgments. As previously discussed, everyone has values and beliefs. Using our personal value system to judge patients' thoughts, feelings, or behaviors is not helpful or productive. For example, if a patient is using drugs or is involved in risky sexual behavior, the nurse recognizes that these behaviors are unhealthy. Rather than labeling these activities as good or bad, the nurse helps the patient explore the thoughts and feelings that influence this behavior. Judgment on the part of the nurse will most likely interfere with further exploration.

The first steps in eliminating judgmental thinking and behaviors are to (1) recognize their presence, (2) identify how or where you learned these responses, and (3) construct alternative ways to view the patient's thinking and behavior. Denying judgmental thinking will only compound the problem.

Helping Patients to Develop Resources. Encouraging patient independence is essential for fostering problem-solving skills, building support networks, and planning for the future. The nurse's role is to support—not take over—the responsibilities that belong to the patient. Consistently encouraging patients to use their own resources reduces feelings of helplessness and dependency. It also validates their ability to bring about change and practice self-advocacy with confidence.

CHAPTER 3

Therapeutic Communication

Humans have an innate need to relate to others. Our advanced ability to communicate with others gives substance and meaning to our lives. Every action, word, and facial expression convey meaning to others—we cannot *not* communicate. Even silence carries meaning and may convey acceptance, anger, or thoughtfulness.

Strong communication is the foundation for happy and productive relationships. On the other hand, ineffective communication can lead to misunderstandings, increased anxiety, and negative emotions. In healthcare settings, poor communication may also contribute to serious errors that impact patient safety.

In the provision of nursing care, communication takes on a new emphasis. Goal-directed and scientifically based communication is referred to as *therapeutic communication*. Therapeutic communication is central to the formation of patient-centered therapeutic relationships. *Patient-centered* refers to the patient as a full partner in care whose values, preferences, and needs are respected. Examples of patient-centered care include:
- Determining levels of pain in a postoperative patient
- Listening as parents express feelings of fear concerning their child's diagnosis
- Understanding, without words, the needs of an intubated patient in the intensive care unit

These are all essential skills in providing quality nursing care.

Ideally, therapeutic communication is a professional ability you learned and practiced early in your nursing education. In psychiatric-mental health nursing, communication skills take on a deeper and more nuanced role. Psychiatric disorders can manifest with physical symptoms (e.g., fatigue, loss of appetite, insomnia) as well as emotional symptoms (e.g., sadness, anger, hopelessness,

---

Box 3.1 Saying the Wrong Thing

Nursing students are often concerned that they may say the wrong thing, especially when learning to apply therapeutic techniques. Will you say the "wrong thing"? Yes, you probably will. That is how we all learn to find more useful and effective ways of helping individuals reach their goals.

Will saying the wrong thing be harmful to the patient? Consider that symptoms of psychiatric disorders—irritability, agitation, negativity, minimal communication, or excessive talkativeness—can be frustrating and may strain relationships with friends and family. As a result, the patient's past interactions may not always have been positive. Patients tend to appreciate a well-meaning person who conveys genuine acceptance, respect, and concern for their situation. Even if you make mistakes in communication it is unlikely that the comments will do actual harm.

---

euphoria), all of which can impact a patient's ability to connect and communicate with others.

It is often during the psychiatric clinical rotation that students appreciate the usefulness of therapeutic communication. They begin to rely on techniques that may have once seemed artificial. For example, restating sounds so simplistic, the student may hesitate to use this technique:

Patient: "At the moment they told me my daughter would never be able to walk like her twin sister, I felt like I couldn't go on."

Student: *(restates the patient's words after a short silence)* "You felt like you couldn't go on."

That technique, and the empathy it conveys, is supportive in such a situation.

Developing therapeutic communication skills takes time, and with continued practice, you will find your own style and rhythm. Eventually, these techniques will become a part of the way you instinctively communicate with others in the clinical setting. Box 3.1 addresses a common concern among nursing students.

VERBAL AND NONVERBAL COMMUNICATION

Verbal Communication

Verbal communication consists of all the words a person speaks. We live in a society of symbols, and our main social symbols are words. Words are the symbols for emotions and mental images. Talking is our link to one another and the primary instrument of instruction. Talking is a need, an art, and one of the most personal aspects of our private lives.

Nonverbal Communication

Have you heard, "It's not what you say but how you say it"? While this expression is not 100% true, it is the nonverbal behaviors that may be sending much of the real message through. Other common examples of nonverbal communication are physical appearance, body posture, eye contact, hand gestures, sighs, fidgeting, and yawning. Table 3.1 identifies examples of nonverbal behaviors.

Vocal quality, or paralinguistics, is an aspect of nonverbal communication. It encompasses voice volume, pitch, rate, and fluency. Speaking in soft and gentle tones is likely to encourage a person to share thoughts and feelings. Speaking in a rapid, high-pitched tone may convey anxiety and create it in the patient. Emphasis on certain words also conveys meaning. Consider, for example, how drastically tonal quality and inflection can affect communication in a simple sentence like "I will see you tonight."

1. "*I* will see you tonight." (I will be the one who sees you tonight.)
2. "I *will* see you tonight." (No matter what happens, or whether you like it or not, I will see you tonight.)
3. "I will see *you* tonight." (Even though others are present, it is you I want to see.)
4. "I will see you *tonight*." (It is definite, tonight is the night we will meet.)

Interaction of Verbal and Nonverbal Communication

Spoken words represent our public selves. They can be straightforward or used to distort, conceal, or disguise true feelings. Nonverbal behaviors include a wide range of human activities, from body movements to facial expressions to physical responses to messages received from others. How a person listens, uses silence, and uses the sense of touch may also convey important information about the private self that is not available from conversation alone.

Table 3.1 **Nonverbal Behaviors**

Behavior	Nonverbal Cues	Example
Body behaviors	Posture, body movements, gestures, gait	The patient is slumped in a chair, face in hands, and occasionally taps the right foot.
Facial expressions	Frowns, smiles, grimaces, raised eyebrows, pursed lips, licking of lips, tongue movements	The patient scowls when speaking to the nurse, but when alone, smiles and giggles.
Eye expression and gaze behavior	Lowering brows, intimidating gaze	The patient's eyes harden with suspicion.
Voice-related behaviors	Tone, pitch, level, intensity, inflection, stuttering, pauses, silences, fluency	The patient talks in a loud voice with pressured speech.
Observable autonomic physiological responses	Increase in respirations, diaphoresis, pupil dilation, blushing, paleness	At the mention of discharge, the patient becomes pale, diaphoretic, and respirations increase.
Personal appearance	Grooming, dress, hygiene	The patient is dressed in a wrinkled shirt, stained pants, and dirty socks, and is unshaven.
Physical characteristics	Height, weight, build, complexion, age	The patient is overweight with poor posture.

Messages are not always simple. They can appear to be one thing when in fact they are another. Often, people have greater conscious awareness of their verbal messages than their nonverbal behaviors. The verbal message is sometimes referred to as the *content* of the message (what is said), and the nonverbal behavior is called the *process* of the message (nonverbal cues a person gives to substantiate or contradict the verbal message).

When the content is congruent with the process, the communication is more clearly understood and is considered healthy. For example, if a student says, "It's important that I get good grades in this class," that is *content*. If the student has bought the books, takes thorough notes, and has a study buddy and/or tutor, that is *process*. In this case, the content and process are congruent and straightforward, and there is a healthy message.

If, however, the verbal message is not reinforced or is in fact contradicted by the nonverbal behavior, the message is confusing. If a student says, "It's important that I get good grades in this class" and does not have the books, skips classes, and does not study, the content and process do not match. The student's verbal and nonverbal behaviors are incongruent.

COMMUNICATION SKILLS FOR NURSES

Therapeutic Communication Techniques

As you establish a therapeutic relationship, you and your patient can identify specific needs and problems. You can then begin to work with the patient on increasing problem-solving skills, learning new coping behaviors, and experiencing more appropriate and satisfying ways of relating to others. Strong communication skills will facilitate your work. These skills are called *therapeutic communication techniques* and include words and actions that help to achieve health-related goals. Some useful techniques for nurses when communicating with their patients are (1) silence, (2) active listening, (3) clarifying techniques, and (4) questions.

Silence

Students and practicing nurses alike may find that when the flow of words stops, they become uncomfortable. They may rush to fill the void with questions or idle conversation. These responses may cut off important thoughts and feelings the patient might be taking time to think about before speaking.

Although there is no specific rule concerning how much silence is too much, silence is worthwhile only as long as it is serving some function and it is not anxiety-provoking to the patient. Knowing when to speak largely depends on the nurse's perception of what is being conveyed through the silence.

Silence may provide meaningful moments of reflection for both participants. It is an opportunity to thoughtfully contemplate what has been said and felt, weigh alternatives, formulate new ideas, and gain a new perspective. When the nurse waits to speak, this allows the patient to break the silence, resulting in the patient sharing thoughts and feelings that may otherwise have been withheld.

Some psychiatric disorders, such as major depressive disorder and schizophrenia, and medications may slow thought processes. Patience and gentle prompting can help patients gather their thoughts. For example, "You were saying that you are worried about the side effects of the new antidepressant."

Active Listening

People want more than just a physical presence in human communication. In active listening, nurses fully concentrate, respond, and remember what the patient is saying verbally and nonverbally. By giving the patient undivided attention, the nurse communicates that the patient is not alone. This kind of intervention enhances self-esteem and encourages the patient to direct energy toward finding ways to deal with problems and promote learning. Serving as a sounding board, the nurse listens as the patient tests thoughts by voicing them out loud.

Clarifying Techniques

Understanding depends on clear communication, which is aided by verifying the nurse's interpretation of the patient's messages. The nurse can request feedback on the accuracy of the message received from verbal and nonverbal cues.

Paraphrasing. Paraphrasing occurs when you restate the basic content of a patient's message in different, usually fewer, words. Using simple, precise, and culturally relevant terms, the nurse may confirm an interpretation of the patient's message. Phrases such as "I'm not sure I understand" or "You seem to be saying …" help the nurse to interpret the message in what may be a bewildering amount of detail. It also helps the patient to feel heard and may provide greater focus. The patient may confirm or deny the perceptions nonverbally by nodding or looking confused or by direct responses: "Yes, that is what I was trying to say" or "No, I meant …"

Restating. Restating is a clarifying strategy that helps the nurse to understand what the patient is saying. It also lets patients know that they are being heard.

Restating differs from paraphrasing in that it involves repeating the same key words the patient has just spoken. If a patient remarks, "My life is empty … it has no meaning," additional information may be gained by restating, "Your life has no meaning?"

Although this is a valuable technique, it should be used sparingly. Patients may interpret frequent and indiscriminate use of restating as inattention or disinterest. Overuse makes restating sound mechanical. To avoid overuse of restating, the nurse can combine restatements with direct questions that encourage descriptions: "What goals do you have for your evening?" "How is your family responding to your illness?"

Reflecting. Reflection assists patients to understand their thoughts and feelings better. Reflecting may take the form of a question or a simple statement that conveys the nurse's observations of the patient. The nurse might briefly provide an interpretation of the patient's verbal and nonverbal behavior. For example, to reflect a patient's feelings about life, a good beginning might be, "You sound as if you have had many disappointments."

When you reflect, you make the patient aware of inner feelings and encourage the patient to own them. For example, you may say to a patient, "You look sad." Perceiving your concern may allow the patient to spontaneously share feelings. The use of a question in response to the patient's question is another reflective technique. For example:

Patient: "Do you think that I really need to be hospitalized?"

Nurse: "What do you think, Kelly?"

Patient: "I'm not sure. Part of me feels like I do, but another part of me is scared."

Exploring. Exploring is a technique that enables the nurse to examine important ideas, experiences, or relationships more fully. For example, if a patient tells you he does not get along well with his wife, you will want to further explore this area. Possible openers include the following:

"Tell me more about your relationship with your wife."

"Give me an example of how you and your wife don't get along."

Table 3.2 summarizes therapeutic communication techniques.

Table 3.2 Therapeutic Communication Techniques

Therapeutic Technique	Description and *Example*
Silence	Gives the person time to collect thoughts or think through a point. *Encouraging a person to talk by waiting for the answers.*
Accepting	Indicates that the person has been understood. An accepting statement does not necessarily indicate agreement but is nonjudgmental. *"Yes." "Uh-huh." "I understand what you are saying".*
Giving recognition	Indicates awareness of change and personal efforts. Does not imply good or bad, right or wrong. *"Good morning, Mr. James." "I see you've eaten your whole lunch."*
Offering self	Offers presence, interest, and a desire to understand. Is not offered to get the person to talk or behave in a specific way. *"I would like to spend time with you." "I'll sit with you awhile."*
Offering general leads	Allows the other person to take direction in the discussion. Indicates that the nurse is interested in what comes next. *"Go on." "And then?" "Tell me about it."*
Giving broad openings	Clarifies that the lead is to be taken by the patient. However, the nurse discourages pleasantries and small talk. *"Where would you like to begin?" "What are you thinking about?"*
Placing the events in time or sequence	Puts events and actions in better perspective. Notes cause-and-effect relationships and identifies patterns of interpersonal difficulties. *"What happened before?" "When did this happen?"*

Making observations	Calls attention to the person's behavior (e.g., trembling, nail-biting, restless mannerisms). Encourages the patient to notice the behavior and describe thoughts and feelings for mutual understanding. *"You appear tense." "I notice you're biting your lips." "You appear nervous whenever John enters the room."*
Encouraging description of perception	Increases the nurse's understanding of the patient's perceptions. Talking about feelings and difficulties can lessen the need to act them out inappropriately. *"What are the voices saying?" "What is happening now?" "Tell me when you feel anxious."*
Encouraging comparison	Brings out recurring themes in experiences or interpersonal relationships. Helps the person clarify similarities and differences. *"Has this ever happened before?" "Is this how you felt ....?" "Was it something like ...?"*
Restating	Repeats the main idea expressed. Gives the patient an idea of what has been communicated. If the message has been misunderstood, the patient can clarify it. **Patient:** *"I can't sleep. I stay awake all night."* **Nurse:** *"You stay awake all night."*
Reflecting	Directs questions, feelings, and ideas back to the patient. Encourages the patient to accept personal ideas and feelings. Acknowledges patients' right to make decisions and encourages patients to think of themselves as capable people. **Patient:** *"What should I do about my husband's affair?"* **Nurse:** *"What do you think you should do?"* *or* **Patient:** *"My brother spends all of my money and then has the nerve to ask for more."* **Nurse:** *"It sounds like this is very frustrating for you."*

(Continued)

Table 3.2 Therapeutic Communication Techniques—cont'd

Therapeutic Technique	Description and *Example*
Focusing	Concentrates attention on a single point; useful when the patient jumps from topic to topic. This technique is not helpful if a person is experiencing a severe or panic level of anxiety. *"You've mentioned many things. Let's go back to your comment of 'ending the pain'."*
Exploring	Involves asking follow-up questions in a way that encourages deeper discussion without making the patient feel pressured. This approach is useful when a patient's response is vague or unclear, or when more specific information is needed. *"Would you describe it more fully?" "Could you talk about how it was that you learned your mom was dying of cancer?"*
Giving information	Helps patients make informed decisions by providing them with the essential facts they need. It offers knowledge that supports decision-making, enables patients to draw their own conclusions, and serves as a valuable teaching tool. *"This medication is prescribed to help with …" "The test will help determine …"*
Seeking clarification	Helps patients clarify their thoughts and maximize mutual understanding between nurse and patient. *"I am not sure I follow you." "Give an example of a time you thought everyone hated you."*
Presenting reality	Indicates what is real. The nurse does not argue or try to convince the patient, just describes personal perceptions or facts in the situation. *"That was Dr. Todd, not a man from the Mafia." "That was the sound of a car backfiring."*
Voicing doubt	Expressing uncertainty regarding the reality of the patient's perceptions or conclusions, especially in hallucinations and delusions. Use with caution and only after rapport has been well established. *"Isn't that unusual?" "Really?" "I wonder if there could be any other explanation for that?"*

Verbalizing the implied	Puts into concrete terms what the patient implies, making the patient's communication more explicit.
	Patient: "I can't talk to you or anyone else. It's a waste of time."
	Nurse: "Do you feel that no one understands?"
Summarizing	Brings together important points of discussion to enhance understanding.
	"Have I got this straight?" "You said that ..." "During the past hour, you and I have discussed ..."
Translating words into feelings	Responds to the feeling expressed, not just the content.
	Patient: "I am dead inside."
	Nurse: "Are you saying that you feel lifeless? That life seems meaningless?"
Formulating of a plan of action	Allows the patient to identify alternative actions for interpersonal situations the patient finds disturbing (e.g., when anger or anxiety is provoked).
	"What could you do to let anger out harmlessly?" "What are some other ways you can approach your boss?"

Adapted from Hays, J. S., & Larson, K. (1963). *Interacting with patients*. Macmillan. Copyright 1963 by Macmillan Publishing Company.

Table 3.3 Nontherapeutic Communication—cont'd

Nontherapeutic	Description and *Example*	More Helpful Response
Excessive questioning	Results in the patient not knowing which question to answer and possibly being confused about what is being asked. *"How's your appetite? Are you losing weight? Are you eating enough?"*	Clarifying: "Tell me about your eating habits since you've been depressed."
Giving approval, agreeing	Implies the patient is doing the *right* thing—and that not doing it is wrong. May lead the patient to focus on pleasing the nurse or clinician. *"I'm proud of you for applying for that job." "I agree with your decision."*	Making observations: "I noticed that you applied for that job." Asking open-ended questions: "What led to that decision?"
Disapproving, disagreeing	Can make a person defensive. *"You really should have shown up for the medication group."*	Exploring: "How did you decide not to come to your medication group?" "How did you arrive at that conclusion?"
Changing the subject	Invalidates the patient's feelings and needs. Leaves the patient feeling isolated and increases feelings of hopelessness. **Patient:** *"I'd like to die."* **Nurse:** *"Did you go to Alcoholics Anonymous like we discussed?"*	Validating and exploring: "This sounds serious. Have you thought of harming yourself?"

Adapted from Hays, J. S., & Larson, K. (1963). *Interacting with patients.* Macmillan. Copyright 1963 by Macmillan Publishing Company.

controlling tactic and may reflect the interviewer's lack of security in allowing patients to tell their own stories. It is better to ask more open-ended questions and then follow the patient's lead. For example:

Excessive questioning: "Why did you leave your wife? Did you feel angry with her? What did she do to you? Are you going back to her?"

More therapeutic approach: "Tell me about the situation between you and your wife."

Giving Approval or Disapproval. We often give our friends and family approval when they do something well, but giving praise and approval becomes more complex in a nurse–patient relationship. Saying, "That is an amazing mask you made in art therapy" is supportive and may, in fact, promote a dialogue about the emotional meaning of the mask. Contrast that comment with, "It makes me happy to see you sitting with Chelsea at lunch." When the patient is doing a behavior to please another person, it is not coming from the individual's conviction. Thus the new response is not a change in behavior as much as an act to win approval and acceptance from another.

Disapproval is the opposite side of the same coin. "I was disappointed that you showed up late for group therapy" or "You should quit smoking" are counterproductive for any therapeutic relationship. Statements such as these will cause negative feelings such as shame or resentment and undermine the patient's recovery process.

Giving Advice. We ask for and give advice all the time. In a way, nurses give advice when they teach (e.g., "Take your medication with food."). The nontherapeutic form is when the advice becomes more personal. "If I were you, I would leave your husband" or even "You should find a new job" interferes with the patient's ability to make personal decisions. When a nurse offers patients solutions, the patients eventually begin to think the nurse does not view them as capable of making effective decisions.

Asking "Why" Questions. "Why" demands an explanation and implies wrongdoing. Think of the last time someone asked you why: "Why didn't you go to the funeral?" or "Why did you pick *that* outfit?" Such questions imply criticism. We may ask our friends or family these questions, and in the context of a solid relationship, the why may be understood more as "What happened?" With people we do not know—especially those who may be anxious or overwhelmed—a why question from a person in authority (e.g., nurse, physician, or teacher) can be experienced as intrusive and judgmental, which serves only to make the person defensive.

ENVIRONMENTAL VARIABLES

Setting

Effective communication can take place almost anywhere. However, the quality of the interaction—whether in a clinic, a clinical unit, an office, or the patient's home—depends on the degree to which the nurse and patient feel safe. Establishing a setting that enhances feelings of security is important to the therapeutic relationship. A healthcare setting, a conference room, or a quiet part of the unit that has relative privacy but is within view of others is ideal.

When care is provided in a home setting, patients may feel safer and more comfortable than in the clinical setting. An additional benefit of a home visit is being able to assess the patient in the context of everyday life.

Nursing care such as counseling, screening, health education, and coordinating services can easily be accomplished in an electronic setting. Benefits to this telehealth include increasing access to care and eliminating the stigma associated with visiting psychiatric facilities. A primary disadvantage of telehealth is the elimination of in-person interaction. Other challenges, such as limited internet access in rural areas, lack of necessary equipment in low-income households, licensing restrictions, and reimbursement policies, can often be addressed through policy changes and technological advancements.

Seating

In settings where there is a physical presence, arrange chairs so that conversation can take place in normal voice volume and so that eye contact can be comfortably maintained or avoided. A nonthreatening physical environment for both nurse and patient includes the following:

- Maintaining equal height by both sitting or both standing.
- Avoiding a face-to-face arrangement when possible. Positioning at a slight angle may be less intense, and the patient and nurse can look away from each other without discomfort.
- Providing safety and psychological comfort in terms of exiting the room. The patient is not seated between the nurse and the door, and the nurse is not seated in such a way that the patient feels trapped in the room.
- Minimizing physical barriers such as desks, which tend to be physical and psychological barriers and also represent a power differential.

Walking while talking may be an alternative to sitting. Some psychiatric disorders result in hyperactivity and agitation, making sitting extremely uncomfortable. Furthermore, activity reduces depressive symptoms and is usually a healthier option for both the patient and the nurse.

Spacing

The use of personal space is a significant variable when communicating with another person. Generally speaking, distance is based on the following in the United States:

- **Intimate distance** (1.5 feet or less) is reserved for those we trust most and with whom we feel most safe.
- **Personal distance** (1.5–4 feet) is for personal communications such as those with friends or colleagues.
- **Social distance** (4–12 feet) applies to strangers or acquaintances, often in public places or formal social gatherings.
- **Public distance** (12 feet or more) relates to public space (e.g., public speaking).

It is important to note that in individuals with some psychiatric conditions, space should be altered. For example, if a person with schizophrenia is experiencing paranoia, personal and social distance should be increased. Likewise, during an episode of mania and agitation, space should also be increased.

IMPROVING COMMUNICATION SKILLS

Clinical Debriefing

A widely used method of providing clinical supervision is through debriefing. Debriefing is an excellent learning method that can be incorporated into all clinical experiences. Debriefing refers to a critical conversation and reflection regarding a recent clinical event that results in growth and learning. Debriefing supports essential learning along a continuum of "knowing what" to "knowing how" and "knowing why."

Process Recordings

A good way to increase communication and interviewing skills is to review your clinical interactions after they occur. Process recordings are written records of a segment of the nurse-patient session that reflects as closely as possible the verbal and nonverbal behaviors of both patient and nurse. Process recordings have some disadvantages because they rely on memory and are subject to distortions. However, you may find them to be useful in identifying communication patterns.

Communication Skills Evaluation

After you have had some introductory clinical experience, you may find the facilitative skills checklist in Table 3.4 useful for evaluating your progress in developing interviewing skills. Note that some of the items might not be relevant for some of your patients (e.g., numbers 11–13 may not be possible when a patient is experiencing psychosis [disordered thought, delusions, and/or hallucinations]). Self-evaluation of clinical skills is a way to focus on therapeutic improvement. Role-playing can help prepare you for clinical experience and practice effective and professional communication skills.

Table 3.4 **Communication Self-Assessment Checklist**

Instructions: Periodically during your clinical experience, use this checklist to identify areas needed for growth and progress made. Think of your clinical patient experiences. Indicate the extent of your agreement with each of the following statements by marking the scale:

SA = strongly agree, A = agree, NS = not sure, D = disagree, SD = strongly disagree

1.	I maintain appropriate eye contact.	SA	A	NS	D	SD
2.	Most of my verbal comments follow the lead of the other person.	SA	A	NS	D	SD
3.	I encourage others to talk about feelings.	SA	A	NS	D	SD
4.	I ask open-ended questions.	SA	A	NS	D	SD
5.	I restate and clarify the person's ideas.	SA	A	NS	D	SD
6.	I paraphrase the person's nonverbal behaviors.	SA	A	NS	D	SD
7.	I summarize in a few words the basic ideas of a long statement made by the person.	SA	A	NS	D	SD
8.	I make statements that reflect the person's feelings.	SA	A	NS	D	SD
9.	I share my feelings relevant to the discussion when appropriate to do so.	SA	A	NS	D	SD
10.	I give feedback.	SA	A	NS	D	SD
11.	At least 75% or more of my responses help enhance and facilitate communication.	SA	A	NS	D	SD
12.	I assist the person in listing some available alternatives.	SA	A	NS	D	SD
13.	I assist the person in identifying some specific and observable goals.	SA	A	NS	D	SD
14.	I assist the person in specifying at least one next step that might be taken toward the goal.	SA	A	NS	D	SD

From Myrick, D., & Erney, T. (1984). *Caring and sharing*. Educational Media Corporation.

Nursing students caring for children and adolescents may refer to other chapters in this manual for general care plans related to other psychiatric disorders.

We begin with an overview of assessment techniques and therapeutic methods that are useful when working with children and adolescents. This overview is followed by associated nursing care for two specific neurodevelopmental disorders, ADHD and ASD.

INITIAL ASSESSMENT

In the initial assessment, the nurse asks the child or adolescent about life at home with parents and siblings and life at school with teachers and peers. Children and adolescents are encouraged to describe current concerns. The nurse then asks questions to gain an understanding of their developmental history. Play activities, such as games, drawing, puppets, and free play, are used for younger children who have difficulty responding to a more direct approach.

An important part of the first interaction is observing interactions between the child, caregiver, and siblings when possible. Other methods of collecting data include gathering medical history and performing screening and testing utilizing various assessment tools and rating scales.

GENERAL INTERVENTIONS WITH CHILDREN

Ideally, the treatment of childhood and adolescent disorders uses a multimodal approach of coordinated care. Close work with schools, remediation services, and mental health professionals who provide behavior modification are all a part of the care.

General interventions include the following:

- Rewarding positive behaviors (e.g., using a point system) to reduce maladaptive behaviors
- Play therapy
- Bibliotherapy
- Expressive arts therapy
- Journaling
- Music therapy
- Managing disruptive behaviors with time out or time in a quiet room

Selected Childhood Disorders

Two disorders commonly seen in children and adolescents are discussed in this chapter. ADHD will be presented first along with associated nursing care. This discussion is followed by an overview of ASD and associated nursing care.

Attention-Deficit/Hyperactivity Disorder

Individuals with ADHD exhibit inattention, impulsiveness, and hyperactivity. It is important to note that some people are inattentive but not hyperactive or impulsive. In the absence of hyperactivity, the diagnosis becomes inattentive-type ADHD, with symptoms such as disorganization, lack of focus, and forgetfulness.

To diagnose an individual with ADHD, symptoms must be present in at least two settings (e.g., at home and school) and occur before the age of 12. The disorder is often initially detected when the child has difficulty adjusting to elementary school. Attention problems and hyperactivity contribute to low frustration tolerance, temper outbursts, labile moods, poor school performance, peer rejection, and low self-esteem.

Peer relationships are strained because of difficulty taking turns, poor social boundaries, intrusive behaviors, and interrupting others. Individuals with inattentive-type ADHD may exhibit high degrees of distractibility and disorganization. They may be unable to complete challenging or tedious tasks, become easily bored, frequently lose things, or require frequent reminders to complete tasks. Children with ADHD are also more likely than their peers to experience enuresis (bed-wetting) along with a similar trend for encopresis (fecal soiling).

Epidemiology

According to a national parent survey, an estimated 7 million— approximately 11.4%—have been diagnosed with ADHD (CDC, 2024). Boys are more likely to receive this diagnosis than girls—nearly 15% and nearly 8%, respectively. The estimated prevalence of ADHD in adults is 4.4%, with more men (5.4%) than women affected (3.2%) (Kessler et al., 2006). The median age of onset is 7 years, although some people may go undiagnosed until functional impairments become noticeable in adulthood.

Risk Factors

ADHD tends to run in families. The concordance rate for identical twins is between 51% and 58% (Ebert et al., 2016). Although certain genes are correlated with the disorder, there have been no absolute connections.

Environmental factors also contribute to ADHD risk. Very low birth weight triples the likelihood of this disorder. Additional risk factors include maternal smoking and alcohol use, child abuse, neglect, neurotoxin exposure such as lead, and infections such as encephalitis.

Assessment Guidelines

Attention-Deficit/Hyperactivity Disorder

1. Gather data from parents, caregivers, teachers, or other adults involved with the child. Ask about the level of physical activity, attention span, talkativeness, frustration tolerance, impulse control, and the ability to follow directions and complete tasks.
2. Assess social skills, friendship history, problem-solving skills, and school performance. Gather this information from the family or caregiver and one or two additional sources.
3. Assess for comorbidities such as anxiety and depressive symptoms.
4. Assess for indicators of learning disorders, ASD, or intellectual disabilities.
5. Ask about eating and sleeping patterns and monitor these regularly, particularly if the child is being treated with stimulants.

Nursing Diagnoses

The International Classification for Nursing Practice (ICNP; International Council of Nurses [ICN], 2019) provides useful nursing diagnoses for individuals with ADHD. A primary focus is *impaired impulse control*, as children and adolescents with ADHD often display impulsive behaviors. Conflict with authority figures, refusal to comply with requests, and inappropriate methods of meeting needs are addressed with *impaired coping*.

Difficulties in forming and maintaining friendships are addressed with *impaired socialization*, while *chronic low self-esteem* reflects interpersonal and academic struggles. Since parental or caregiver involvement is crucial in therapeutic programs, *impaired family process* is also a key diagnosis.

Intervention Guidelines

Help the child or adolescent in reaching their full potential by fostering developmental competencies and coping skills:

1. Protect from harm and provide for physical and emotional needs.
2. Provide immediate feedback for both acceptable and unacceptable behaviors.
3. Encourage the use of interpersonal skills to build and maintain satisfying relationships with adults and peers.
4. Increase the child's or adolescent's ability to control impulses through structured guidance and reinforcement.
5. Use role-playing to practice appropriate responses to frustration.
6. Foster the development of a realistic self-identity and self-esteem based on achievements and the formation of realistic goals.
7. Offer support, education, and guidance to parents and caregivers to enhance their ability to assist the child effectively.

Nursing Care for Attention-Deficit/Hyperactivity Disorder

Impaired Impulse Control

Related to
- Biochemical alterations in the brain
- Distractibility
- Lack of self-restraint
- Difficulty in delaying gratification

Desired Outcome The patient will demonstrate improved impulse control.

Assessment/Interventions and *Rationales*

1. Implement techniques for managing disruptive behaviors (Table 4.1). *These techniques are effective in connecting with the child, diffusing potential outbursts, keeping the child safe, and teaching appropriate behaviors.*

2. Set clear, consistent limits in a calm, nonjudgmental manner. Remind the patient of the consequences of acting out. *Patients gain a sense of security with clear limits and calm adults who consistently follow through.*

3. Avoid power struggles and repeated negotiations about rules and limits. *Provides clear, consistent expectations, reducing frustration and promoting a structured, supportive environment for better self-regulation.*

4. Use strategic removal if the patient cannot respond to limits (e.g., time out in a quiet room). *Removal allows the patient to regain self-control in a less stimulating environment.*

5. Process incidents with the patient to make it a learning experience. *Reality testing, problem-solving, and testing new behaviors are necessary to foster cognitive growth.*

6. Use behavioral methods that reward the patient for seeking help with handling feelings and controlling impulses to act out. *Consistently reinforcing positive responses results in improved social behavior and increased self-esteem.*

7. Redirect expressions of disruptive feelings into non-destructive, age-appropriate behaviors such as physical activities. *Learning how to modulate the expression of feelings and use anger constructively are essential for self-control.*

8. Teach mindfulness techniques to increase the patient's ability to remain in the here-and-now rather than jumping from activity to activity. *Mindfulness techniques improve focus, self-regulation, and impulse control.*

9. Encourage feelings of concern for others and remorse for the results of impulsive actions. *The development of empathy promotes thinking before acting.*

10. Provide prescribed medication and encourage the patient to be involved in monitoring symptoms, side effects, and improvement. *Patients who are actively involved in their care feel empowered and are more likely to adhere to a medication regimen.*

Table 4.1 **Techniques for Managing Disruptive Behaviors in Children**

Technique	Description
Planned ignoring	When behaviors are determined by staff to be attention seeking and not dangerous, they may be ignored.
Use of signals or gestures	Use a word, gesture, or eye contact to remind the child or adolescent to use self-control.
Behavioral contract	A verbal or written agreement between the patient and nurse or other parties (e.g., family, treatment team, teacher) about behaviors, expectations, and needs.
Additional affection	Involves giving a child planned emotional support for a specific problem or engaging in an enjoyable activity.
Use of humor	Use well-timed appropriate kidding as a diversion to help the child or adolescent save face and relieve feelings of guilt or fear.
Collaborative and proactive solutions	Identifies and defines problematic behaviors and specific triggers, and develops a collaborative method for creating mutually agreeable solutions to the specific situation or trigger.
Counseling	Verbal interactions, role-playing, and modeling to teach, coach, or maintain adaptive behavior and provide positive reinforcement.
Clarification as intervention	Help the child or adolescent understand the situation and motivation for the behavior.
Restructuring	Changing the activity in a way that decreases the stimulation or the frustration (e.g., shorten a story or change to a physical activity).
Modeling	Learning behaviors or skills by observation and imitation that can be used in a wide variety of situations.
Role-playing	Acting out a specified script or role to enhance the child's understanding of that role and to learn and practice new behaviors, skills, and specific situations.
Limit setting	Giving direction, stating an expectation, or telling a child what to do or where to go.
Redirection	Used after an undesirable or inappropriate behavior to engage or re-engage an individual in an appropriate activity.

(Continued)

Table 4.1 Techniques for Managing Disruptive Behaviors in Children—cont'd

Technique	Description
Simple restitution	After a behavioral disruption, the child is required or expected to correct the adverse environmental or relational effects of misbehavior (e.g., apologizing to the people harmed, setting up the chairs that are overturned).
Time out in a quiet room	A quiet environment away from other people allows the child or adolescent time to regroup and manage feelings and behavior.
Seclusion and restraint	During extreme circumstances, after less restrictive responses have failed, the child may need protection from impulses to act out or hurt themselves or others.

Impaired Coping

Related to
- Biochemical alterations in the brain
- Low level of self-confidence
- Fear of failure/humiliation
- Disturbance in ability to release tension
- Highly reactive and difficult to comfort temperament
- Disturbed relationship with parent or caregiver (e.g., lack of trust, abuse, neglect, conflicts, inadequate role models, disorganized family system)
- Deficient support system

Desired Outcome The patient will demonstrate improved coping.

Assessment/Interventions and *Rationales*
1. Use one-to-one or an appropriate level of observation to monitor rising levels of frustration and determine emotional/situational triggers. *External controls are needed for emotional support and to prevent tantrums and rage reactions.*
2. Intervene early to calm the patient, problem solve, and defuse a potential outburst. *Learning can take place before the patient loses control. New solutions and compromises can be proposed.*
3. Avoid power struggles and no-win situations. *Therapeutic goals are lost in power struggles.*

4. Use behavioral techniques to reward tolerating frustration, delaying gratification, and responding to requests and behavioral limits. *Rewarding the patient's efforts will increase positive behaviors and help with the development of self-control.*

5. Allow the patient to question reasonable requests or limits while providing a simple, clear rationale to promote understanding and cooperation. *Discussion allows the patient to maintain some sense of autonomy and power.*

6. Use medication if indicated to reduce anxiety, rage, and aggression and to stabilize mood. *Medication may help the patient to better engage in therapy, social interactions, daily activities.*

7. When feasible, negotiate an agreement on the expected behaviors. Avoid bribes or allowing the patient to manipulate the situation. *An agreement on expected behavior will result in improved compliance. However, constant negotiations can result in increased manipulation and testing of limits.*

Impaired Socialization

Related to
- Biochemical alterations in the brain
- Lack of appropriate role models
- Poor impulse control, frustration tolerance, or empathy for others
- Disturbed relationship with parents or caregivers
- Identification with aggressive/abusive models
- Loss of friendships due to disruptions in family life and living situation

Desired Outcome The patient will demonstrate improved socialization.

Assessment/Interventions and *Rationales*

1. Use the one-to-one relationship to engage the patient in a working relationship. *A one-to-one relationship provides a secure, supportive interaction that builds trust, enhances communication skills, and encourages positive socialization.*

2. Monitor for negative behaviors and identify maladaptive interaction patterns. *Negative behaviors are identified and targeted for replacement with age-appropriate social skills.*

3. Provide early, constructive feedback and tech alternative social strategies to help the patient develop appropriate communication and interaction skills. *Children learn from feedback and early intervention prevents rejection by peers and provides immediate ways to cope.*
4. Use therapeutic play to teach social skills such as sharing, cooperation, realistic competition, and manners. *Learning new ways to interact with others through play allows the development of satisfying friendships and improved self-esteem.*
5. Use role-playing, stories, and therapeutic games to practice skills. *Enjoyable activities support the practice of new skills in a safe environment.*
6. Support the patient in building connections with peers through one-on-one play while modeling social skills and assisting with peer conflict resolution. *Building connections helps children with poor social skills develop confidence, improve communication, and foster meaningful relationships.*
7. Help the patient develop peer relationships with honest and appropriate expression of feelings and needs. *When patients can identify personal feelings and needs, they are better prepared to use more direct communication rather than manipulation and/or intimidation.*

Chronic Low Self-Esteem

Related to
- Perceived lack of belonging
- Perceived lack of respect from others
- Lack of success in role functioning
- Disturbed relationship with parent or caregiver
- Bullied by peers

Desired Outcomes The patient will demonstrate an improved self-esteem:
- Describe self in positive ways.
- Fulfill personally significant roles.
- Engage in meaningful interaction with others.

Assessment/Interventions and *Rationales*
1. Give unconditional positive regard without reinforcing negative behaviors. *Demonstrating basic acceptance of and respect for a person regardless of what they say or do is essential for healthy development.*

2. Reinforce the patient's self-worth with time and attention. *Fosters a sense of belonging, validation, and confidence, which can improve emotional well-being and social engagement.*
3. Help the patient identify positive qualities and accomplishments. *An accurate appraisal of accomplishments can help reduce unrealistic expectations.*
4. Help the patient identify behaviors needing change and set realistic goals. *To change, the patient needs goals and knowledge of new behaviors.*
5. Use behavioral techniques that rewards the patient for practicing new behaviors and evaluates results. *Rewarding the patient's efforts will increase positive behaviors and foster the development of increased self-esteem.*

Impaired Family Process

Related to
- Biochemical alterations in the brain
- Disruptive symptoms of ADHD in the child
- Limited understanding of ADHD (e.g., biological origins and treatment)
- Role strain or overload
- Relationship disturbance in the caregivers
- Disability in the parent(s)
- History of being abused or history of being abusive
- Lack of parent or caregiver fit with the child

Desired Outcome The family will demonstrate improved family processes.

Assessment/Interventions and *Rationales*
1. Explore the impact of ADHD on the life of the family. *Helps identify challenges, improve understanding, and develop coping strategies that promote a supportive and structured home environment.*
2. Assess the parent's or caregiver's knowledge of childhood growth and development and parenting skills. *Problem identification and analysis of learning needs are necessary before intervention begins.*
3. Assess the parent's or caregiver's understanding of the child's diagnosis and treatment. *Knowledge will increase parental or caregiver participation, motivation, and satisfaction.*

4. Help the parent or caregiver identify the child's physical, emotional, and social needs. *Adequate parenting involves being able to identify the child's age-appropriate needs.*

5. Involve the parent or caregiver in identifying a realistic plan for how these needs will be met. *Parents or caregivers have the opportunity to learn the skills necessary to meet the child's needs.*

6. Work with the parent or caregiver to set realistic behavioral goals. *Mutually setting goals provides continuity and prevents the child from using splitting or manipulation to sabotage treatment.*

7. Teach behavioral principles and give the parent or caregiver support in using them and evaluating their effectiveness. *Education and follow-up support are key to a successful treatment program.*

8. Assess the parent or caregiver support system and provide referrals to strengthen resources and assistance as needed. *Self-help groups and special programs such as respite care can increase the caregiver's ability to cope.*

9. Provide information on legal rights and available resources that can assist in advocating for services for the child. *The parent or caregiver commonly lacks information on how to secure services for the child.*

TREATMENT FOR ATTENTION-DEFICIT/HYPERACTIVITY DISORDER

Biological Treatments

Pharmacotherapy

Stimulants and nonstimulants are used to treat ADHD See Chapter 21 for medications used in the treatment of ADHD. To manage aggressive behaviors, other pharmacological agents—including mood stabilizers, alpha-adrenergic agonists, and antipsychotics—are used.

Psychological Therapies

Treatment for ADHD includes behavior modification, special education programs for academic difficulties, and psychotherapy and play therapy for concurrent emotional problems. Cognitive–behavioral therapy (CBT) is used to change patterns of impulsivity by fostering the development of internal control. Mindfulness meditation may also help individuals with ADHD to self-observe and to develop different responses to stressful experiences. Chapter 29 provides more information on these treatment modalities.

AUTISM SPECTRUM DISORDER

ASD is a complex neurobiological and developmental disability that typically appears during the first 3 years of life. ASD affects the normal development of social interaction and communication skills. It ranges in severity from mild to moderate to severe.

Symptoms associated with ASD include deficits in social relatedness with deficits in developing and maintaining relationships. Other behaviors include stereotypical repetitive speech, obsessive focus on specific objects, rigid adherence to routines or rituals, hyperreactivity or hyporeactivity to sensory input, and resistance to change. The symptoms first occur in childhood and cause impairments in everyday functioning.

Epidemiology

The prevalence of ASD is 1 in 36 children (CDC, January 2024). The prevalence is four times higher in boys. ASD has no racial, ethnic, or social boundaries and is not influenced by family income, educational levels, or lifestyles. There is a genetic component to autism. The concordance rate for monozygotic (identical) twins is 70% to 90%, meaning that most of the time if one twin is affected, the other is as well.

Assessment Guidelines

Autism Spectrum Disorder

1. Assess for developmental delays, uneven development, or loss of acquired abilities. Use baby books and diaries, photographs, videotapes, or anecdotal reports from nonfamily caregivers.
2. Assess the child's verbal and nonverbal communication, sensory, social, and behavioral skills including the presence of any aggressive or self-injurious behaviors.
3. Assess the parent-child relationship for evidence of bonding, anxiety, tension, and fit of temperaments.
4. Assess for physical and emotional signs of possible abuse since children with behavioral and

developmental problems are at increased risk for abuse.
5. Ensure that screening for comorbid intellectual disability has been completed.
6. Assess the need for community programs with support services for parents and children, including parent education, counseling, and after-school programs.

Nursing Diagnoses

Several ICNP (ICN, 2019) nursing diagnoses are relevant to ASD. In ASD, the severity of the impairment is demonstrated by the child's lack of responsiveness to or interest in others, a deficiency of empathy or sharing with peers, and little or no cooperative or imaginative play with peers. Therefore, *impaired socialization* is always present. Language delay or absence of language and the unusual stereotyped or repetitive use of language are other areas for nursing, making *impaired communication* a useful focus.

Stereotyped and repetitive motor movements include behaviors such as head banging, face slapping, and hand biting. The child's apparent indifference to pain can result in serious self-injury, so *risk for injury* can become a priority. Individuals with ASD often lack an interest in activities outside of self, and they frequently disregard bodily needs. These deficiencies interfere with the development of a personal identity, so *disturbed personal identity* might also be the focus for care.

Nursing Care for Autism Spectrum Disorders

Impaired Socialization

Related to
- Biochemical alterations in the brain
- Self-concept disturbance (e.g., immaturity or developmental deviation)
- Absence of available significant others or peers
- Disturbed thought processes
- Disturbance in response to external stimuli
- Disturbance in attachment or bonding with the parent or caregiver

Desired Outcomes The patient will demonstrate improved socialization.

Assessment/Interventions and *Rationales*

1. Ensure consistent staff for one-on-one interactions to foster trust, stability, and engagement in a therapeutic relationship. *Consistent one-on-one interactions with the same staff build trust, reduce anxiety, and create a stable environment.*

2. Monitor for signs of anxiety or distress and intervene early to provide comfort. *Anticipating the need for assistance in managing stress will enhance the patient's feelings of security.*

3. Provide emotional support and guidance for activities of daily living (ADLs) and other activities. Use a system of rewards for attempts and successes. *Behavior change occurs through meaningful social interactions involving imitation, modeling, feedback, and reinforcement.*

4. Set up social interactions beginning with parallel play and moving toward cooperative play. *Learning to play with peers is sequential.*

5. Facilitate opportunities for the patient to find a special friend. *A connection with one other person may lead to connections with others.*

6. Role model social interaction skills (e.g., interest, empathy, sharing, and taking turns speaking). *Role modeling facilitates the development of necessary social and emotional skills.*

7. Reward attempts to interact and play with peers and the use of appropriate emotional expressions. *Behaviors that are rewarded are repeated.*

8. Role-play situations that involve conflicts in social interactions to teach reality testing, cause and effect, and problem-solving. *These cognitive skills are needed for successful social and emotional reciprocity.*

Impaired Communication

Related to
- Biochemical alterations in the brain
- Physiological conditions and/or emotional conditions
- Disturbance in attachment or bonding with the parent or caregiver

Desired Outcome The patient will demonstrate improved communication.

Interpersonal consistency provides for the development of trust needed for a sense of safety and security.

2. Use names and descriptions of others to reinforce their separateness. *Consistent reinforcement will help connect the patient to others.*

3. Draw the patient's attention to the activities of others and events that are happening in the environment. *Interrupts the patient's self-absorption and stimulates outside interests.*

4. Limit self-stimulating and ritualistic behaviors by providing alternative play activities or by providing comfort during times of stress. *Redirecting the patient's attention to favorite or new activities increases interaction and personal identity.*

5. Foster self-concept development by reinforcing identity and body boundaries through drawing, stories, and play activities. *Learning body parts strengthens self-identity by helping the individual distinguish themselves from others and develops a sense of personal awareness.*

6. Help the patient distinguish body sensations and how to meet bodily needs by picking up on cues and using ADLs to promote self-care. *The lack of self-awareness contributes to problems with self-care, especially toileting.*

7. Provide play opportunities for the patient to identify the feelings of others (e.g., stories, puppet play, and peer interactions). *Consistent feedback about the feelings of others helps with self-differentiation and the development of empathy.*

TREATMENT FOR AUTISM SPECTRUM DISORDERS

Biological Treatments

Pharmacotherapy

Medications are used to target specific symptoms. They may be used to improve relatedness and decrease anxiety, compulsive behaviors, or agitation. The second-generation antipsychotics risperidone (Risperdal) and aripiprazole (Abilify) have US Food and Drug Administration approval for treating children with ASD beginning at 5 and 6 years of age, respectively. See Chapter 22 for more information on these drugs.

Stimulant medications may be used to target hyperactivity, impulsivity, or inattention (see Chapter 21). Selective serotonin reuptake inhibitors (SSRIs) are used for people with ASD to improve mood and reduce anxiety (see Chapter 24).

Psychological Therapies

Behavioral intervention strategies focus on social communication skill development, especially when the child would naturally be gaining these skills. In higher functioning individuals, CBT may help to address the anxiety associated with ASD. See Chapter 29 for behavioral therapy and CBT. For some children, occupational and speech therapy may be useful.

Applied Behavior Analysis (ABA) encourages positive behaviors and discourages negative behaviors. The Early Intensive Behavioral Intervention (EIBI) is a long-term, intensive approach that improves language and cognitive skills. The Early Start Denver Model (ESDM) is also evidence based in the treatment of individuals with ASD.

👪 NURSE, PATIENT, AND FAMILY RESOURCES

American Academy of Child and Adolescent Psychiatry
The mission of AACAP is to promote the healthy development of children, adolescents, and families through advocacy, education, and research, and to meet the professional needs of child and adolescent psychiatrists throughout their careers.
www.aacap.org

American Psychiatric Nurses Association (search child)
A member-driven community that advances the science and education of psychiatric-mental health nursing.
www.apna.org

The Association for Autism and Neurodiversity (AANE)
The AANE helps Autistic and other Neurodivergent people build meaningful, connected lives, and provides individuals, families, and professionals with education, community, and support.
www.aane.org

Autism Resources
Created by the father of a child with autism to provide information and links for developmental disabilities.
www.autism-resources.com

Autism Society
The Autism Society connects people to the resources they need through education, advocacy, support, information and referral, and community programming.
www.autism-society.org

Children and Adults With Attention-Deficit/Hyper-activity Disorder (CHADD)
CHADD empowers people affected by ADHD by providing evidenced-based information; supporting individuals, families, and professionals who assist them throughout their journeys; and advocating for equity, inclusion, and universal rights.
www.chadd.org

CHAPTER 5

Schizophrenia Spectrum Disorders

Schizophrenia spectrum disorders are disorders that share features with schizophrenia. These disorders are characterized by psychosis, which refers to disorganized thinking, delusions (false thoughts), and hallucinations (false sensory input).

DELUSIONAL DISORDER

Delusional disorder is characterized by delusions that have lasted 1 month or longer. The delusions tend to be grandiose, persecutory, somatic, and referential (these terms are defined in later paragraphs). The delusions in delusional disorder are not usually severe enough to impair functioning.

BRIEF PSYCHOTIC DISORDER

Brief psychotic disorder involves the sudden onset of at least one of the following: delusions, hallucinations, disorganized speech, and disorganized or catatonic (severely decreased motor activity) behavior. The symptoms must last longer than 1 day but no longer than 1 month, with the expectation of a return to normal functioning.

SCHIZOPHRENIFORM DISORDER

The essential features of schizophreniform disorder are exactly like those of schizophrenia, except that the symptoms have lasted less than 6 months. Beyond 6 months, schizophrenia is diagnosed. Also, impaired social or occupational functioning may not be apparent. After an acute episode, some people return to their previous level of functioning, whereas others develop a persistent or recurrent psychosis.

SCHIZOAFFECTIVE DISORDER

Individuals with schizoaffective disorder experience symptoms of schizophrenia, such as delusions and hallucinations, along with a continuous period of illness that includes major depressive or manic episodes. These mood symptoms occur concurrently with schizophrenia-related symptoms and are not caused by substance use or another medical condition.

SUBSTANCE-INDUCED PSYCHOTIC DISORDER AND PSYCHOTIC DISORDER RELATED TO ANOTHER MEDICAL CONDITION

Illicit drugs, alcohol, medications, or toxins can induce delusions or hallucinations. Delusions or hallucinations can also be caused by a general medical condition such as delirium, neurological problems, and hepatic or renal diseases. Substance use and medical conditions are ruled out before making a primary diagnosis of schizophrenia or other psychotic disorders.

SCHIZOPHRENIA

Schizophrenia is a potentially devastating brain disorder. It is often considered the cancer of mental illness. Schizophrenia affects more than 1% of adults (3.2 million people in the United States) and can be among the most disruptive and disabling of psychiatric disorders. Schizophrenia often first appears in people in their teens or early 20s at the beginning of their productive lives. The onset is typically 15 to 25 years of age for males and 25 to 35 years of age for females.

Schizophrenia may be the result of multiple inherited genetic abnormalities in combination with other factors. Viral infections, birth injuries, environmental stressors, prenatal malnutrition, and trauma have been associated with this disorder. Abnormal neural pruning that alters brain development or function has also been associated with schizophrenia.

Some people with schizophrenia can function well with the aid of medications and social support. Others are more disabled and need a higher level of assistance in terms of housing, health maintenance, financial aid, and daily functioning. A large percentage of people with schizophrenia are homeless. The longer the psychosis remains untreated, the poorer the prognosis. About 95% of affected individuals experience the disorder throughout their lifetime. People who develop paranoid features usually have a later age of onset. Although schizophrenia is a biologically based illness, stressful life events can trigger an exacerbation or relapse of the illness.

Phases of Schizophrenia

Schizophrenia usually progresses through predictable phases, although the presenting symptoms during a given phase and the length of the phase may vary. The phases are as follows:

- **Prodromal:** Before acute symptoms of schizophrenia occur, people may experience mild changes in thinking, reality testing, and mood. Speech and thoughts may be odd, and anxiety, obsessive thoughts, and compulsive behaviors may be present. The person may feel "not right" or that "something strange" is happening. Symptoms typically appear 1 to 12 months before the first full episode of schizophrenia.
- **Acute:** Symptoms vary, from few and mild to many and disabling. Hallucinations, delusions, apathy, social withdrawal, diminished effect, anhedonia, disorganized behavior, and impaired judgment and cognition result in functional impairment. The person can have difficulty coping, and symptoms become apparent to others. This phase can last several months, even with treatment. Increased support and additional treatment or hospitalization may be required.
- **Stabilization:** In this phase, symptoms are stabilizing and diminishing, and there is movement toward a previous level of functioning. This phase can last for months. Care in an outpatient mental health center or a partial hospitalization program may be needed. The person may receive care in a residential crisis center (similar to a mental health unit but based in the community) or a staff-supervised residential group home or apartment.

Cognitive Symptoms

Cognitive symptoms are perhaps the most crucial because they interfere with the person's ability to function in all areas of life such as learning, holding a job, and having friends. Cognitive symptoms that are altered in schizophrenia include:
1. Working memory
2. Attention and vigilance
3. Verbal learning and memory
4. Reasoning and problem-solving
5. Speed of processing
6. Social learning and cognition

Affective Symptoms

Affective symptoms involve an altered experience and expression of emotions. Mood may be unstable, erratic, labile (i.e., changing rapidly and easily), or incongruent (i.e., emotional responses that are not would be expected for the circumstances). Co-occurring major depressive disorder is a common complication in people with schizophrenia, as are substance-use disorders, both of which alter affect.

Assessment Guidelines

Positive Symptoms

1. Assess for command hallucinations (e.g., voices telling the person to harm self or another). If present, ask the following:
   a. Do you plan to follow the command?
   b. Do you believe the voices are real?
2. Assess for delusions. Determine whether the patient has a fragmented, poorly organized, well-organized, systematized, or extensive system of beliefs that are not supported by reality. If so, follow-up is necessary.
   a. Assess whether delusions have to do with someone trying to harm the patient and whether the patient is planning to retaliate against a person or organization.
   b. Assess whether precautions need to be taken.
   c. Assess for suspiciousness about everyone and their actions (paranoia)—for example, whether the patient is:
      i. On guard, hyperalert, vigilant

ii. Blaming others for consequences of own behavior

iii. Hostile, argumentative, or threatening in verbalization or behavior.

Negative Symptoms

Assess for negative symptoms of schizophrenia including affective blunting, alogia, avolition/apathy, asociality, and anhedonia.

Cognitive Symptoms

1. Assess the severity of cognitive symptoms.
2. Assess how the cognitive symptoms impact the patient's functioning.

Affective Symptoms

1. Assess for the depressive symptoms and the potential for self-harm.
2. Assess for anger and agitation and the potential for harm to others.

Mood is an essential component of any nursing assessment, particularly due to the potential for self-harm with depressive symptoms and the potential for other-directed violence with angry or aggressive symptoms. The affective symptoms are particularly problematic with schizophrenia when combined with altered judgment and the possibility of persecutory delusions.

Nursing Diagnoses

The International Classification for Nursing Practice (ICNP; International Council of Nurses [ICN], 2019) provides useful nursing diagnoses for individuals with schizophrenia. Communicating with people with schizophrenia can be a challenge, especially in the acute phase. The diagnosis of *impaired verbal communication* addresses this challenge. Another related nursing diagnosis pertains to interacting and social skills is addressed with *impaired socialization*. Hearing voices that seem to originate either inside or outside of the person is addressed with the diagnosis of *hallucinations*. Because of delusions and disorganized thinking, *distorted thinking* is a focus. Due to uncomfortable and often intolerable side effects, coupled with the belief that medication is unnecessary, the diagnosis *nonadherence to medication regime* provides direction for useful interventions. Finally, *impaired family process* addresses the exhaustive needs of families dealing with symptoms of schizophrenia.

Nursing Care for Schizophrenia

Impaired Verbal Communication

Related to
- Biochemical alterations in the brain
- Negative symptoms (i.e., alogia, attentional impairment)
- Positive symptoms (i.e., delusions, hallucination, disorganized thought)
- Medication side effects (i.e., sedation, dry mouth, extrapyramidal symptoms)

Desired Outcomes The patient will demonstrate improved communication.

Assessment/Interventions and *Rationales*
1. Assess whether communication problems are chronic or the result of a current acute episode with an exacerbation of symptoms. *Establishing a baseline facilitates the development of realistic goals, the cornerstone for planning effective care.*
2. Determine whether the patient is currently on antipsychotic medication and assess the duration of treatment. *Assessing antipsychotic medication use and duration helps determine whether communication difficulties stem from untreated or undertreated schizophrenia, medication side effects (such as sedation or tardive dyskinesia), or an acute exacerbation of symptoms, guiding appropriate interventions.*
3. Plan short, frequent meeting periods with the patient throughout the day. *Short periods are less stressful, and periodic meetings give the patient a chance to develop familiarity and safety.*
4. Use simple words and keep directions simple. *The patient might have difficulty processing and responding to even simple sentences.*
5. Keep your voice low and speak slowly. *A high-pitched or loud tone of voice can raise anxiety levels, while a slow, calm speech pattern enhances comprehension.*
6. When you do not understand a patient, ask for clarification (e.g., "I want to understand what you

are saying, but I am having difficulty"). *Asking for clarification demonstrates respect, encourages effective communication, and helps the patient feel heard, while also ensuring accurate understanding and reducing frustration.*

7. Use therapeutic techniques to try to understand the patient's concerns (e.g., "Are you saying…?" "You mentioned demons. Are you feeling frightened?"). *Even if the words are hard to understand, try getting to the feelings behind them.*

8. Focus on and direct the patient's attention to concrete aspects of the environment. *Helps draw focus away from delusions and focus on an objective reality.*

9. Keep the environment quiet and as free of stimuli as possible. *Helps to prevent anxiety from escalating and may reduce confusion, hallucinations, and delusions.*

10. Use simple, concrete, and literal explanations. *Minimizes the patient misunderstanding and incorporating those misunderstandings into delusional systems.*

11. Encourage methods to lower anxiety and minimize voices and "worrying" thoughts. Take time out, read out loud, seek out another supportive person, listen to music, replace irrational thoughts with rational statements, replace negative thoughts with constructive thoughts, and practice deep breathing. *Helping the patient use tactics to lower anxiety can enhance functional speech.*

Impaired Socialization

Related to
- Negative symptoms (i.e., alogia, avolition/apathy, anhedonia/asociality, attentional impairment)
- Positive symptoms (i.e., hallucinations, delusions, disorganized thought)
- Negative self-concept
- Inappropriate or inadequate emotional responses
- Feeling threatened in social situations

Desired Outcomes The patient will demonstrate improved socialization.

Assessment/Interventions and *Rationales*
1. Structure times each day to include brief interactions and activities with the patient on a one-on-one basis.

Helps to develop a sense of connection to another and eventual connection with peers.

2. Communicate the expectation that the patient stays in shared areas rather than the patient's room during most of the day. *Patients often find it easiest to isolate in their rooms, thereby eliminating the potential for interaction with others.*

3. Encourage attendance at group meetings, educational groups, and therapies. You may even suggest, "How about I walk with you to the next meeting?" *Even if the patient does not participate in group activities, simply being with others is a good first step toward socialization.*

4. Review the patient's evaluation of the group experience and the patient's participation in the group. *Reviewing the patient's perception of the group allows for debriefing, support for concerns, and positive reinforcement for participation.*

5. Administer antipsychotic medication as ordered. *Antipsychotic medication helps to reduce psychotic symptoms, thereby supporting interaction with others.*

6. Engage other patients and significant others in social interaction and activities with the patient (e.g., card games, ping-pong, singing, group outings) at the patient's level. *External support helps the patient to feel safe and competent in a graduated hierarchy of interactions.*

7. Provide social skills training to learn adaptive skills such as using good eye contact, appropriate personal space, and a moderate voice tone. *Social skills training helps patients adapt, function more effectively in society, and improve their quality of life by building self-confidence and fostering positive social interactions.*

8. Recognize and acknowledge positive steps the patient takes in increasing social skills and appropriate interactions with others. *Recognition and acknowledgment go a long way toward sustaining and increasing a specific behavior.*

Hallucinations

A change in the amount or patterning of incoming stimuli accompanied by a diminished, exaggerated, distorted, or impaired response to such stimuli.

Related to

- Biochemical alterations in the brain

- Positive symptoms of schizophrenia
- Environmental stressors

Desired Outcome The patient will report a cessation of auditory hallucinations.

or

The patient will manage auditory hallucinations effectively.

Assessment/Interventions and *Rationales*

1. If auditory hallucinations are suspected, ask the patient directly about hearing something that you cannot hear. *Because hearing voices is a subjective experience and not measurable, directly asking about hallucinations is necessary.*

2. Evaluate the nature of the hallucinations: Is the content of the hallucination positive (e.g., offering reassurance or praise) or negative (e.g., degrading or angry)? *Evaluating the nature of hallucinations helps determine their emotional impact, guiding interventions to reduce distress, enhance coping strategies, and ensure safety if the hallucinations are threatening.*

3. Assess whether the voices are commanding the patient to engage in self-harm or to harm others. *Understanding the impact of hallucinations on the patient's feeling of safety or the safety of others is essential in planning precautions.*

4. Reassure the patient that while the voices may feel real to them, you are unable to hear them. *Instilling reasonable doubt as to the reality of the voices is supportive when presented carefully.*

5. Explore methods of distraction to reduce the voices-including singing, listening to music, reading, or a hobby such as gardening. *Distraction is an important part of managing auditory hallucinations.*

6. Teach thought-stopping techniques such as simply using the word "Stop!" to break the thought cycle with auditory hallucinations. *Self-help methods such as thought-stopping can help the patient regain a sense of control.*

7. Help the patient identify the times that the hallucinations are most prevalent and frightening. Keeping a diary of the voices and exploring the impact of stressors on their frequency may help some patients. *Anxiety has been implicated in provoking auditory*

hallucinations. Identifying triggers provides points of intervention.

8. Decrease environmental stimuli when possible. *Reduces the potential for anxiety that might trigger hallucinations.*

9. Encourage the patient to test reality by validating hallucinations with trusted others. *Validation provides reassurance and grounding.*

10. Discuss medication management. Identify potential adherence issues and encourage the patient to take on the role of self-advocate in this treatment. *Medication adherence is an essential part of reducing auditory hallucinations. Ownership of the illness, its symptoms, and its treatment is essential for recovery.*

11. Educate family and significant others about ways to deal with a patient who is experiencing hallucinations. *Educating others in the patient's environment provides an additional level of safety and security for the patient.*

Distorted Thinking

A disruption in mental activities in which a person experiences disturbance in thinking, reality orientation, problem-solving, and judgment.

Related to
- Biochemical alterations in the brain
- Positive symptoms of schizophrenia
- Environmental stressors

Desired Outcome The patient will demonstrate improved thinking.

Assessment/Interventions and *Rationales*

1. Initiate safety measures to protect the patient and others if the patient feels threatened by others. *During the acute phase of psychosis, delusional thinking might put others at risk. External controls may be needed.*

2. Explore the personal significance of the patient's false beliefs, as their delusions may provide insight into underlying fears and emotional distress. *Help to identify the patient's underlying fears and concerns, allowing for more effective communication, targeted interventions, and compassionate support.*

3. Be aware that delusions represent the way that the patient experiences reality. *Identifying the patient's experience allows the nurse to understand the patient's feelings.*
4. Help the patient identify and express feelings associated with their delusions, as acknowledging their emotions can reduce distress. *When patients feel understood, anxiety might lessen.*
5. Do not argue with the patient's beliefs or try to correct false beliefs using facts. *Arguing will reinforce false beliefs and will result in the patient feeling even more isolated and misunderstood.*
6. Do not touch the patient unless necessary for care activities (e.g., blood pressure). *Individuals with psychosis may misinterpret touch as threatening, making it essential to respect their need for increased personal space to reduce anxiety and prevent agitation.*
7. Use distraction to minimize the focus on delusional thoughts. For example, attempt to engage the patient in cards, simple board games, and arts and crafts projects. *When thinking is focused on reality-based activities, the patient is free from delusional thinking during that time. This helps focus attention externally.*
8. Encourage healthy habits to optimize functioning, such as maintaining a regular sleep pattern, abstaining from alcohol and drug use, maintaining self-care, and adhering to the medication regimen. *Psychotic illness interferes with sleep, results in self-medication, reduces the completion of activities of daily living (ADLs), and reduces medication adherence.*
9. Teach the patient coping skills that minimize troubling thoughts, including talking to a trusted person, phoning a helpline, going to a gym, and using thought-stopping techniques. *Self-care strategies promote recovery.*

Nonadherence to Medication Regime

Lack of follow-through with an agreed-upon medication regimen

Related to
- Anosognosia [ano·sog·no·sia] (i.e., the inability to realize one is ill—an inability caused by the illness itself)
- Side effects of medication

- Inability to acquire medication (e.g., transportation, lack of access)
- Financial limitations
- Disagreement with medication regimen

Desired Outcome The patient will demonstrate adherence to the medication regime.

Assessment/Interventions and *Rationales*

1. Evaluate the medication response and side effects. *Identify medications and dosages that have increased therapeutic value and decreased side effects.*
2. Convey empathy and support while providing education about how to manage side effects so that they are less disruptive. *Reduces distress and resulting resistance caused by side effects, increasing the patient's sense of control.*
3. Address anosognosia. Do not try to convince them that they are ill, rather talk about their goals, such as keeping a job or living on their own. *Patients may begin to take medications if they will help them to achieve their goals. Once they begin taking medication, they may experience greater insight into their illness.*
4. Explore the benefits of medications in meeting goals (e.g., eliminate or decrease hallucinations). *Seeing that medication helps the patient to achieve goals will increase the motivation for treatment.*
5. Include the patient as a partner in planning for the medication regime. The most important person in the treatment plan is the patient. *If medication choices, doses, and dosing are unacceptable, there is a strong possibility for nonadherence.*
6. Discuss the possibility of long-acting injectables to eliminate the need for remembering to take medication or to remember if they have already taken it. *Patients may unintentionally not adhere to the medication regimen because they forget to take medications or forget whether they have already taken them.*
7. Explore using technology such as electronic reminders and monitoring systems linked to electronic medication dispensers to enhance adherence. *Technology may support individuals who are unintentionally nonadherent in remembering to take medication.*

8. Discuss your recommendations regarding potential medication changes with the patient's prescriber to promote adherence and improve quality of life. *Patient advocacy and functioning as part of a team are primary nurse roles. Nurses usually have more interaction with patients and are aware of medication benefits and side effects.*
9. Explore social services and community support in securing medication if access and transportation are problems. *Barriers to access to medication can be addressed by social supports to improve adherence.*

Impaired Family Process

Related to
- Biochemical alterations in a family member
- Deterioration of the health status of a family member
- Situational crisis or transition
- Developmental crisis or transition

Desired Outcome The family will demonstrate an improved family process.

Assessment/Interventions and *Rationales*
1. Evaluate the family's ability to cope by assessing their experience of loss, caregiver burden, and need for additional support. *The family's needs must be addressed to stabilize the family unit.*
2. Provide an opportunity for the family to discuss feelings and identify their immediate concerns. *Nurses and staff can best intervene when they understand the family's experience and needs.*
3. Assess the family's current knowledge about schizophrenia and medications used for treatment. *The family might have misconceptions and misinformation about schizophrenia and treatment, or little knowledge at all.*
4. Provide information regarding schizophrenia and treatment strategies at the family's level of knowledge. *Providing information at the family's level of understanding empowers them to manage the condition effectively, reduces misinformation, enhances coping skills, and promotes a supportive environment for the patient.*
5. Provide teaching in understandable terms verbally and in written form. Topics include the purpose of medication therapy, the dose, the importance of a schedule and adherence, managing side effects, and monitoring for potential serious side effects. *Understanding the*

disorder and its treatment encourages greater family support and patient adherence.

6. Provide information on patient and family community resources after discharge, such as support groups, organizations, day treatment programs, educational programs, and respite centers. *Schizophrenia is an overwhelming disorder for both the patient and family. Patient and family community resources can help.*

7. Teach the patient and family the warning symptoms of relapse including insomnia, social withdrawal, difficulty concentrating, loss of interests, increasing paranoia, and hallucinations. *Recognizing relapse symptoms and getting help early can help prevent a more severe episode.*

TREATMENT FOR SCHIZOPHRENIA SPECTRUM DISORDERS

Biological Treatments

Pharmacotherapy

Antipsychotic medications are the primary treatment for psychotic disorders, including schizophrenia. The first of these drugs became available in the 1950s, revolutionizing care. Before their widespread use, individuals with schizophrenia often spent months or years in state or private hospitals, placing significant emotional and financial costs to patients, families, and society. Today, a combination of antipsychotic medication and psychosocial support helps manage symptoms, enabling most individuals to receive treatment and live with in their communities. See Chapter 22 for information about antipsychotic medications.

Psychological Therapies

Advanced practice mental health professionals are trained to provide individual and group psychotherapy, including cognitive behavioral therapy (CBT). Cognitive symptoms of schizophrenia can be addressed with cognitive remediation or enhancement therapy. These therapies enhance memory, attention, and problem-solving skills to reduce cognitive impairment. By addressing cognitive impairments, these strategies support better daily functioning and overall quality of life.

Family therapy is also important. Families often experience considerable distress related to living with individuals who have acute or residual symptoms of schizophrenia. Direct caregivers and caregivers who are subjected to hostility are in special need of outside support. In family therapy sessions, fears, faulty communication patterns, and distortions are identified. Communication, symptom management, and problem-solving skills are taught, healthier alternatives to conflict are explored, and guilt and anxiety can be lessened. In some cases, therapists may recommend alternate living arrangements such as a group home or assisted living.

The Recovery Model

The recovery model is supported by the National Alliance on Mental Illness (NAMI), the leading mental health consumer support and advocacy organization in the United States. Nurses play a key role in supporting recovery by providing care that promotes independence, social engagement, and overall quality of life. Patients with schizophrenia or other serious mental illnesses will benefit from this type of care and also as they adopt the model as a way of life for themselves.

Important aspects of the recovery model include:

- Emphasizes the person and the future rather than the illness and the present
- Involves an active partnership between the individual (also known as the mental health consumer) and care providers
- Focuses on strengths and abilities rather than dysfunction and disability
- Encourages independence and self-determination.
- Focuses on achieving goals of the individual's choosing rather than care providers' choosing
- Emphasizes staff working collaboratively with clients, building on strengths to help consumers achieve the highest possible quality of life
- Aims for increasingly productive and meaningful lives for individuals with serious mental illness (SMI)

👪 NURSE, PATIENT, AND FAMILY RESOURCES

Brain and Behavior Research Foundation
The Brain & Behavior Research Foundation is committed to alleviating the suffering caused by mental illness by

awarding grants that will lead to advances and break-throughs in scientific research.
www.bbrfoundation.org

I Am Not Sick, And I Don't Need Help

Xavier Amador's essential book about anosognosia and poor insight was inspired by his success in helping his brother, who developed schizophrenia, accept treatment.
https://leapinstitute.org/leap-books/

National Alliance on Mental Illness (NAMI)

NAMI is the National Alliance on Mental Illness, the nation's largest grassroots mental health organization dedicated to building better lives for the millions of Americans affected by mental illness. Educational materials and support for individuals with mental illness and their families.
www.nami.org

National Institute of Mental Health

Learn about schizophrenia, including onset & symptoms, risk factors, treatments and therapies, how to help a loved one, and resources for more information.
https://www.nimh.nih.gov/health/topics/schizophrenia

Overcoming Schizophrenia Blog Spot

This blog is about educating and empowering peers, caregivers, and loved ones with hope for recovery.
https://overcomingschizophrenia.blogspot.com/

Schizophrenia and Psychosis Action Alliance

A global impact organization moving individuals, families, and policies forward to improve and save lives.
https://sczaction.org/

Schizophrenia.com

An internet community dedicated to providing high-quality information, support, and education to the family members, caregivers, and individuals whose lives have been impacted by schizophrenia.
www.schizophrenia.com

CHAPTER 6

Bipolar Disorders

Bipolar spectrum disorders are among the most serious of the psychiatric disorders. The extreme symptoms may result in the loss of partners, families, friendships, employment, and financial security.

According to the American Psychiatric Association (APA) (2022), bipolar disorders consist of diagnoses that are characterized by one or more episodes of mania or hypomania and usually one or more depressive episodes.

- Mania is a period of intense mood disturbance with persistent elevation, expansiveness, irritability, and extreme goal-directed activity or energy. These periods last at least 1 week for most of the day, every day. An acute manic phase usually requires hospitalization to protect and stabilize the patient.
- Hypomania refers to a low-level and less dramatic mania. The hypomania of bipolar II disorder tends to be euphoric and often increases functioning. Psychosis is never present in hypomania, and hospitalization is rarely necessary. Table 6.1 contrasts the differences between mania and hypomania.
- A major depressive episode is a sustained (2 weeks or more) depressed mood and/or a loss of interest or pleasure in everyday activities. Concentration and decision-making are usually impaired. People with depression feel empty, hopeless, anxious, worthless, guilty, and/or irritable. Depression in people with bipolar disorder can be profound and dangerous because of suicidal ideation and the potential for psychotic symptoms.

EPIDEMIOLOGY

The lifetime risk, or the percentage of the population who experience bipolar disorder sometime in their lives, is 4.4% for adults and 2.9% for adolescents (National Institute of

Table 6.1 Characteristics of Hypomania and Acute Mania

Hypomania	Acute Mania
Communication	
1. Talks and jokes incessantly, life of the party, gets irritated when not center of attention.	1. Mood is labile—may change suddenly from elation to anger or sadness.
2. Far more outgoing and sociable than usual.	2. Inappropriate demands of people's attention, intrusive.
3. Talk is often sexual and can be obscene; inappropriate propositions to strangers.	3. Speech may contain profanities and crude sexual remarks.
4. Jumps from one topic to the next, pressured speech.	4. Flight of ideas, jumps from topic to topic, complains of racing thoughts.
Affect and Thinking	
1. Full of energy and humor, feelings of euphoria, sociability.	1. Humor gives way to irritability, hostility, and short-lived periods of rage, especially when not getting the patient's way or when limits are set for behaviors. Mood may shift from hostile to calm.
2. Increase in goal-directed activity and planning, may be more creative.	2. Delusional thinking may result in grandiose plans and schemes or paranoid plans for protection.
3. Judgment often poor, but usually not severe enough for hospitalization.	3. Judgment is so poor that hospitalization is often necessary.
4. May write large quantities of mail or make calls to famous people regarding schemes.	4. May attempt to contact famous people. Severe mania may interfere with planning.
5. Decreased attention span to internal and external cues.	5. Decreased attention span and distractibility are intensified.
Physical Behavior	
1. Overactive, distractible, buoyant, occupied with grandiose plans, goes from one activity to the next.	1. Extremely restless and chaotic. May have outbursts such as throwing things. May be dangerous, disoriented, and agitated.

Table 6.1 Characteristics of Hypomania and Acute Mania—cont'd

Hypomania	Acute Mania
2. Hypersexual, desire, sexually irresponsible, indiscreet. Unplanned pregnancies in females with hypomania. Sexually transmitted disease may be contracted.	2. No time for sex—too busy. Poor concentration. Distractibility and restlessness are severe.
3. May have voracious appetite, eat on the run, or gobble food during brief periods.	3. Too distracted and disorganized to eat.
4. May go without sleeping or feel rested after 3 hours of sleep. However, may be able to take short naps.	4. No time for sleep— Psychomotor activity too high to sleep.
5. Financially extravagant, goes on spending sprees, gives money and gifts away freely, can easily go into debt.	5. Same as in hypomania, but in the extreme.

Mental Health, 2024). Many factors increase the risk for bipolar disorder, including a genetic predisposition. Other risk factors include an imbalance in neurotransmitters; neurological dysfunction in regions such as the prefrontal cortex, hippocampus, and hypothalamic-pituitary-thyroid-adrenal (HPTA) axis; and environmental stress and adverse experiences.

The APA (2022) identifies bipolar spectrum as consisting of three main disorders: (1) bipolar I, (2) bipolar II, and (3) cyclothymic disorder. Separate diagnostic categories categorize bipolar disorders that are caused by other factors such as substances, medications, and other medical conditions.

BIPOLAR I

Bipolar I is the most severe bipolar disorder, characterized by at least one manic episode. The manic episode must last for at least 1 week for most of the day, every day. Before or after the manic episode, individuals may experience a hypomanic or major depressive episode. Some individuals with manic episodes may also experience psychosis, which includes disorganized thinking, false beliefs, and/or hallucinations.

Considerable impairment in social, occupational, and interpersonal functioning exists with bipolar I. Symptoms of mania are so severe that this state may be a psychiatric emergency. Hospitalization is often required to protect the person from the consequences of poor judgment and hyperactivity.

BIPOLAR II

Individuals with bipolar II disorder have experienced at least one hypomanic episode *and* at least one major depressive episode. Psychosis is never present in hypomania but may be a feature of the depressive episode. The hypomanic episode lasts at least 4 days, while the major depressive episode lasts at least 2 weeks.

CYCLOTHYMIC DISORDER

In cyclothymic disorder, symptoms of hypomania alternate with symptoms of mild to moderate depression for at least 2 years in adults and 1 year in children. Hypomanic and depressive symptoms do not meet the criteria for either bipolar II or major depressive disorder, yet the symptoms are disturbing enough to cause social and occupational impairment.

Phases of Bipolar Disorder

Bipolar I disorder symptoms are categorized by acute and maintenance phases:

1. The acute phase begins with the onset of a new manic or hypomanic episode. Hospitalization is usually indicated for patients in the acute manic phase of bipolar disorder. Hospitalization protects patients from harm (e.g., exhaustion, financial loss) and allows time for medication stabilization.
2. During the maintenance phase, the most acute symptoms have been controlled. The longer-term maintenance phase begins after the resolution of an acute episode. The goal now is the prevention of future cycles of mania or hypomania.

Many of the interventions discussed in this chapter focus on the acute phase, as this phase often requires hospitalization. Immediate, complex interventions are essential during mania to manage impulsivity, agitation, and potential risks. For strategies specific to major depressive episodes in bipolar disorders, see Chapter 7.

ASSESSMENT

Signs and Symptoms

- Euphoric mood (i.e., intense feelings of well-being, overly joyous mood)
- Periods of hyperactivity (e.g., pacing, restlessness, accelerated actions)
- Overconfident, exaggerated view of own abilities
- Decreased need for sleep, no acknowledgment of fatigue, increased energy
- Poor social judgment, engages in reckless and self-destructive activities (e.g., risky business ventures, hypersexuality, spending sprees)
- Rapid speech, pressured speech, loud talking, rhyming, punning
- Brief attention span, easily distractible, flight of ideas, loose associations
- Expansive, irritable, paranoid behaviors
- Impatient, uncooperative, abusive, sexually crude, manipulative

ASSESSMENT TOOLS

The Altman Self-Rating Mania Scale is a five-item scale to assess the presence or severity of symptoms of mania over the past 7 days. The individual can complete the scale or, if the patient is too impaired to complete the form, a knowledgeable friend, family member, or clinician can do so. See Table 6.2 for the rating scale.

Assessment Guidelines

Manic Phase

1. Assess whether the patient is a danger to self or others
   - Patients with mania can exhaust themselves.
   - The patient might not eat or sleep for days at a time.
   - Poor impulse control might result in harm to self or others.

7. Provide structured solitary activities. Tasks that take minimal concentration are best.
8. Avoid groups and stimulating activities until the patient can tolerate that level of activity.
9. Spend time with the patient if psychosis or anxiety is present. Consider providing staff for one-on-one observation.
10. Provide frequent rest periods.
11. Provide high-calorie fluids and finger foods frequently throughout the day.
12. Monitor the following:
    • Sleep pattern
    • Food intake
    • Elimination (constipation is a common problem)
13. Provide the patient and family with education about the illness, along with written information regarding the illness and medications.
14. Provide the patient and family with information on supportive services in their community for further information and support.

Nursing Care for Mania

The following sections identify primary nursing diagnoses for use with a patient who is experiencing mania, particularly in the acute and severe manic phases of the illness.

Risk for Injury

Related to
• Biochemical alterations in the brain
• Cognitive, affective, and psychomotor factors
• Alteration in cognitive functioning
• Alteration in psychomotor functioning
• Compromised nutrition
• Malnutrition
• Alteration in affective orientation

Desired Outcome The patient will be free from injury.

Assessment/Interventions and *Rationales*
1. Maintain a low level of stimuli in the patient's environment (e.g., away from loud noises, bright lights, and people). *Helps decrease the escalation of anxiety.*

2. Provide structured solitary activities with a nurse or an aide. *Helps to reduce overstimulation, improve focus, ensure safety, and promote emotional regulation by channeling excessive energy into a controlled, calming environment.*

3. Provide frequent high-calorie fluids. *Nutritional status may be compromised due to lack of interest in food and liquids. Regularly offering fluids increases the success of acceptance.*

4. Provide frequent rest periods in a darkened room even if sleep is not possible. *Prevents exhaustion even if sleep is not achieved.*

5. Redirect aggressive behavior and encourage exercise. *Physical exercise can decrease tension and provide focus.*

6. Provide prescribed scheduled and as-needed medications. *Medication helps reduce excessive physical activity, preventing exhaustion, dehydration, sleep deprivation, and increased confusion.*

7. If on lithium, observe for signs of lithium toxicity. *There is a narrow margin of safety between therapeutic and toxic doses.*

8. Hold valuables in the hospital safe or send them home. *Protect the patient from giving away or losing money and possessions.*

Risk for Violence

Related to
- Biochemical alterations in the brain
- Alteration in cognitive functioning
- Impulsiveness
- Excessive energy and agitation
- Delusional thinking

Desired Outcome The patient will refrain from assaultive, combative, or destructive behaviors toward others.

Assessment/Interventions and *Rationales*

1. Use a calm and firm approach. *Provides structure and control for a patient who is out of control.*

2. Use short, concise explanations or statements. *A short attention span limits comprehension to small bits of information.*

3. Maintain a consistent approach, employ consistent expectations, and provide a structured environment. *Clear and consistent limits and expectations minimize the potential for the patient to manipulate the staff.*

4. Remain neutral and avoid power struggles and value judgments. *The patient can use inconsistencies and value judgments as justification for arguing, which may escalate mania.*

5. Decrease environmental stimuli by minimizing loud music and noises, people, and bright lights. *A calm environment helps prevent escalating anxiety and manic symptoms.*

6. Assess the patient's behavior frequently (e.g., every 15 minutes) for signs of increased agitation and hyperactivity. *Early detection and intervention of escalating mania might help prevent harm to the patient or others and decrease the need for seclusion.*

7. Redirect agitation with physical outlets in areas of low stimulation (e.g., punching bag, exercise bike). *Relieves agitation and muscle tension.*

8. Alert staff if the potential for restraint or seclusion appears imminent. The usual priority of interventions is (1) setting limits, (2) encouraging time out, (3) offering as-needed medication, and (4) restraint or seclusion. *A team approach to aggression is essential Always use the least restrictive intervention when intervening with a patient exhibiting potentially violent behavior.*

9. Document patient behaviors, interventions, triggers for agitation, effective calming strategies, administration and effects of as-needed medications, and what proved most helpful. *Documentation provides staff with valuable information for debriefing and guidelines for future interventions.*

Impaired Impulse Control

Related to
- Biochemical alterations in the brain
- Alteration in cognitive functioning
- Mania

Desired Outcome The patient will demonstrate self-restraint of impulsive behaviors.

Assessment/Interventions and (Rationales)
1. Administer prescribed scheduled and as-needed medications, and evaluate for efficacy, side effects, and toxic effects. *Bipolar spectrum disorders are caused by*

biochemical imbalances in the brain. Medication is effective in stabilizing dysregulated mood.

2. Observe for destructive behavior toward self or others. Intervene in the early phases of escalation of manic behavior. *Hostile verbal behaviors, poor impulse control, and violent acting out against others or property are seen in acute mania. Early detection and intervention can prevent harm to the patient or others in the environment.*

3. Send valuables, credit cards, and cash home with family or secure them in the hospital safe until the patient is discharged. *During manic episodes, individuals may give away valuables and money indiscriminately to strangers, often leaving themselves in debt.*

4. Maintain a firm, calm, and neutral approach at all times. Avoid power struggles and arguing. *Professional behavior by the staff will reduce the chance of conflict and escalation.*

5. Provide hospital legal service when and if a patient is involved in making or signing important legal documents during an acute manic phase. *Judgment and reality testing are both impaired during acute mania. Patients might need legal advice and protection against making important decisions that are not in their best interest.*

6. Assess and recognize early signs of manipulative behavior and intervene appropriately. *Consistently setting limits is important when intervening in manipulative behaviors.*

Distorted Thinking

Related to
- Biochemical alterations in the brain
- Mania
- Disruption in cognitive operations and activities
- Sleep deprivation

Desired Outcomes The patient will experience reduced distortion in thinking processes.

    or

The patient will experience clarity in thinking processes.

Assessment/Interventions and *Rationales*
1. Meet with the patient for short periods each day. *Short, consistent meetings help establish contact and decrease anxiety.*

2. Attempt to understand the significance of false beliefs to the patient. *Important clues to underlying fears and issues can be found in the patient's seemingly illogical delusions.*

3. Acknowledge that delusions represent the way that the patient experiences reality. *Identifying the patient's experience allows the nurse to understand the patient's feelings.*

4. Help the patient to identify feelings related to delusions. *When patients feel understood, anxiety might lessen.*

5. Do not argue with the patient's beliefs or try to correct false beliefs using facts. *Arguing will reinforce false beliefs. This will result in the patient feeling even more isolated and misunderstood.*

6. Assess the content of hallucinations. *Understanding the content of auditory hallucinations helps to determine whether they are dangerous (e.g., command hallucinations telling the patient to harm someone).*

7. Reduce environmental stimuli by monitoring agitation cues and removing triggers. A private room may help create a calmer, more controlled setting. *Reducing a stressful environment will help to decrease agitation and confusion.*

8. Reinforce reality by talking about actual events and topics such as unit activities, *Helping the patient in reality and present issues can increase a here-and-now focus.*

Self-Care Deficit

Related to
- Biochemical alterations in the brain
- Alteration in cognitive functioning
- Hyperactivity

Desired Outcome The patient will conduct optimal self-care activities based on personal abilities.

Assessment/Interventions and *Rationales*
Insufficient Nutritional Intake

1. Monitor intake and output. *Minimizes dehydration and supports interventions for adequate fluid and caloric intake.*

2. Encourage frequent high-calorie protein drinks and finger foods (e.g., sandwiches, fruit, milkshakes). *Fluid and calorie replacement are needed. Since the patient might be too active to sit at meals, finger foods allow for "eating on the run."*

3. Frequently remind the patient to eat (e.g., "Tom, finish your milkshake." "Skylar, eat this banana."). *The patient is unaware of bodily needs, is easily distracted, and requires supervision to eat.*

Sleep Pattern Disturbance

1. Encourage frequent rest periods during the day. *Lack of sleep can lead to exhaustion and worsen manic symptoms.*
2. Keep the patient in areas of low stimulation. *Promotes relaxation and reduces manic behavior.*
3. In the evening, encourage warm baths, soothing music, and medication when indicated while avoiding caffeine. *Promotes relaxation, rest, and sleep.*

Dressing or Grooming Problems

1. Supervise clothing choices as needed to prevent inappropriate, bizarre, or sexually suggestive attire, ensuring dignity and appropriateness. *Helps maintain the patient's dignity, prevent inappropriate social interactions, and reduce the risk of drawing negative attention or exploitation.*
2. Give simple step-by-step reminders for hygiene and dress (e.g., "Here is your razor. Shave the left side … now the right side." "Here is your toothbrush. Put the toothpaste on the brush."). *Distractibility and poor concentration are countered by simple, concrete instructions.*

Constipation

1. Monitor bowel habits, encourage fluid and high-fiber food intake, assess the need for a laxative, and remind the patient to use the bathroom regularly. *Promotes regular toileting. Prevents fecal impaction resulting from dehydration and decreased peristalsis.*
2. Encourage physical activity as appropriate. *Movement stimulates peristalsis and can help prevent constipation.*

Impaired Socialization

Related to

- Biochemical alterations in the brain
- Disturbance in thought processes
- Excessive hyperactivity and agitation
- Mania

Desired Outcome The patient will demonstrate improved socialization.

Assessment/Interventions and *Rationales*

1. When possible, provide an environment with minimal stimuli (e.g., quiet, soft music; dim lighting). *Reduction in stimuli lessens distractibility*.
2. Initially, suggest solitary activities that require a short attention span with mild physical exertion (e.g., writing, painting [finger painting, murals], woodworking, or walks with staff). *Solitary activities minimize stimuli. Mild physical activities release tension constructively*.
3. When mania lessens, encourage the patient to join one or two other patients in quiet, nonstimulating activities (e.g., board games, drawing, cards). Avoid competitive games. *As mania subsides, involvement in activities that provide focus and social contact becomes more appropriate. Competitive games can stimulate aggression and increase psychomotor activity*.

TREATMENT FOR BIPOLAR DISORDERS

Biological Treatments

Pharmacotherapy

Patients with bipolar disorder often resist medication, as they may enjoy the increased energy, creativity, and confidence. Unfortunately, if left untreated, the high progresses into a more disastrous mania or painful depression. Chapter 23 provides an overview of mood stabilizers along with treatment for bipolar depression.

Neuromodulation Therapy

Electroconvulsive therapy (ECT) is useful when a patient is unable to wait until a medication starts to become effective, cannot tolerate one of the first-line medications, or does not respond to the first-line medications. ECT is most commonly used with patients who have bipolar disorder with severe depressive episodes. ECT may also be considered for mania, mixed, and depressed states of bipolar disorder, as well as in maintenance treatment.

Transcranial magnetic stimulation (TMS) and repetitive transcranial magnetic stimulation (rTMS) are noninvasive neuromodulation techniques. They work through repeated magnetic pulses targeting hypoactive or hyperactive cortical areas. In 2020 the first TMS device received a Food and Drug Administration (FDA) breakthrough device designation for bipolar depression. This designation specifies its use for adult patients with bipolar I or II disorders with treatment-resistant depression. See Chapter 30 for more information about brain stimulation therapies.

Psychological Therapies

Many patients with bipolar disorder have strained interpersonal relationships, marriage and family problems, academic and occupational problems, and legal or other social difficulties. Psychotherapy provided by an advanced practice professional can help them work through these difficulties, decrease some of the psychic distress, and increase self-esteem. Psychotherapy can also help patients improve their functioning between episodes and attempt to decrease the frequency of future episodes.

A combination of psychological therapies along with pharmacotherapy can reduce the morbidity and mortality associated with bipolar disorder. Cognitive behavioral therapy (CBT) is typically used as an adjunct to pharmacotherapy in many psychiatric disorders. Depression and manic-type states impair a person's ability to interact with others. Interpersonal and social rhythm therapy can be helpful for this. Family-focused therapy helps improve communication among family members. See Chapter 29 for descriptions of psychological treatments.

NURSE, PATIENT, AND FAMILY RESOURCES

Bipolar Disorder Guide
Includes articles and fact sheets reviewed by psychiatrists from Verywell Mind, whose mission is to help prioritize mental health and find balance.
www.bipolar.about.com

Bipolar Disorder Page
Mentalhelp.net provides accurate and up-to-date information available in the field of addiction medicine and behavioral health and has enlisted an acclaimed team of authors, treatment professionals, and editorial experts to write, review, and update content to check that it meets our high editorial standards.
www.mentalhelp.net (search Bipolar)

Depression and Bipolar Support Alliance (DBSA)
DBSA provides help, support, and education to improve the lives of people who have mood disorders.
www.dbsalliance.org

National Alliance on Mental Illness (NAMI)
NAMI is the National Alliance on Mental Illness, the nation's largest grassroots mental health organization dedicated to building better lives for the millions of Americans affected by mental illness. Educational materials and support for individuals with mental illness and their families.
www.nami.org

National Institute of Mental Health
Learn about bipolar disorder, including onset & symptoms, risk factors, treatments and therapies, how to help a loved one, and resources for more information.
www.nimh.nih.gov

CHAPTER 7

Depressive Disorders

Sadness and unhappiness are natural responses to challenging life events. However, when feelings of sadness, grief, or hopelessness become overwhelming and persist for an extended period, they may signal the presence of a depressive disorder. This condition can profoundly impact one's daily functioning and overall quality of life, making it vital to recognize and address its signs. Distinguishing between temporary emotional responses and clinical depression is crucial for seeking support and treatment.

Depressive symptoms are common among individuals who have other psychiatric conditions such as anxiety disorders, eating disorders, personality disorders, and schizophrenia. Major depressive disorder is also highly comorbid with individuals who have experienced abused (e.g., physical, psychological, or sexual). Additionally, depressive symptoms often coexist with alcohol or substance use disorders. Depression may also emerge as a critical symptom of other medical conditions, including hepatitis, mononucleosis, multiple sclerosis, dementia, cancer, diabetes, or chronic pain.

The two depressive disorders discussed in this chapter are major depressive disorder and persistent depressive disorder (American Psychiatric Association, 2022).

MAJOR DEPRESSIVE DISORDER

In major depressive disorder, a severely depressed mood, usually recurrent, causes clinically significant distress or impairment in social, occupational, or other important areas of the person's life. The depressed mood can be distinguished from the person's usual functioning and might occur suddenly or gradually.

People with major depressive disorder may experience additional symptoms, such as:

- Anxious distress: feelings of tension, restlessness, fear (e.g., anticipating something bad might happen or lose control), excessive worry, poor concentration
- Psychotic features: delusions or hallucinations
- Catatonia: unusual voluntary movements, motor immobility, purposeless motor activity, echolalia, or echopraxia
- Melancholic features: severe symptoms, loss of pleasure, worsening symptoms in the morning, early morning awakening, significant weight loss, excessive guilt
- Peripartum onset: during pregnancy or within 4 weeks after delivery
- Seasonal pattern: most prominent during certain seasons (e.g., winter or summer). With increased prevalence in regions with longer periods of darkness in a 24-hour cycle

Epidemiology

In the United States, approximately 5 million adolescents, or 19.5% of all adolescents, experienced at least one major depressive episode in 2022 (Substance Abuse and Mental Health Services Administration [SAMHSA], 2023). Among adults aged 18 or older, 8.8% or 22.5 million people had a major depressive episode that same year. The prevalence was highest among young adults aged 18 to 25 (20.1%, or 7.0 million people) and lowest among adults aged 50 or older (4.6%, or 5.5 million people). The rate of major depression in women is twice that of men.

Untreated depressive episodes of major depressive disorder can last anywhere from 6 to 12 months. About 20% of cases become chronic (lasting more than 2 years). While depression may begin with a single episode, most people experience recurrent episodes. Recurrence occurs within the first year about 50% of the time and up to 85% over a lifetime.

The high variability in symptom manifestation, treatment response, and illness course support the belief that major depressive disorder is the result of a complex interaction of factors. For example, a genetic predisposition to depression combined with childhood stress may lead to significant neurochemical changes that contribute to the development of depression. Risk factors for major depressive disorder are listed in Box 7.1.

> **Box 7.1 Primary Risk Factors for Major Depressive Disorder**
>
> - Female sex (higher prevalence in females)
> - Adverse childhood experiences (e.g., abuse, neglect, trauma)
> - Stressful life events (e.g., loss of a loved one, financial difficulties, relationship problems)
> - Family history of major depressive disorder (first-degree relatives)
> - Personality traits such as neuroticism (i.e., a negative personality trait characterized by anxiety, fear, moodiness, worry, envy, frustration, jealousy, and loneliness)
> - Cooccurring psychiatric disorders (e.g., substance use, anxiety, personality disorders)
> - Chronic or disabling physical conditions (e.g., chronic pain, autoimmune diseases

Data from Substance Abuse and Mental Health Services Administration. (2023). *Key substance use and mental health indicators in the United States: Results from the 2022 National Survey on Drug Use and Health* (HHS Publication No. PEP23-07-01-006, NSDUH Series H-58). Retrieved from https://www.samhsa.gov/data/report/2022-nsduh-annual-national-report.

To diagnose major depressive disorder, symptoms must be present nearly every day for at least two weeks. Symptoms must be severe enough to cause significant distress and impairment in daily functioning. These symptoms include:

A. Depressed mood most of the day
B. Markedly reduced interest or pleasure in all or nearly all activities
C. Weight loss when not dieting or weight gain of more than 5% of body weight
D. Insomnia or hypersomnia
E. Psychomotor retardation or agitation
F. Fatigue or loss of energy
G. Feelings of worthlessness or excessive guilt
H. Poor concentration and indecisiveness
I. Recurrent thoughts of suicide or death

A diagnosis of major depressive disorder with mixed features may be given if the individual has experienced subclinical hypomania. However, if the depressive episode occurs in someone who has previously experienced a full manic or hypomanic episode, the diagnosis will be bipolar I disorder or bipolar II disorder, respectively (see Chapter 6).

TREATMENT FOR MAJOR DEPRESSIVE DISORDERS

Biological Treatments

Pharmacotherapy

Major depressive disorder is a recurring condition, and most people will go on to have multiple episodes. However, antidepressants make depression one of the most treatable psychiatric disorders. Medication can improve poor self-concept, degree of withdrawal, vegetative signs of depression, and activity level. See Chapter 24 for a discussion of pharmacotherapy used in the treatment of major depressive disorder.

Neuromodulation Therapies

Neuromodulation therapies, also known as brain stimulation therapies, are becoming increasingly popular and available. Before 2008, there was only one brain stimulation therapy, electroconvulsive therapy (ECT). ECT has US Food and Drug Administration (FDA) approval for depressive symptoms associated with major depressive disorder or bipolar disorder in patients aged 13 years and older. In 2008 and 2009, respectively, repetitive transcranial magnetic stimulation (rTMS) and vagus nerve stimulation (VNS) were approved for treatment-resistant depression. Deep brain stimulation (DBS) involves surgically implanting electrodes to stimulate brain regions that are underactive in depression. It is used without specific FDA approval (i.e., off-label) for major depressive disorder. Chapter 30 provides more information regarding neuromodulation therapies.

Integrative Therapies

Light therapy is a first-line treatment for seasonal affective disorder (SAD), along with or without medication. It uses full-spectrum wavelength light to help regulate mood in individuals who live in climates with significant seasonal variations in daylight. Seasonal variations in mood disorders in the Southern Hemisphere are the reverse of those in the Northern Hemisphere. Light therapy may also serve as a useful adjunct to medications for individuals with chronic major depressive disorder or dysthymia that worsens during certain seasons.

Non-FDA-approved integrative pharmacological approaches are also used in the treatment of major depressive disorder. Herbal therapies such as St. John's Wort and S-adenosylmethionine (SAMe) are commonly used over-the-counter drugs. Refer to Appendix B for integrative therapies used in the treatment of major depressive disorder.

Exercise is a healthy and highly effective approach to reducing depressive symptoms, with biological, social, and psychological benefits. Regular physical activity promotes the release of endorphins and other mood-enhancing neurotransmitters, reduces stress, and provides opportunities for social interaction and a sense of accomplishment.

Psychological Therapies

Cognitive behavioral therapy (CBT), interpersonal therapy (IPT), time-limited focused psychotherapy, and behavioral therapy are particularly effective in the treatment of depression. However, only CBT and IPT demonstrate superiority in the maintenance phase, where the goal is the prevention of new episodes or recurrences. CBT helps individuals restructure negative thought patterns and behaviors, leading to lasting mood improvements. IPT focuses on addressing ongoing relationship issues that may contribute to depression. Group therapy is a widespread modality for the treatment of depression and provides many benefits, particularly in helping individuals to feel "not alone" with their symptoms. See Chapter 29 for more information about psychological models of therapy.

NURSE, PATIENT, AND FAMILY RESOURCES

Depressed Anonymous
Depressed Anonymous is a fellowship of people who share their experiences, strengths, and hopes with each other so that they may solve their common problem and help others to recover from depression.
www.depressedanon.com

Depression and Bipolar Support Alliance
DBSA in-person and online support groups give people living with depression and bipolar disorder a safe, welcoming

place to share experiences, discuss coping skills, and offer each other hope
www.dbsalliance.org

Families for Depression Awareness
Families for Depression Awareness helps families recognize and cope with depression and bipolar disorder to get people well and prevent suicides.
https://www.familyaware.org/#

Internet Mental Health
We are a health technology company guiding people towards self-understanding and connection. Our platform offers reliable resources, accessible services, and nurturing communities.
www.mentalhealth.com

Medline Plus
MedlinePlus is a service of the National Library of Medicine (NLM), the world's largest medical library, which is part of the National Institutes of Health (NIH). Provides high-quality, relevant health and wellness information that is trusted, easy to understand, and free of advertising, in both English and Spanish. Anywhere, anytime, on any device—for free.
https://medlineplus.gov/depression.html

Mental Health America
Mental Health America advances the mental health and well-being of all people living in the United States through public education, research, advocacy, public policy, and direct service.
https://mhanational.org/about-us

Mom's Mental Health Matters
Depression and anxiety can happen during pregnancy or after birth. Learn the signs and how to get help.
https://www.nichd.nih.gov/ncmhep/initiatives/moms-mental-health-matters/moms

National Alliance on Mental Illness (NAMI)
National Alliance on Mental Illness (NAMI) is a nonprofit grassroots group originally founded by family members of people diagnosed with mental illness. NAMI identifies its mission as providing advocacy, education, support,

and public awareness so that all individuals and families affected by mental illness can build better lives. Its vision is promoting a world where all people affected by mental illness live healthy, fulfilling lives supported by a community that cares. Local branches are available in most communities.
www.nami.org

National Institute of Mental Health (NIMH): Depression
The National Institute of Mental Health (NIMH) is the lead federal agency for research on mental disorders. NIMH is one of the 27 Institutes and Centers that make up the National Institutes of Health (NIH), the largest biomedical research agency in the world. NIH is part of the U.S. Department of Health and Human Services (HHS).
https://www.nimh.nih.gov/health/topics/depression

CHAPTER 8

Anxiety and Obsessive–Compulsive Disorders

Anxiety is a fundamental human experience, ranging from mild unease to overwhelming distress. In this chapter, we explore two groups of psychiatric disorders where anxiety takes center stage: anxiety disorders and obsessive–compulsive disorders (OCDs). We begin by defining anxiety and examining its manifestations across a continuum from mild to severe. Next, we delve into specific disorders, highlighting their unique characteristics and challenges. Finally, we provide practical guidance through the nursing process, offering strategies for compassionate, effective care.

ANXIETY

Anxiety is a universal human experience and one of our most basic emotions. It is a feeling of apprehension, uncertainty, or dread triggered by a real or perceived threat. Normal anxiety is a healthy, adaptive response—an evolutionary strategy for survival.

LEVELS OF ANXIETY

Peplau (1968) developed a widely recognized model of anxiety that consists of four levels: mild, moderate, severe, and panic. The boundaries between these levels are not distinct, and the behaviors and characteristics of individuals experiencing anxiety may and often do overlap. Recognizing an individual's general level of anxiety is essential in selecting appropriate and effective nursing interventions.

Mild Anxiety

Mild anxiety is a common part of everyday life and helps individuals perceive reality with greater clarity. A person experiencing a mild level of anxiety sees, hears, and processes more information, enhancing problem-solving abilities. Physical signs of mild anxiety may include slight discomfort, restlessness, or mild tension-relieving behaviors such as nail-biting, foot- or finger-tapping, or fidgeting.

Moderate Anxiety

As anxiety increases, the perceptual field narrows, causing some details to be overlooked. The person sees, hears, and processes less information and may exhibit selective inattention, focusing only on certain aspects of the environment unless others point out what is missed. Clear thinking becomes more difficult, though learning and problem-solving can still occur, albeit less effectively. Activation of the sympathetic nervous system leads to an increased pulse, increased respiratory rates, and perspiration. Mild somatic symptoms such as gastric discomfort, headache, and urinary urgency are also common with moderate anxiety.

Severe Anxiety

A person experiencing severe anxiety experiences a greatly reduced perceptual field. The individual's focus may narrow to one particular detail or become scattered on unrelated details. Other environmental stimuli are often disregarded, even when pointed out by others. Learning and problem-solving are nearly impossible. In this state, behavior is automatic and aimed at reducing or relieving anxiety. Symptoms commonly include trembling, a pounding heart, hyperventilation, and a sense of impending doom or dread. Somatic symptoms such as headache, nausea, and dizziness tend to intensify.

Panic Anxiety

Panic is the most extreme level of anxiety and results in significantly dysregulated behavior. Someone in a state of panic is unable to process their surroundings and may lose touch with reality. Behaviors range from pacing, running, or screaming to complete withdrawal. Patients report a sense of impending doom or danger or feelings of unreality or detachment.

Physical symptoms may include a racing heart, sweating, chills, hot flashes, trembling, shortness of breath, weakness, dizziness, and tingling and or numbness of the hands. Other somatic symptoms, such as include headache, nausea, abdominal cramping, and chest pain, are also common.

ANXIETY DISORDERS

Anxiety disorders are among the most common of all psychiatric conditions. Individuals with these disorders experience anxiety to such a degree that it interferes with personal, occupational, or social functioning. The American Psychiatric Association ([APA], 2022) identifies the following types of anxiety disorders:

- Separation anxiety disorder
- Specific phobia
- Social anxiety disorder
- Panic disorder
- Agoraphobia
- Generalized anxiety disorder

Separation Anxiety Disorder

Separation anxiety is a normal part of infant development that begins around 8 months of age, peaks at about 18 months, and then begins to decline. However, people with separation anxiety disorder exhibit developmentally inappropriate levels of concern over being away from a significant other. There may also be fear that something horrible will happen to the other person and that it will result in permanent separation. The anxiety is so intense that it interferes with normal activities and causes sleep disruptions and nightmares. Physical symptoms, such as gastrointestinal disturbances and headaches, are also common.

Although this disorder is most often associated with children, it can also affect adults. This disorder is characterized by harm avoidance, excessive worry, shyness, uncertainty, fatigability, and a lack of self-direction. Fear of separation from a significant other (e.g., a parent or spouse) causes extreme discomfort and disability that can impair educational, social, and occupational functioning.

Separation anxiety disorder is typically diagnosed before the age of 18, following at least one month of symptoms. Lifetime prevalence rates in children and adults are 4.1% and 6.6%, respectively (Shear et al., 2006). Approximately one-third (about 36%) of childhood cases persist into adulthood, while the majority (78%) of adult cases have onsets in adulthood. It is the most common anxiety disorder in children. Females are more likely to be affected.

Specific Phobia

A specific phobia is a persistent irrational fear of a specific object, activity, or situation. This fear leads to a desire to avoid or actual avoidance of the object, activity, or situation. Phobias compromise a person's daily functioning, since people with phobias are consumed with avoiding the feared object or situation.

Humans may be hardwired to develop certain phobias as an evolutionary protective mechanism. Common and potentially protective phobias include arachnophobia (fear of spiders and other arachnids), ophidiophobia (fear of snakes), acrophobia (fear of heights), and cynophobia (fear of dogs).

The twelve-month prevalence rate for specific phobias is 9.1%, with higher rates in females (12.2%) than in males (5.8%) (NIMH, 2024). Phobic reactions tend to run in families. Having a first-degree relative with a specific phobia puts one at greater risk of having the same specific phobia. Negative and traumatic experiences with the feared objects or situations often precede the phobia.

Social Anxiety Disorder

Social anxiety disorder, formerly called social phobia, is characterized by severe anxiety or fear. This response is provoked by social or performance situations that have the potential for negative evaluations by others. Social anxiety triggers include the fear of saying the wrong thing in a public setting, eating or drinking in front of others, or speaking in public. These fears lead to extreme avoidance of these situations. When avoidance is not possible, individuals endure the situation with intense anxiety and emotional distress. Fear of public speaking is the most common manifestation of social anxiety disorder.

Young children with this disorder may be mute and nervous and may hide behind their parents. Older children and adolescents may be paralyzed by fear of speaking in class due to worry of saying the wrong thing or being criticized. Conversely, younger people may act out to compensate for this fear, making an accurate diagnosis more difficult. Physical complaints are often used to avoid social situations, particularly school.

The 12-month prevalence of social anxiety disorder is 7.1% (NIMH, 2024). Females are more likely to be affected. Risk factors for social anxiety disorder include childhood mistreatment and adverse childhood experiences. Shyness, a strongly heritable trait, also plays a role. Children with shy parents face a double risk due to both genetic predisposition and the influence of parental modeling.

Panic Disorder

Panic attacks are the key feature of panic disorder. A panic attack is the sudden onset of extreme apprehension or fear, usually associated with feelings of impending doom. During a panic attack, normal functioning is suspended, the perceptual field is severely limited, and misinterpretation of reality may occur. People feel like they are losing their minds or are having a heart attack. Typically, panic attacks come on suddenly, last a matter of minutes, and then subside. A secondary disability occurs when people who experience these attacks begin to "fear the fear" and become so preoccupied with the possibility of future episodes that they avoid what could be pleasurable activities.

The 12-month prevalence for panic disorder is 2.7% in adults and is higher in females than males (NIMH, 2024). About **2% of adolescents aged 13–18** experience panic disorder and an additional 2.3% face severe impairment at least once in their lifetime. Research suggests that panic disorder has a complex genetic basis, likely influenced by both genetic variations and environmental factors. So far, no single gene has been consistently identified as a definitive cause of the disorder.

Agoraphobia

The term agoraphobia is derived from the Greek words agora ("open space") and phobia ("fear"). This term refers to excessive anxiety or fear about being in places or situations from which escape might be difficult or embarrassing or where help might be unavailable. The feared places or situations may be avoided altogether to control anxiety. People with agoraphobia often have a fear of being alone, traveling (e.g., in a car, bus, or airplane), being on a bridge, and riding in an elevator. These situations may be more tolerable when accompanied by another person.

About 1% of adults experience agoraphobia each year, with females and males being almost equally affected (NIMH, 2024). Some children may experience agoraphobia, but it typically begins in late adolescence or early adulthood.

Generalized Anxiety Disorder

The key pathological feature of generalized anxiety disorder is excessive worry. Children, teens, and adults may experience this worry, which is out of proportion to the true impact of events or situations.

Common concerns in generalized anxiety disorder are inadequacy in interpersonal relationships, job responsibilities, finances, and the health of family members. Because of this worry, huge amounts of time are spent preparing for activities. Putting things off and avoidance are key symptoms, which may result in lateness or absence from school or employment and overall social isolation. Family members and friends are overtaxed as the person seeks constant reassurance and perseverates about meaningless details.

Sleep disturbances are common due to worrying about the day's real or imagined mistakes, reviewing past problems, and anticipating future difficulties. Fatigue is a side effect of sleep deprivation.

The 12-month prevalence rate of generalized anxiety disorder is nearly 1% in adolescents and nearly 3% in adults (APA, 2024). Over a lifetime, the risk of this disorder is 9%. The ratio of affected females to males is 2:1.

Parental overprotection and adverse experiences are associated with anxiety disorders. Genetics accounts for about a third of the risk of developing generalized anxiety disorder.

OBSESSIVE–COMPULSIVE DISORDERS

OCDs are a group of anxiety-related disorders that all have obsessive–compulsive characteristics. Obsessions are thoughts, impulses, or images that persist and recur. They cannot be dismissed even though the individual attempts to do so. Obsessions often seem senseless to the individual who experiences them (referred to as egodystonic), and their presence causes severe anxiety.

Compulsions are ritualistic behaviors individuals feel driven to perform as the result of obsessions. They are an attempt to reduce anxiety or prevent an imagined calamity. Performing the compulsive act temporarily reduces anxiety, but because the relief is only temporary, the compulsive act must be repeated again and again.

OCDs include the following:

- Obsessive–compulsive disorder
- Body dysmorphic disorder
- Hoarding disorder
- Trichotillomania (hair-pulling) disorder
- Excoriation (skin-picking) disorder

Obsessive–Compulsive Disorder

Obsessive–compulsive behavior exists along a continuum. Most of us experience mild obsessive–compulsive symptoms, such as nagging doubts as to whether a door is locked or if the stove is turned off. These doubts may compel us to go back to check the door or stove. Mild obsessions with timeliness, orderliness, and reliability are valued traits in US society.

At the pathological end of the continuum is OCD, with symptoms that occur daily and may involve issues of sexuality, violence, contamination, illness, or death. Pathological obsessions or compulsions cause marked distressing feelings such as humiliation and shame. Rituals are time-consuming and interfere with normal routines, social activities, and relationships. Severe OCD occupies so much of the individual's mental process that cognition is impaired.

The 12-month prevalence of OCD is 1.2% (APA, 2024). Females are slightly more affected, but males have an earlier age of onset (about 25% before age 10). Onset after age 35 is rare.

Sexual and physical abuse or trauma in childhood increases the risk of this disorder. Some children develop OCD as a postinfectious autoimmune syndrome. Genetics are strongly associated with this disorder. First-degree relatives have twice the risk. Early-onset OCD results in a 10 times greater risk of the disorder appearing in first-degree relatives.

Body Dysmorphic Disorder

Individuals with body dysmorphic disorder are commonly seen in psychiatric, cosmetic surgery, and dermatological settings. Although these individuals tend to have a normal appearance, their preoccupation with an imagined flaw results in obsessional thinking and compulsive behavior such as mirror checking and camouflaging. People may be aware that their thoughts are distorted, or they may be convinced of the existence of the defect.

The prevalence of body dysmorphic disorder is slightly higher in females (2.5%) than in males (2.2%) (APA, 2024). The incidence is higher among individuals seeking cosmetic surgery, dermatology treatment, adult orthodontia, and oral/maxillofacial surgery.

Risk factors for this disorder are backgrounds of abuse and neglect. Body dysmorphic disorder is closely related to OCD, with first-degree relatives often sharing one or both of these conditions.

Hoarding Disorder

Hoarding disorder results in the over-accumulation of belongings with little or no value. This hoarding interferes with everyday functioning. Belongings may cover every available surface and fill every drawer, cupboard, and closet. Animal hoarding is particularly insidious and may result in disease, starvation, and death of the pets.

Family members and other guests may be unwilling or unable to visit due to the conditions. Hoarding behaviors may progress to the point where the home is nearly uninhabitable due to unsafe and unsanitary conditions. Individuals with hoarding disorder may have limited awareness of the problem and the extent to which their collecting has consumed their lives and strained relationships.

Hoarding disorder occurs in an estimated 2% to 6% of the population (APA, 2024). This disorder may be more common in males than in females. Three times as many older adults aged 55 to 94 years are affected by hoarding disorder when compared with adults aged 34 to 44 years old.

Stressful life events seem to precede the onset of symptoms. The disorder has a strong genetic component, with a twin concordance rate of 50%, indicating a 50% likelihood that one twin will be affected if the other has the disorder.

Trichotillomania Disorder and Excoriation Disorder

Two types of OCDs fall under the category of body-focused repetitive behaviors:trichotillomania (hair-pulling disorder) and excoriation disorder (skin-picking disorder). These disorders can cause significant distress, often leading to varying degrees of disability, social stigma, and noticeable changes in appearance. The compulsive behaviors are egodystonic—unwanted and inconsistent with the individual's self-image—prompting many affected individuals to go to great lengths to hide their actions

The common expression, "I was so annoyed I wanted to pull my hair out" reflects the anxiety-related nature of trichotillomania (tricho·til·lo·ma·nia). While scalp hair is most often targeted, individuals may pull hair from other areas, including the eyebrows, eyelashes, pubic region, axillae, and limbs. The extent of hair removal in trichotillomania varies, ranging from small, patchy areas to completely bare skin. For some individuals, the pain associated with hair-pulling can temporarily reduce anxiety, like the relief some experience with cutting, another form of self-injurious behavior. Individuals may not be aware of the behavior until they notice a nearby wad of hair in their hand.

Trichotillomania appears to have a genetic component, as it often runs in families. Individuals with relatives who have OCD are at an increased risk of developing trichotillomania, suggesting a potential hereditary link between the two disorders.

The 12-month prevalence of trichotillomania in adolescents and adults is 1% to 2% (APA, 2024). Females are disproportionately affected at a ratio of 10:1. While some infants engage in hair-pulling, this behavior typically resolves with age. In most cases, however, the disorder begins around puberty and often develops into a chronic, long-term condition.

Excoriation disorder (ex·co·ri·ay·shun) often involves skin-picking behaviors that may serve as a way to relieve anxiety, though some individuals engage in the behavior automatically, without conscious awareness. Fingers and fingernails are the usual implements, but nail cutters, tweezers, and even teeth may also be involved. The most common areas of focus are the face, head, cuticles, back, arms and legs, and hands and feet. Complications can include pain, sores, scarring, and infections, which may further contribute to distress and social discomfort.

Genetic factors play a significant role in the development of excoriation disorder, with research suggesting potential genetic overlaps across the broader OCD spectrum. These shared genetic influences may contribute to the similar compulsive behaviors seen in related disorders.

The lifetime prevalence of this usually chronic problem is 1.4% (APA, 2024). About 75% of those affected are female. The onset is in adolescence and frequently begins with conditions such as acne.

Assessment

People with anxiety disorders rarely need hospitalization unless they have suicidal thoughts or have behaviors with the potential for injury, such as severe avoidance and hazardous hoarding. Most individuals with anxiety and OCD disorders are encountered incidentally in community settings rather than inpatient care. For instance, a person may arrive at the emergency department with symptoms resembling a myocardial infarction, only to learn they are experiencing a panic attack.

Signs and Symptoms

- Narrowed perceptual field, difficulty concentrating, ineffective problem solving
- Elevated vital signs (e.g., blood pressure, pulse, and respiration), muscle tension, sweating, pupil dilation
- Palpitations, urinary urgency or frequency, nausea, throat tightness, unsteady voice
- Complaints of persistent fatigue, disrupted sleep patterns, irritability, disorganization
- Panic attacks, obsessions, compulsions, phobias, compulsive hoarding, or free-floating anxiety that interferes with everyday functioning
- A sense of impending doom or the feeling of dying

Assessment Tools

Objectively, a variety of scales are available to measure anxiety and anxiety-related symptoms. There are specific measures for phobias, panic symptoms, and obsessive thoughts and behaviors. The Severity Measure for

Generalized Anxiety Disorder in Adults is a popular tool for measuring anxiety (Fig. 8.1). High scores may indicate generalized anxiety disorder or panic disorder, although it is important to note that high anxiety scores may also indicate major depressive disorder. Another measure, with identical assessment items, is available for people 11 to 17 years of age.

Assessment Guidelines

It is essential to determine whether anxiety is the primary problem, as in an anxiety disorder, or secondary to another cause, such as physical condition or substance use.

A. Assess for a history of childhood abuse.

B. Assess for the potential for self-harm. Severe anxiety disorder is associated with suicide as well as misuse of medications or illicit drugs.

C. Assess the patient's community for clinics, groups, and counselors who offer anxiety-reduction techniques.

D. Be aware that differences in culture can affect how anxiety is manifested.

PROMIS Emotional Distress—Anxiety—Short Form

In the past SEVEN (7) DAYS....		Never	Rarely	Sometimes	Often	Always	Use Item Score
1.	I felt fearful.	❏ 1	❏ 2	❏ 3	❏ 4	❏ 5	
2.	I felt anxious.	❏ 1	❏ 2	❏ 3	❏ 4	❏ 5	
3.	I felt worried.	❏ 1	❏ 2	❏ 3	❏ 4	❏ 5	
4.	I found it hard to focus on anything other than my anxiety.	❏ 1	❏ 2	❏ 3	❏ 4	❏ 5	
5.	I felt nervous.	❏ 1	❏ 2	❏ 3	❏ 4	❏ 5	
6.	I felt uneasy.	❏ 1	❏ 2	❏ 3	❏ 4	❏ 5	
7.	I felt tense.	❏ 1	❏ 2	❏ 3	❏ 4	❏ 5	
						Total Score	

Fig. 8.1 Severity measure for generalized anxiety disorder in adults.

Nursing Diagnoses

Not surprisingly, the nursing diagnosis *anxiety* is most often used to address these disorders. When focusing on this diagnosis, the nurse needs to clarify the level of anxiety, because different levels call for different intervention strategies. *Impaired coping* is another common nursing diagnosis, because high levels of anxiety interfere with the ability to work, disruptrelationships, and impair one's ability to interact satisfactorily with others.

The nursing diagnosis *lack of knowledge of the treatment regimen* indicates a need for increased understanding of the anxiety disorder, its symptoms, and symptom management. Since people with anxiety often experience difficulty falling asleep, difficulty maintaining sleep, and early-morning awakening. Sleep disruptions can impair functioning at work, at school, and in social situations. Therefore the problem of *impaired sleep* is an essential nursing diagnosis when caring for this population.

Intervention Guidelines

When medications are used in conjunction with therapy, patients and their significant others can benefit from thorough teaching. Give written information and instructions to the patient and family.

A. Use counseling, milieu therapy, promotion of self-care activities, pharmacotherapy, biological, and health teaching interventions.
B. Guide patients through relaxation techniques such as progressive muscle relaxation.
C. Identify community resources that can offer the patient specialized treatment proven to be highly effective for people with a variety of anxiety disorders.
D. Identify community support groups for people with specific anxiety disorders and their families.

Nursing Care for Anxiety and Obsessive–Compulsive Disorders

Anxiety

Related to

- Biochemical alterations in the brain
- External stressors (e.g., economic, job loss, housing problems)

- Internal stressors (e.g., illness, altered self-concept)
- Deficient resources
- Substance use
- Crisis (situational, maturational, adventitious)
- Exposure to phobic object or situation
- Ritualistic behavior
- Fear of panic attack
- Intrusive, unwanted thoughts

Desired Outcome The patient will experience decreased anxiety.

Assessment/Interventions and *Rationales*
1. Promote a calm environment by reducing environmental stimuli, such as noise, activity, and visual distractions. *A quiet, structured environment helps decrease sensory overload, which can intensify anxiety and make it more difficult to focus or self-regulate.*
2. Provide reassurance that you will help the patient reduce anxiety. *A sense of connection and safety can ease feelings of fear and vulnerability and can reduce anxiety.*
3. Help the patient to reduce anxiety from severe or panic to mild or moderate through slow, deep breathing or medication if prescribed. *Reducing anxiety to mild or moderate levels is necessary for learning to take place.*
4. Encourage the patient to talk about feelings and concerns. *When concerns are stated out loud, problems can be discussed, and feelings of isolation reduced.*
5. Help the patient to reframe the problem in a way that is solvable. Provide a new perspective and correct distorted perceptions. *Correcting distortions increases the possibility of finding workable solutions to a realistically defined problem.*
6. Assist the patient in identifying thoughts or feelings before the onset of anxiety: "What were you doing or thinking right before you started to feel anxious?" *Recognizing the thoughts, feelings, or situations that trigger anxiety provides insight into its origins. This recognition helps the patient understand why these triggers feel so distressing, paving the way for more effective coping strategies.*
7. Teach relaxation techniques (e.g., deep breathing exercises, meditation, progressive muscle relaxation). *Learning to reduce physiological arousal helps patients*

manage anxiety more effectively and improves their ability to assess situations and apply problem-solving skills.

8. Help the patient to identify negative self-talk or messages (e.g., "I'll never be able to do this right." "This means I'll never succeed in anything."). Recognizing negative thought patterns allows the patient to reframe their thinking, promoting more constructive problem-solving and reducing anxiety.

9. Refer the patient and significant others to support groups, self-help programs, or advocacy groups when appropriate. *Patients with specific problems greatly benefit from being around others who are grappling with similar issues. This provides the patient with information and support and decreases feelings of isolation in stressful and difficult situations.*

10. Administer medications or obtain an order for medications when appropriate. *Medications can lower symptoms of anxiety to a level that allows the patient to learn and better use coping mechanisms.*

Impaired Coping

Related to

- Severe to panic levels of anxiety—panic attack, generalized anxiety disorder
- Excessive negative beliefs about self
- Presence of obsessions and compulsions
- Avoidance behavior
- Compulsive hoarding

Desired Outcome The patient will verbally demonstrate the ability to cope effectively with anxiety.

Assessment/Interventions and *Rationales*

1. Monitor and reinforce the patient's use of positive coping skills. *Identifies what does and does not work for the patient. The patient learns to build upon strengths.*

2. Explore new coping skills to substitute for ineffective ones. *Provides more adaptive options.*

3. At the patient's level of understanding, explain the fight-or-flight response and the relaxation response of the autonomic nervous system. Address how breathing can be used to bring about the relaxation response. *Understanding the physiological aspects of anxiety and that individuals have some degree of control*

6. Role-play and rehearse alternative coping strategies that can be used in threatening or anxiety-provoking situations. *Gives the patient a chance to be proactive, giving the patient a choice of alternatives instead of the patient using the usual unsatisfactory automatic reactions.*

7. Encourage the patient to keep a daily journal of thoughts and situations that seem to precede anxiety and the coping strategies used. *Allows the patient to monitor triggers and evaluate coping strategies over time.*

8. Teach the patient to rate anxiety levels on a scale from 1 to 10, with 1 the lowest and 10 the highest. *Using a rating scale helps the patient develop self-awareness of anxiety fluctuations, identify triggers, and assess the effectiveness of coping strategies over time.*

9. Encourage the patient to keep a journal to record anxiety levels, triggers, and the situations in which anxiety occurs. *Journaling provides insight into anxiety patterns, helps identify triggers, and allows the patient to track progress and evaluate the effectiveness of coping strategies.*

10. Review the journal with the patient to identify which strategies were effective and which were not. *Analyzing journal entries helps the patient recognize successful coping techniques, adjust ineffective ones, and maintain motivation during challenging periods.*

11. Review the patient's progress and acknowledge their efforts. *Positive feedback reinforces learning,* boosts confidence, and encourages continued use of effective coping strategies.

12. Review stress-reduction techniques with the patient, family, and significant others during teaching sessions, andencourage regular practice of relaxation techniques. *Anxiety can be communicated interpersonally, and involving family members helps create a supportive environment.*

13. Provide printed materials that explain and demonstrate stress-reduction techniques. *Written resources serve as a reference for patients and their families, reinforcing learning and supporting the consistent practice of stress-management strategies.*

14. Refer the patient to community support groups with individuals facing similar challenges. *Support groups provide a sense of belonging, reduce feelings of isolation, and offer positive reinforcement, which can enhance self-esteem and encourage adherence to coping strategies.*

15. Refer family members and significant others to community resources such as family therapy, couples counseling, financial counseling, support groups, or relaxation classes. *Providing support for family and significant others helps them develop effective coping strategies, reduces stress, and fosters a healthier environment for both the patient and their support system.*

Impaired Sleep

Related to Provide written material
- Biochemical alterations in the brain
- Fear
- Anxiety
- Inadequate sleep hygiene
- Obsessive thoughts

Desired Outcome The patient will report satisfaction with falling asleep, maintaining sleep, and time upon awakening.

Assessment/Interventions and *Rationales*

1. Assess the patient's sleep patterns, changes that have occurred, and whether there was a precipitating event around the onset of the sleep problem or whether it is chronic. *Understanding the baseline sleep pattern provides direction for addressing the impaired sleep.*

2. Identify the patient's usual sleep habits, including bedtime rituals, time of retiring, time of rising, use of alcohol or caffeine before bedtime, and use of sleep aids (prescribed or over-the-counter medications.) *Establishing a baseline helps to determine useful interventions.*

3. Promote a sleep relaxation routine using techniques such as self-hypnosis, progressive muscle relaxation, and guided imagery. *Engaging in both physical and mental relaxation helps reduce anxiety, calm the nervous system, and promote restful sleep.*

4. Demonstrate and rehearse relaxation techniques with the patient until they are able to confidently practice them at bedtime. *Repeated practice builds confidence and increases the likelihood of successfully using these techniques to promote relaxation and improve sleep.*

activity. Another noninvasive option is cranial electrotherapy stimulation (CES), which delivers low-level, pulsed electrical currents through electrodes placed on the head. CES is FDA-cleared for the treatment of anxiety and insomnia.

A more invasive but reversible surgical treatment for OCD is deep brain stimulation (DBS). The FDA has approved DBS as an add-on treatment for adults with treatment-resistant OCD who have not responded to at least three SSRI trials. The procedure involves surgically placing electrodes in both sides of the subthalamic nucleus of the brain. A pulse generator implanted in the chest then delivers a low-dose electrical current over a set period, sometimes lasting several months. Chapter 30 discusses brain stimulation therapies in more depth.

Integrative Care

Appendix B identifies complementary practices or integrative therapies that people use to cope with anxiety.

Psychological Therapies

Psychiatric-mental health advanced practice registered nurses, like other advanced practice psychiatric professionals, are qualified to conduct individual and group psychotherapy. Two important forms of therapy for anxiety disorders are behavioral therapy and cognitive behavioral therapy. Examples of these types of therapies include:

- Cognitive restructuring
- Breath restraining and muscle relaxation
- Modeling techniques
- Systematic desensitization or graduated exposure
- Flooding (implosion therapy)
- Teaching self-monitoring for panic and other symptoms
- In vivo (real life) exposure to feared objects or situations

Nonpharmacologic therapies seem to be particularly useful for OCDs. They include:

- Exposure and response prevention
- Flooding

See Chapter 29 for more discussion on psychotherapeutic models.

👫 NURSE, PATIENT, AND FAMILY RESOURCES

Anxiety and Depression Association of America (ADAA)
ADAA is an international nonprofit organization dedicated to the prevention, treatment, and cure of anxiety, depression, OCD, PTSD, and cooccurring disorders through aligning research, practice, and education.
www.adaa.org

Body Dysmorphic Disorder (BDD) Foundation
The BDD Foundation aims to relieve the suffering of people with BDD while advancing research, treatments, and awareness of the condition.
www.bddfoundation.org/

International OCD Foundation
Provides up-to-date education and resources, strengthens community engagement, delivers quality professional training, and advances groundbreaking research.
www.iocdf.org

Mental Help Net
Mentalhelp.net provides accurate and up-to-date information available in the field of addiction medicine and behavioral health and has enlisted an acclaimed team of authors, treatment professionals, and editorial experts to write, review, and update content to check that it meets our high editorial standards.
www.mentalhelp.net

Medline Plus: Panic Disorder
Medline Plus links to health information from the National Institutes of Health, other Federal government agencies, and non-government websites.
www.nlm.nih.gov/medlineplus/panicdisorder.html

Panic/Anxiety Disorders Guide
Includes articles and fact sheets reviewed by psychiatrists from Verywell Mind, whose mission is to help prioritize mental health and find balance.
www.panicdisorder.about.com

TLC Foundation for Body-Focused Repetitive Behavior
A health-related human services organization dedicated
to supporting the 1-in-20 individuals experiencing body-
focused repetitive behaviors (BFRBs) through advocacy,
awareness, connection, health education, celebration, and
equitable access to effective evidence-based treatments.
www.bfrb.org/

CHAPTER 9

Trauma-Related Disorders

Traumatic life events can leave deep and lasting imprints on both the mind and body. From witnessing distressing events to enduring interpersonal violence, sexual abuse, physical harm, or severe neglect, trauma takes many forms. Experiences like repeated abandonment or the sudden, tragic loss of a loved one—whether in childhood, adolescence, or adulthood—can disrupt a person's sense of safety and profoundly affect mental and physical health.

Understanding of the long-term physiological and psychological effects of trauma has grown significantly, and effective treatments are now available. Trauma-informed care is a treatment framework that involves recognizing and responding to the effects of all types of trauma. Integrating trauma-informed care is a framework that helps healthcare professionals recognize and respond to the effects of trauma. Integrating this approach into healthcare settings can reduce trauma's pervasive and damaging impact.

The American Psychiatric Association's (APA) *Diagnostic and Statistical Manual of Mental Disorders, fifth edition, text revision* ([DSM-5-TR] APA, 2022) categorizes the following trauma- and stressor-related disorders:

- Reactive attachment disorder: Occurs in children whose trauma leaves them unable to respond emotionally to caregivers.
- Disinhibited social engagement disorder: Occurs in children whose trauma causes them to bond superficially and indiscriminately with unfamiliar adults.
- Adjustment disorder: Emotional or behavioral symptoms develop in response to stress and are out of proportion to the stressor.
- Prolonged grief disorder: May be diagnosed one year after the death of someone close, there is a deep

longing for the person and a fixation on them, resulting in impaired functioning.

This chapter focuses on two other trauma-related disorders: acute stress disorder (ASD) and posttraumatic stress
disorder (PTSD). Both conditions develop after exposure to
an extremely traumatic event, typically outside the range
of normal experience. The key difference between ASD and
PTSD is timing: ASD symptoms appear within 1 month of
the traumatic event and usually resolve within that time. If
symptoms persist beyond 1 month, the diagnosis changes
from ASD to PTSD. A summary of ASD and PTSD is presented in Table 9.1.

ASD may develop after exposure to a traumatic event.
It can arise following direct exposure to a life-threatening
situation, serious injury, or sexual violence. ASD may
also occur after witnessing such events or learning that a
traumatic event has happened to a close family member or
friend. Repeated exposure to traumatic events may result
in ASD. First responders who collect human remains,
healthcare workers exposed to descriptions of child abuse,
and police officers who hear horrific details about crimes
are examples of those at risk.

The onset of ASD is typically within three days to
four weeks after a traumatic event. It is characterized by
symptoms such as intense fear, helplessness, or horror,
often accompanied by distressing memories, flashbacks,
or dreams related to the event. Traumatic events that may
trigger ASD include, but are not limited to:

- Military experiences: Combat, prisoner-of-war situations, or being taken hostage.
- Criminal events: Bombings, assaults, muggings, or
  sexual violence (e.g., rape).
- Natural disasters: Floods, tornadoes, hurricanes, and
  earthquakes.
- Accidents: Automobile crashes, airline and train accidents, or industrial accidents.
- Medical trauma: Being diagnosed with or witnessing a
  loved one with a life-threatening illness or undergoing
  intense medical treatment, particularly in an intensive
  care unit (ICU) setting.

Individuals with ASD may experience intrusive memories, dissociative symptoms, negative mood, avoidance
behaviors, heightened arousal, and difficulties with daily
functioning. Early intervention and appropriate therapeutic

support are crucial for a person using ASD as preventing its progression into a more chronic condition, such as PTSD.

To receive an ASD diagnosis, a person must exhibit at least nine of the following symptoms during or after the traumatic event:

1. Intrusive distressing memories of the event
2. Recurrent distressing dreams
3. Dissociative reactions, such as flashbacks, in which the person feels as if the traumatic event is recurring
4. Intense, prolonged psychological distress
5. Persistent negative mood, including an inability to experience joy
6. Altered sense of reality regarding one's surroundings
7. Inability to remember an important part of the event
8. Attempts to avoid distressing memories or feelings associated with the event
9. Attempts to avoid external reminders, such as people, places, and objects that are reminders of the trauma
10. Sleep disturbances
11. Hypervigilance
12. Irritable anger/behavior
13. Exaggerated startle response
14. Difficulty concentrating

POSTTRAUMATIC STRESS DISORDER

For individuals aged 6 and over, posttraumatic stress disorder (PTSD) is characterized by the persistent reexperiencing of a highly traumatic event. This event typically involves actual or threatened serious injury to oneself or others. These symptoms can begin or increase post, helplessness, or fear. This can occur after any traumatic event that fits the criteria. While ASD and PTSD is diagnosed when symptoms persist for at least one month, however, it is not uncommon for symptoms to be delayed for months or even years after the event.

In both adults and children, the common features of PTSD include one or more of the following (APA, 2022):

1. Intrusive, distressing memories of the event
2. Recurrent distressing dreams
3. Dissociative reactions or flashbacks in which the trauma seems to be recurring

Table 9.1 Comparison of Acute Stress Disorder and Posttraumatic Stress Disorder

Condition	Onset	Duration	Symptoms	Treatment
Acute stress disorder	0–28 days after the trauma occurs	3 days to 1 month	Dissociative symptoms	Short-term psychotherapy and antidepressant medications
Posttraumatic stress disorder	At least one month after the trauma occurs	1 month to years	Reexperiencing, avoidance, heightened arousal, marked changes in mood and cognition	Long-term psychotherapy, medication, and eye movement desensitization and reprocessing (EMDR) therapy

support are crucial for managing ASD and preventing its progression into more chronic conditions, such as PTSD.

To receive an ASD diagnosis, an individual must exhibit at least nine of the following symptoms during or after the traumatic event:

1. Intrusive distressing memories of the event
2. Recurrent distressing dreams
3. Dissociative reactions (flashbacks) in which the trauma seems to be recurring
4. Intense, prolonged distress or physical reactivity
5. Persistent negative mood and reduced ability to experience joy
6. Altered sense of reality regarding oneself or surroundings
7. Inability to remember important parts of the event
8. Attempts to avoid distressing memories or feelings associated with the trauma
9. Attempts to avoid external cues such as people, places, and objects that serve as reminders of the trauma
10. Sleep disturbances
11. Hypervigilance
12. Irritable, angry, or aggressive behavior
13. Exaggerated startle response
14. Difficulty concentrating

POSTTRAUMATIC STRESS DISORDER

For individuals aged 6 years and older, posttraumatic stress disorder (PTSD) is characterized by the persistent reexperiencing of a highly traumatic event. This event typically involves actual or threatened death or serious injury to oneself or others. The individual may experience intense fear, helplessness, or horror. PTSD may occur after any traumatic event that is outside the range of usual experience, as described in the previous section on ASD. PTSD is diagnosed when symptoms persist for at least one month; however, it is not uncommon forsymptoms to be delayed for months or even years after the event.

In both adults and children, the major features of PTSD include one or more of the following (APA, 2022):

1. Intrusive, distressing memories of the event
2. Recurrent distressing dreams
3. Dissociative reactions (flashbacks) in which the trauma seems to be recurring

4. Intense, prolonged distress or physical reactivity
5. Heightened physiological reactions to cues that resemble an aspect of the trauma

Other symptoms relate to avoidance, as exhibited by one or both of the following:

1. Avoiding distressing thoughts, feelings, or memories related to the event
2. Avoidance of external reminders (e.g., people, places, activities) that are associated with the traumatic event

Negative changes in mood or thinking are reflected by two or more of the following:

1. Gaps in memory related to important aspects of the traumatic event
2. Persistent negative beliefs about oneself, others, and the world
3. Ongoing self-blame or blaming others for the cause or consequences of the trauma
4. Negative emotions such as fear, anger, or guilt
5. Diminished interest in usual activities
6. A sense of detachment from other people
7. Difficulty experiencing positive emotions, such as happiness or satisfaction

Changes in reactivity following the traumatic event are evidenced by two or more of the following:

1. Irritability and outbursts of angry verbal or physical aggression
2. Self-destructive or reckless behavior
3. Hypervigilance
4. Exaggerated startle response
5. Difficulty with concentration
6. Sleep problems, such as trouble falling asleep, staying asleep, or experiencing restlessness sleep

The APA (2022) distinguishes PTSD diagnostic criteria for preschool children due to their developing cognitive and verbal skills, requiring more behaviorally based indicators. A primary symptom in preschool children may manifest as a reduction in play. Other symptoms include reenactment of aspects of the traumatic event, social withdrawal, and negative emotions such as fear, guilt, anger, horror, sadness, shame, or confusion. Children may blame themselves for the traumatic event. In addition, they may experience feelings of detachment or estrangement from others and show less interest or participation in significant activities.

Epidemiology

About 70% of individuals experience at least one traumatic in their lifetime (National Council for Mental Well-Being, 2022). Men are more likely to experience physical assaults, accidents, disasters, combat, and witness injury or death. Women are more likely to experience childhood sexual abuse or become victims of sexual assault. Estimates of PTSD prevalence range from 3.5% to as high as 26.9% of the population at some time in their lives (Schein et al., 2021).

Not everyone who experiences trauma develops PTSD. An individual's response to a disturbing event varies widely, depending on factors such as age, developmental stage, coping skills, support system, cognitive abilities, and preexisting neural physiology.

Assessment

Assessment involves evaluating the onset, frequency, course, and severity of symptoms. It is also important to assess the level of distress and degree of functional impairment. Additional factors to consider include suicidal or violent thoughts, family and social supports, insomnia, social withdrawal, current life stressors, medication, past medical and psychiatric history, and a mental status exam.

A commonly used screening tool for PTSD in adults is the Primary Care PTSD Screen for DSM-5 (PC-PTSD-5) (Prins et al., 2015). See Box 9.1.

Nursing Care for Trauma-Related Disorders

After a comprehensive trauma assessment, priority nursing diagnoses are identified (International Council of Nurses [ICN], 2019). The most common nursing diagnosis for both children and adults is *posttrauma response*, which directly applies to both ASD and PTSD. *Anxiety* is also a key nursing diagnosis for this population. *Anxiety* levels may be levels of moderate, severe, and panic and are triggered by intrusive memories, distressing dreams, and flashbacks. Anxiety can also cause symptoms such as avoidance, hypervigilance, and an exaggerated startle response.

Posttrauma Response

Related to
- Biochemical alterations in the brain

Box 9.1 **Primary Care PTSD Screen for DSM-5**

Sometimes things happen to people that are unusually or especially frightening, horrible, or traumatic. For example:

- A serious accident or fire
- A physical or sexual assault or abuse
- An earthquake or flood
- A war
- Seeing someone be killed or seriously injured
- Having a loved one die through homicide or suicide

Have you ever experienced this kind of event?

If no, screen total = 0. Please stop here

If yes, please answer the questions below.

In the past month, have you:

1. Had nightmares about the event(s) or thought about the event(s) when you did not want to?
   Yes   No
2. Tried hard not to think about the event(s) or went out of your way to avoid situations that reminded you of the event(s)?
   Yes   No
3. Been constantly on guard, watchful, or easily startled?
   Yes   No
4. Felt numb or detached from people, activities, or your surroundings?
   Yes   No
5. Felt guilty or unable to stop blaming yourself or others for the event(s) or any problems the event(s) may have caused?
   Yes   No

Scoring: Patients screen positive if they answer "yes" to three or more items and should receive further evaluation for PTSD.

PTSD, Posttraumatic stress disorder.
From Prins, A., Bovin, M. J., Kimerling, R., Kaloupek, D. G, Marx, B. P., Pless Kaiser, A., & Schnurr, P. P. (2015). *The primary care PTSD screen for DSM-5   (PC-PTSD-5)*. https://www.ptsd.va.gov/professional/assessment/screens/pc-ptsd.asp.

- Physical, psychological, or sexual abuse
- Neglect
- Assault and violence
- Man-made or natural disasters
- Motor vehicle or industrial accidents
- Terrorism, military combat, prisoner-of-war experiences, or torture

- Near-death medical experiences
- Witnessing traumatic event(s)
- Learning about trauma involving family or friends
- Repeated or extreme exposure to trauma-related details

Desired Outcome The patient will report and demonstrate a return to the pretrauma level of functioning.

Assessment/Interventions and *Rationales*

1. Assess for suicidal or homicidal thoughts. *The highest priority is ensuring the safety of the patient and others, and nursing interventions should focus on immediate risk reduction.*

2. Assess the patient's anxiety level. *This assessment helps determine the appropriate level of intervention needed to prevent or minimize anxiety escalation.*

3. Assess for alcohol or drug use and, if present, evaluate the patient's readiness for substance use therapies (e.g., support groups, counseling). Offer referrals if the patient is ready. *Patients cannot effectively participate in learning coping skills, processing traumatic memories, or making positive changes while impaired.*

4. Identify the patient's symptoms and clarify that they are anxiety-related rather than caused by a physical condition (e.g., chest tightness, headaches, dizziness, numbness). *Rule out physical causes before attributing symptoms to psychiatric factors as patients with PTSD may also have cooccurring medical conditions, such as cardiac issues, that require attention.*

5. Identify and document psychiatric symptoms (e.g., shock, anger, withdrawal, panic, confusion, psychosis, emotional instability, nightmares, flashbacks). *This information helps guide intervention strategies, as different symptoms require tailored approaches.*

6. Identify and refer the patient to support groups with others who have experienced similar trauma. *Support groups provide a safe, healing environment for individuals to express their feelings and connect with others who understand their experiences.*

7. Spend time with the patient, allowing the patient to set the pace when describing present or past traumatic events. *Feelings and memories of trauma are often buried. It takes time and trust for a person to open up to a stranger or discuss a topic that has not been shared with anyone before.*

8. Monitor your own emotional responses to the patient's experience. *Hearing traumatic stories can be distressing and may trigger personal reactions that could affect therapeutic effectiveness.*

9. Avoid interrupting, minimizing the painfulness of events, or over-identifying with the patient's experience. *These behaviors can undermine the patient's sense of safety, invalidate their feelings, and disrupt the therapeutic process.*

10. Therapeutic communication is important when working with patients who have experienced significant trauma. Remain nonjudgmental in your interactions with patients who have experienced trauma. *Patients who have experienced trauma often blame themselves and feel guilt and are extremely sensitive to disapproval. Nurses are most supportive when they monitor their responses and avoid reinforcing blame, shame, and guilt.*

11. Listen actively and attentively as the patient describes traumatic events. *Sharing their pain in a supportive environment can be a crucial first step toward healing.*

12. Encourage the expression of feelings through talking, writing, crying, role-playing, or other ways in which the patient is comfortable. *The description of the events and the expression of feelings associated with the event are essential to the healing process.*

13. Teach cognitive and behavioral strategies to manage symptoms of emotional and physical reactivity. These strategies include deep breathing, relaxation exercises, cognitive techniques, desensitization, assertive behavior, thought-stopping techniques, and stress-reduction techniques. *These strategies help patients reduce distress, regain a sense of control, and improve their ability to cope with trauma-related symptoms in daily life.*

14. Assess the family and social support system to determine the need for family interventions or counseling. *Family members often experience confusion, fear, anger, or hopelessness when coping with trauma-related symptoms, and external support can improve understanding and resilience.*

15. Provide education for the patient and family on the signs and symptoms of PTSD. *Understanding the signs and symptoms of PTSD helps patients and their families recognize distressing patterns, respond appropriately, and seek timely support, promoting better coping and recovery outcomes.*

Anxiety (Moderate or Severe)

Related to
- Biochemical alterations in the brain
- Dysregulation of the hypothalamic-pituitary-adrenal axis
- Traumatic event
- Intrusive recurrent memories
- Flashbacks
- Recurrent distressing dreams
- Exaggerated negative beliefs
- Sleep disturbance

Desired Outcome The patient will report decreased anxiety.

Assessment/Interventions and *Rationales*
1. Spend time with the patient and provide a calm, reassuring presence. *Your presence can offer a sense of safety and comfort, helping to reduce anxiety and promote emotional stability.*
2. Be conscious of the patient's need for increased personal space, especially during episodes of hypervigilance. *Patients experiencing hypervigilance may feel easily threatened, and respecting their space can help reduce anxiety.*
3. Observe the patient's nonverbal cues, such as leaning back or backing away, to gauge their comfort with physical proximity. *Nonverbal behaviors can provide insight into the patient's level of distress and the space they need to feel safe.*
4. Acknowledge the patient's anxiety with a statement such as, "I understand that you have been going through a rough time and that you've been anxious. How would you describe your level of anxiety now?" *Discussing anxiety symptoms out loud and identifying the level of anxiety provide empathy to the patient and help guide interventions.*
5. Encourage the use of a quiet environment such as the patient's room during periods of acute anxiety. *External stimuli and unit noise increase anxiety levels.*
6. If the patient is agitated or restless, offer to walk together with them as you talk. *Walking while talking can help reduce agitation by providing a physical outlet for*

excess energy, promoting relaxation, and facilitating more open communication in a less confrontational setting.

7. Provide clear, immediate guidance if anxiety becomes severe or appears to be escalating. "Molly, take a deep breath in through your nose… now exhale slowly through your mouth. Let's do that again." *Sow, deep breathing helps reduce the body's stress response and provides a calming point of focus during moments of intense anxiety.*

8. If guidance does not reduce the patient's anxiety, offer as-needed medication if ordered. If no medication is available, consult the care provider to discuss this option. *During acute exacerbation, medication can provide essential relief, allowing patients to engage more effectively in nonpharmacological interventions once anxiety decreases.*

9. Ask the patient what calming measures have worked in the past, such as "What usually helps you feel less anxious?" *Reinforcing previously successful coping strategies providesreassurance and encourages the patient to use familiar, effective techniques during periods of heightened anxiety.*

10. As anxiety decreases ask what was happening immediately before the onset of anxiety symptoms. *Understanding triggers for anxiety is the first step in addressing the problem. The patient may be unaware of thoughts, feelings, or events that set the anxious feelings in motion.*

11. When the patient's anxiety decreases to a moderate or mild level, explore behavioral techniques (e.g., progressive muscle relaxation) and cognitive strategies (e.g., challenging exaggerated, negative thoughts) to manage future anxiety. *Learning and practicing these skills can help patients recognize early signs of anxiety and apply effective techniques to prevent escalation.*

TREATMENT FOR TRAUMA-RELATED DISORDERS

Biological Approaches

Pharmacotherapy

Medications can play a key role in the treatment of PTSD. Antidepressants are commonly prescribed to help alleviate symptoms of depression and anxiety, as well as improve sleep and concentration. The selective serotonin reuptake inhibitors (SSRIs) **sertraline (Zoloft)** and **paroxetine (Paxil)** are approved by the US Food and Drug Administration (FDA) for the treatment of PTSD.

Other antidepressants that are prescribed off-label include fluoxetine (Prozac) and venlafaxine (Effexor). Nefazodone (Serzone), imipramine (Tofranil), and phenelzine (Nardil) are suggested if other medications are ineffective (U.S. Department of Veterans Affairs and Department of Defense, 2017). See Chapter 24 for more information on antidepressants.

Psychological Therapies

Advanced practice psychiatric professionals, including advanced practice psychiatric-mental health registered nurses, are qualified to provide individual and group psychotherapy. Trauma-focused psychotherapy is the most effective approach for treating PTSD. Trauma-focused psychotherapy uses various techniques to help patients process traumatic experiences. Some methods involve visualizing, talking, or thinking about the traumatic memory, while others focus on reframing unhelpful beliefs about the trauma. This type of therapy typically lasts 8 to 16 sessions."

Eye movement desensitization and reprocessing (EMDR) therapy is a first-line treatment for PTSD. During EMDR, the patient briefly focuses on the traumatic memory while engaging in bilateral stimulation, such as side-to-side eye movements or hand tapping. See Chapter 29 for more information on these psychological therapies.

Trauma-focused cognitive behavioral therapy (TF-CBT) is another first-line intervention for treating PTSD in adults, adolescents, and children. In TF-CBT, patients are encouraged to reevaluate their thinking patterns and identify unhelpful distortions. This approach often includes techniques such as cognitive restructuring, exposure therapy, and stress inoculation training to help patients process traumatic experiences and develop healthier coping mechanisms.

👪 NURSE, PATIENT, AND FAMILY RESOURCES

International Society for Traumatic Stress Studies
The International Society for Traumatic Stress Studies is dedicated to sharing information about the effects of trauma and the discovery and dissemination of knowledge about policy, program, and service initiatives that seek to reduce traumatic stressors and their immediate and long-term consequences.
www.istss.org

National Alliance on Mental Illness [PTSD]
NAMI is the National Alliance on Mental Illness, the nation's largest grassroots mental health organization dedicated to building better lives for the millions of Americans affected by mental illness.
www.nami.org

National Center for PTSD
The U.S. Department of Veterans Affairs is a leading research and educational center of excellence on PTSD and traumatic stress.
www.ptsd.va.gov

David Baldwin's Trauma Information Pages
This website primarily focuses on emotional trauma and traumatic stress, including PTSD and dissociation, whether following individual traumatic experience(s) or a large-scale disaster. This site provides information for clinicians and researchers in the traumatic stress field.
www.trauma-pages.com

Trauma Survivors Network
The Trauma Survivors Network is a community for survivors and their families to connect and rebuild after a traumatic physical injury.
https://www.traumasurvivorsnetwork.org

CHAPTER 10

Eating Disorders

Eating disorders cause significant disruption in normal eating patterns and distortions in the perception of body shape and weight. These disorders can be severe and disabling, often requiring long-term care and follow-up for successful treatment. Compared to most other psychiatric conditions, eating disorders can cause substantial physical damage, disability, and may even fatality.

This chapter focuses on anorexia nervosa, bulimia nervosa, and binge-eating disorder. Three additional feeding problems—pica, rumination disorder, and avoidant/restrictive food intake disorder—are briefly discussed.

PICA

Pica is the persistent ingestion of substances with no nutritional value, such as dirt or paint. Consuming nonfood items can interfere with proper nutrition and pose serious health risks. For example, paint that contains lead can result in brain damage. Ingesting objects like stones may cause intestinal blockage, while sharp items, such as tacks or open paper clips, may result in intestinal lacerations. Bacteria from dirt or other contaminated materials can contribute to tooth decay or serious systemic infection. In pregnant individuals, maternal pica may result in intrauterine toxicity.

Pica typically begins in early childhood or during pregnancy and often resolves spontaneously. However, pica that is associated with intellectual disability and developmental disorders such as autism may persist for years.

Patient education on the risks of ingesting nonnutritive substances is essential. In children, monitoring eating behavior is an important aspect of treating this problem. Behavioral interventions, such as rewarding healthy eating are helpful in managing this condition.

RUMINATION DISORDER

Rumination disorder is characterized by the repeated regurgitation of food, which is then re-chewed, re-swallowed, or spit out. Regurgitation involves recently eaten food. Rumination is probably an unconscious process. However, the voluntary relaxation of the diaphragm becomes a learned habit over time. This process is similar to the typical belching reflex, but instead of expelling gas, the reflex causes the regurgitation of actual food.

Rumination symptoms tend to occur after a triggering event, such as a viral illness or a stressful event. Even after the illness or stressor resolves, regurgitation may persist after most meals. While symptoms may remit spontaneously, they can become habitual, leading to complications such as esophageal erosion, malnutrition, and, in severe cases, death. Rumination disorder is associated with intellectual disability and is also linked to neglect.

This rare disorder typically occurs in infants between the ages of 3 and 12 months of age. In individuals with intellectual disability disorder, onset can occur at any age but typically emerges around age 6. Interventions include repositioning infants and young children during feeding. Improving the interaction between the caregiver and child and making mealtimes a pleasant experience often reduces rumination. Distracting the child when rumination begins can also be effective. For individuals with intellectual disability, behavioral therapy may be beneficial, and family therapy can provide additional support.

AVOIDANT/RESTRICTIVE FOOD INTAKE DISORDER

Avoidant/restrictive food intake disorder is characterized by a lack of interest in food and an aversion to the sensory experience of eating. Unlike anorexia nervosa, there are no concerns with body shape or weight. This disorder may result in nutritional deficiencies, weight loss, growth retardation, and interference with emotional and social functioning.

Avoidant/restrictive food intake disorder typically begins in infancy or early childhood and may continue into adulthood. This disorder is more common in adults who focus on specialized diet trends that eliminate one or more food groups. Risk factors include anxiety, depression, and obsessive–compulsive traits. Additionally, a history of gastrointestinal problems such as reflux is also associated with this feeding disorder.

Children with avoidant/restrictive food intake disorder may fail to meet their nutritional or energy, leading to deviations from normal growth patterns. As a result, aggressive treatment is often necessary. Family-based therapy focuses a nonblaming, compassion approach while empowering parents to support weight restoration. Monitoring progress through detailed food diaries and weekly weight graphs help track improvements and reinforce treatment goals.

Cognitive behavioral therapy (CBT) is useful in uncovering unrealistic automatic thoughts and replacing them with realistic responses. Anxiety and depressive symptoms may be treated off-label with second-generation antipsychotics (e.g., olanzapine) and selective serotonin reuptake inhibitors (SSRIs) (e.g., fluoxetine). Additionally, appetite stimulants such as cyproheptadine (Periactin), an antihistamine, have also been used as a treatment approach for this disorder.

ANOREXIA NERVOSA

Individuals with anorexia nervosa have an intense fear of gaining weight. A common misconception is that individuals with anorexia refuse to eat despite being hungry. However, evidence suggests that people with anorexia experience significant differences in sensation of taste, appetite, and satiety, which help to perpetuate the disorder (Kerr et al., 2016).

Individuals with anorexia may engage in compensatory behaviors to counteract food intake or to mitigate previous consumption (National Eating Disorder Association, 2018). Purging, aa common compensatory behavior, involves eliminating food from the body of food to prevent weight gain. Methods of pursing include self-induced vomiting, laxative abuse or diuretic abuse, enemas, and excessive exercise.

Anorexia nervosa is challenging to treat, with a 1-year relapse rate of approximately 50%. Even after 4 years, up to 40% of individuals continue to meet some criteria for anorexia (Harrington et al., 2015). Recovery is viewed as a dynamic process rather than a fixed outcome. Key factors influencing recovery include the percentage of weight restoration, the degree to which self-worth is tied to body shape and weight, and functional impairment in the patient's personal life.

Epidemiology

The estimated lifetime prevalence of anorexia nervosa is 0.6%, (NIMH, 2024). However, actual prevalence may be higher, as many individuals conceal symptoms. Research suggests that less than half of individuals with anorexia seek help for the disorder (Rosenvinge & Petterson, 2015). This disorder typically emerges adolescence or early adulthood, with an onset before puberty or after age 40 being rare.

Risk Factors

The relationship between a lack of tryptophan and its impact on serotonin, anxiety, and dysphoria is implicated. Individuals with anorexia nervosa have less gray and white matter in the central nervous system (Zipfel et al., 2015). They exhibit decreases in the size and/or function of portions of the hypothalamus, basal ganglia, and somatosensory cortex. Regions of the insula, amygdala, and dorsolateral prefrontal cortex appear larger or experience greater activation in comparison to observations in healthy controls (Brownell & Walsh, 2018).

Anxious and perfectionistic temperaments are linked to a heightened need for control and an unrealistic ideal of thinness. Culture factors also play a significant role in shaping self-concept and body satisfaction. Anorexia nervosa is more prevalent in cultures that value thinness, reinforcing distorted body image perceptions and restrictive eating behaviors.

Assessment

Signs and Symptoms

Psychological
- Intense fear of gaining weight.
- Difficulty with social adjustment.
- Preoccupation with thoughts of food.
- Self-image is heavily tied to weight.
- Mood and/or sleep disturbances.
- Obsessive focus on food.

- Perceiving self as overweight even when emaciated.
- Perfectionistic tendencies.

Behavioral
- Compulsive food behaviors
- Food restriction
- Calorie counting
- Excessive exercise
- Binge-eating
- Purging (e.g., laxatives, diuretics, enemas)
- Chewing and spitting out food
- Hiding or throwing away food
- Drinking water before weigh-ins
- Complaining about weight
- Avoiding eating in public
- Engaging in food rituals (e.g., arrangement of food on plates, order of eating food in a certain order, cutting food into tiny pieces, eating slowly)
- Constant mirror checking

Physiological
- Body mass index (BMI): 17+ (mild), 16–17 (moderate), 15–16 (severe), <15 (extreme)
- Cardiovascular abnormalities (hypotension, bradycardia, heart failure)
- Abnormal laboratory test values (low triiodothyronine, low thyroxine levels)
- Neurological changes (abnormal computed tomography [CT] scans, electroencephalogram [EEG] changes)
- Impaired renal function
- Hypoglycemia (glucose <60 mg/dL)
- Cold extremities
- Hypokalemia (<3.5 mEq/L)
- Electrolyte imbalance
- Dehydration
- Peripheral edema
- Muscle weakening
- Dry, yellowish skin
- Amenorrhea (loss of menstruation)
- Lanugo (fine, downy hair on face, chest, shoulders, arms)
- Constipation

Assessment Guidelines

1. Determine the patient's perception of the problem and obtain a verbatim chief complaint.

2. Perform a comprehensive nursing assessment, including orthostatic vital signs, review of systems, and general appearance.
3. Gather a psychosocial history, including screening for suicide or self-harm behaviors.
4. Assess the patient's nutritional pattern and fluid intake.
5. Assess daily activities, including exercise.
6. Review laboratory testing, including the following:
   a. Electrolyte levels
   b. Glucose level
   c. Thyroid function tests
   d. Complete blood count
   e. Electrocardiogram (ECG)
   f. Dual-energy x-ray absorptiometry (DXA) to measure bone density
   g. Erythrocyte sedimentation rate (ESR)
   h. Creatine phosphokinase (CPK)
7. Determine the patient's goals for treatment.

Nursing Diagnoses

The main characteristic of anorexia is a significantly low BMI, making *impaired low nutritional intake* a top safety priority. Individuals with anorexia nervosa also tend to view themselves as overweight even while emaciated. The nursing diagnosis *disturbed body image* is an important focus.

Intervention Guidelines

1. Acknowledge the patient's desire for thinness and sense of control.
2. Conduct a self-assessment and be aware of reactions that might limit your ability to help the patient. Some nurses might experience the following:
   • Feeling shock or disgust toward the patient's behavior or appearance
   • Resenting the patient, believing that the disorder is self-inflicted
   • Feeling helpless to influence the patient's behavior, leading to anger and frustration
   • Becoming overwhelmed by the patient's problems, leading to feelings of hopelessness
   • Engaging in power struggles with the patient, which can result in angry feelings toward the patient

3. Limit discussions of food.
4. Monitor laboratory values and report any abnormal findings to the care provider.

Nursing Care for Anorexia Nervosa

Impaired Low Nutritional Intake

Related to

- Biochemical alterations in the brain
- Psychological factors
- Restricting caloric intake or refusing to eat
- Excessive fear of weight gain
- Excessive physical exertion
- Self-induced vomiting
- Laxative, diuretic, or enema use

Desired Outcome By discharge (inpatient) or after 2 weeks (outpatient) the patient's nutritional intake will be sufficient.

Assessment/Interventions and *Rationales*
Severely Malnourished Patients: Nutritional Rehabilitation

1. In cases of severe malnutrition and refusal of nourishment, tube feedings may be necessary, either alone or in conjunction with oral or parenteral nutrition. *Tube feedings may be the only means available to maintain the patient's life. The patient may not tolerate solid foods at first. The use of nasogastric tube feedings decreases the chance of vomiting.*

2. Tube feedings or parenteral nutrition is often given at night. *Nighttime administration helps diminish drawing attention or sympathy from other patients and allows the patient to participate more fully in daytime activities.*

3. After completion of nasogastric tube feeding, supervise the patient for 90 minutes initially, and gradually reduce the time to 30 minutes. *Helps minimize the patient's chance of vomiting or siphoning off feedings.*

4. Assess vital signs at least three times daily until stable, and then daily. Regularly review electrocardiogram (ECG) and laboratory tests (e.g., electrolytes, acid-base balance, liver enzymes, albumin). *As the patient's weight begins to increase, cardiovascular status improves to within normal range, and less frequent monitoring is needed.*

5. Administer tube feedings in a matter-of-fact manner. *Being consistent and enforcing limits lowers the chance of manipulation and power struggles.*

6. Encourage the patient to consume foods or liquid supplements orally whenever possible, using tube feedings only to supplement inadequate intake. *Allows the patient some control over the need for tube feedings.*

7. Weigh the patient weekly or biweekly at the same time of day, following these guidelines:
   a. Weigh before the morning meal
   b. Weigh after the patient has voided
   c. Ensure the patient wears only a hospital gown and undergarments.
   Patients with eating disorders often experience intense anxiety about weight gain and may attempt to manipulate weigh-ins by consuming excess fluids, avoiding voiding, or adding extra weight, making standardized procedures essential for accurate and consistent measurements.

8. Maintain a neutral stance, avoiding expressions of approval or disapproval. Maintain a neutral stance, avoiding expressions of approval or disapproval. *Separate health concerns from issues of validation, emphasizing that weight gain or loss is a medical matter, not a reflection of staff satisfaction or disapproval.*

Less Severely Malnourished Patients: Nutritional Maintenance

1. Whenever possible, develop a contract with the patient regarding treatment goals and outcome criteria. *Involving the patient in goal-setting, increases their commitment and improves the likelihood of successful outcomes.*

2. Create a pleasant, calm atmosphere during mealtimes by structuring the meal, informing the patient of the specific time and duration (e.g., 30 minutes). *Mealtimes become episodes of high anxiety, and knowledge of regulations decreases tension in the milieu, particularly when the patient has given up so much control by entering treatment.*

3. Monitor the patient during meals to prevent hiding or discarding food, accompany them to the bathroom if purging is suspected, and observe them for at least 1 hour after meals and snacks to prevent purging. *These behaviors are difficult for the patient to control independently. Providing external supervision helps ensure*

*safety and support until the patient develops more internal
resources to manage these behaviors on their own.*

4. Observe the patient closely for the use of physical
   activity to control weight. *Patients are discouraged from
   engaging in exercise until their weight reaches 85% of their
   ideal body weight.*
5. Closely monitor and record the following:
   a. Fluid and food intake
   b. Vital signs
   c. Elimination pattern, while discouraging the use of
      laxatives, enemas, or suppositories
   *Maintaining fluid and electrolyte balance is essential for
   the patient's well-being and safety, and any. abnormal data
   should prompt staff to recognize potential physical crises.*
6. Continue to weigh the patient as described previously.
   Objectively monitors progress.
7. As the patient approaches the target weight, gradually
   encourage personal choices for menu selection. *Fosters
   a sense of control and promotes recovery.*
8. Link privileges to weight loss . If weight loss occurs,
   privileges should be reduced, with the focus shifted
   to understanding the circumstances and emotions
   behind the weight loss. *Reducing privileges in response
   to weight loss provides a clear consequence, while focusing
   on the underlying emotional and situational factors helps
   address the root causes of the behavior, promoting long-term
   recovery.*
9. Link privileges to weight gain. If weight gain occurs,
   privileges should be increased. *The patient receives positive reinforcement for healthy outcomes and behaviors.*

Nutritionally Stabilized Patients: Maintenance of Recovery
1. Continue offering a supportive, empathetic approach
   as the patient works to maintain their target weight.
   *For patients with anorexia, eating regularly, even within the
   framework of restoring health, is extremely difficult.*
2. The weight maintenance phase of treatment challenges
   the patient. This is the ideal time to address more of
   the issues underlying the patient's attitude toward
   weight and shape. *At a healthier weight, the patient is
   cognitively better prepared to examine emotional conflicts
   and themes.*
3. Use a cognitive-behavioral approach to address the
   patient's expressed fears about weight gain. Identify
   and challenge dysfunctional thoughts such as, "If I

gain weight, I am a failure." *Confronting dysfunctional thoughts and beliefs is crucial to changing eating behaviors.*

4. Emphasize the social aspect of eating. Encourage conversations that focus on topics other than food during mealtimes. *Eating is a social activity and participating in conversation serves both as a distraction from obsessional preoccupation and as a pleasurable event.*

5. Focus on the patient's strengths, including progress in normalizing weight and eating habits. *The patient has achieved a major accomplishment. Explore activities unrelated to eating as sources of gratification.*

6. Encourage the patient to apply the knowledge, skills, and gains made from the various individual, family, and group therapy sessions. *Intensive therapy (cognitive behavioral) and education provide tools and techniques useful for maintaining healthy eating and living behaviors.*

7. Teach and role model assertiveness, helping the patient learn to express their needs appropriately. *The patient learns to get needs met appropriately, which helps reduce anxiety and acting-out behaviors.*

Stabilized Patients: Follow-Up Care

1. Involve the patient's family and significant others in teaching, treatment, and discharge planning, including education on nutrition, medication, and the dynamics of the illness. *Family involvement plays a crucial role in the patient's recovery, as family dynamics often contribute to both the illness and the patient's distress. Engaging the family enhances support and promotes better outcomes.*

2. Plan for follow-up therapy for both the patient and family as part of the discharge process. *Family involvement is crucial to the patient's recovery, as family dynamics often contribute to the illness and distress, and engaging the family enhances support, leading to better outcomes.*

3. Offer referrals in-person and/or virtual support groups for the patient and family. (See the list at the end of the chapter for suggestions.) *Support groups offer emotional encouragement, resources, and important information, helping to minimize feelings of isolation while fostering healthier coping strategies.*

Disturbed Body Image

Related to

- Biochemical alterations in the brain
- Cognitive and perceptual factors

- Psychosocial factors
- Negative perception of body
- Morbid fear of obesity
- Low self-esteem

Desired Outcome By discharge (inpatient) or within 2 weeks (outpatient), the patient will verbalize a report of a positive body image.

Assessment/Interventions and *Rationales*

1. Establish a therapeutic alliance with the patient. *Patients with anorexia often resist giving up unhealthy eating behaviors. Building a trusting relationship with the nurse is a crucial first step toward recovery.*

2. Give the patient feedback about their low weight and impaired health, without arguing or challenging their perceptions. *Focus on health-related benefits helps encourage change while respecting the patient's perceptions.*

3. Recognize that the distorted image is real to the patient. Avoid minimizing the patient's perceptions while, at the same time, challenging distortions (e.g., "I understand you see yourself as fat. I do not see you that way.") *This approach acknowledges the patient's perception, which helps them to feel understood, even if your view differs*

4. Encourage expression of feelings regarding how the patient thinks and feels about self and body. *Promotes a clear understanding of the patient's perceptions and lays the groundwork for future interventions.*

5. Assist the patient in distinguishing between thoughts and feelings. Challenge and reframe statements such as "I feel fat." *It is important for the patient to differentiate between their feelings and actual facts, as they often present emotional experiences as reality.*

6. Use a cognitive behavioral approach to help the patient to journal their thoughts and feelings, teaching them how to identify and challenge irrational beliefs. *Cognitive behavioral approaches can be effective in helping the patient challenge irrational beliefs about self and body image. Journaling allows the patient to reflect on thoughts, feelings, and behaviors and facilitates sharing with the nurse.*

7. Encourage the patient to identify positive aspects of their personal appearance. *Helps the patient refocus on strengths and actual physical and other attributes. Disrupts negative rumination.*

8. Educate the family regarding the patient's illness and encourage attendance at family sessions. *The reactions of family members may be triggers of emotional responses and distorted perceptions.*

9. Encourage family therapy for both the family and significant others. *Families and significant others need assistance in learning how to communicate with and relate to a patient who has anorexia.*

TREATMENT MODALITIES

Treatment for anorexia may occur in inpatients, day treatment programs, and outpatient environments. Regardless of setting, treatment typically includes psychosocial interventions, pharmacotherapy, psychotherapy, nutrition, and medical intervention.

Biological Treatments

Pharmacotherapy

No medications have been approved by the US Food and Drug Administration (FDA) for the treatment of anorexia nervosa, as research does not support pharmacological agents for addressing core symptoms. As a result, pharmacotherapy is typically used to manage associated symptoms of cooccurring disorders. Medications commonly used include SSRIs, antianxiety agents, second-generation antipsychotics, and mood stabilizers.

Integrative Care

Individuals with anorexia nervosa may benefit from integrative approaches that complement traditional eating disorder treatment. These approaches can include yoga, massage, acupuncture, and light therapy, which may help support overall well-being and enhance recovery.

Psychological Therapies

There is no empirical evidence to support any specific psychotherapy model in adults with anorexia nervosa. The National Eating Disorders Association (NEDA, n.d.) identifies the Maudsley model of anorexia nervosa treatment for adults (MANTRA) and cognitive remediation therapy

(CRT) as being beneficial. Other standard types of psycho-therapy that have been explored and found to be helpful for eating disorders in general include acceptance and commitment therapy (ACT), integrated cognitive affective therapy (ICAT), dialectical behavior therapy (DBT), exposure and response prevention (ERP), family therapy, and psychodynamic psychotherapy.

Young people with anorexia nervosa may also benefit from adolescent-focused therapy (AFT). This model focuses on self-monitoring of eating and weight gain that is supported by the therapeutic relationship with the advanced practice nurse or other therapist. CBT, which helps to identify automatic negative thoughts and to challenge them, has also been used with success in this population. See Chapter 29 for more information on psychological therapies.

BULIMIA NERVOSA

Individuals with bulimia nervosa engage in repeated episodes of binge eating at least once a week for 3 months. Binge eating involves consuming an amount of food that is larger than what most people would eat in a certain period (e.g., 2 hours). These episodes are followed by compensatory behaviors, such as self-induced vomiting, misuse of laxatives diuretics, or other medications, fasting, or excessive exercise.

This disorder is characterized by a significant disturbance in the perception of body shape and weight. A sense of loss of control accompanies the consumption of large amounts of food, which is typically done in secret. After a binge, individuals often experience intense guilt, depression, or disgust with themselves. A sense of loss of control accompanies the consumption of large amounts of food, which is typically done in secret. After a binge, individuals often experience intense, depression, or disgust with themselves.

Epidemiology

The 12-month prevalence of bulimia nervosa is 0.3%. The lifetime incidence of bulimia nervosa is 1%, with women being five times more likely to be affected than men (NIMH, 2024). Bulimia typically begins in later adolescence, with prevalence peaking in young adulthood. Onset of bulimia nervosa is rare in children younger than 12 years of age and adults over the age of 40.

Risk Factors

Increased frequency of bulimia nervosa is found in first-degree relatives of people with this disorder. Cycles of binging and purging may be associated with neurotransmitters, specifically serotonin and dopamine.

Corticostriatal circuits in individuals with bulimia nervosa, compared to healthy controls, do not function normally. These circuits include the orbitofrontal, prefrontal, and insular cortices (Donnelly et al., 2018).

The psychological roots of bulimia nervosa have been explained by some theorists as stemming from poor early attachment with parents and later difficulties inattachment within friendships and intimate relationships. Parents of affected offspring have been described as negative and unsupportive of their children's independence.

Internalization of a thin body ideal increases the risk for weight concerns, which in turn heightens the risk for bulimia nervosa. There is also some connection between the disorder and childhood sexual or physical abuse. In some cases, traumatic events and environmental stress may serve as contributing factors.

Assessment

Signs and Symptoms

Psychological
- Obsessive thoughts about food
- Feels out of control during binge episodes
- Self-evaluates based on body shape and weight
- Dissatisfaction with body image
- Feelings of dissociation during binge episodes
- Shame about eating habits and attempts to conceal the behavior
- Binge episodes are preceded by negative emotions self-evaluation

Behavioral
- Compulsive food behaviors
- Binge eating large amounts of food within a discrete period (e.g., 2 hours) at least once a week for 3 months
- Eating to the point of discomfort

- Engaging in compensatory behaviors (e.g., self-induced vomiting, use of laxatives, diuretics, enemas, fasting, and excessive exercising)
- Disappearing after meals
- Eating in isolation and secrecy

Physiological
- Normal to slightly low body weight
- Parotid gland swelling
- Dental caries and tooth erosion
- Scars on knuckles (Russell's sign) from self-induced vomiting
- Chronic hoarseness and sore throat
- Cardiovascular abnormalities
- Gastric rupture
- Electrolyte imbalance (e.g., hypokalemia, hypochloremia, hyponatremia)
- Seizures

Assessment Guidelines

1. Determine the patient's perception of the problem and a verbatim chief complaint.
2. Perform a complete nursing assessment, including vital signs, review of systems, and general appearance.
3. Gather a psychosocial history.
4. Assess the patient's nutritional pattern and fluid intake.
5. Assess the patient's binging and purging patterns with direct questions.
6. Assess the patient's daily activities, including exercise.
7. Review the patient's laboratory tests, including the following:
   a. Electrolyte levels
   b. Glucose level
   c. Thyroid function tests
   d. Complete blood count
   e. ECG
8. Determine the patient's goals for treatment.

Nursing Diagnoses

Nursing diagnoses that relate to the disordered eating and weight-control behaviors in bulimia nervosa. The most applicable nursing diagnosis is *compulsive eating behavior*.

This bulimia-specific diagnosis is defined as behaviors related to an insatiable craving for food, excessive appetite, and episodes of binge eating followed by self-induced vomiting, associated with depression and self-deprivation. Also, given the out-of-control symptoms that individuals with bulimia nervosa experience, *powerlessness* is an essential nursing diagnosis with which to frame nursing care.

Disturbed body image is another priority focus. Interventions previously identified with anorexia nervosa may be modified in the care of individuals with bulimia nervosa.

Intervention Guidelines

1. Coexisting disorders, such as major depressive disorder, substance use, and personality disorders, often complicate the clinical picture and require additional treatment and interventions.
2. Cognitive behavioral techniques have been shown to be effective in managing symptoms.
3. Group therapy with other individuals who have bulimia is often part of successful therapy.
4. Because anxiety and feelings of stress often precede binging, alternative ways of dealing with anxiety and alternative coping strategies to lessen anxiety are useful tools.
5. Family therapy is helpful and encouraged.

Nursing Care for Bulimia Nervosa

Compulsive Eating Behavior

Related to

- Biochemical alterations in the brain
- Uncontrollable binge–purge cycles
- Inadequate coping mechanisms for dealing with anxiety and stress
- Poor impulse control

Desired Outcome By discharge (inpatient) or within 2 weeks (outpatient), the patient will report and demonstrate regulated eating behavior.

Assessment/Interventions and *Rationales*

1. Assess for suicidal thoughts and other self-destructive behaviors. Patients with bulimia often feel out of

control and have a negative self-evaluation. *Ensuring physical safety is the priority nursing intervention.*

2. Educate the patient about the negative effects of self-induced vomiting (i.e., dental erosion, low potassium level, cardiac problems). *Health teaching is essential for helping the patient understand the insidious and often unseen effects of purging behavior.*

3. Educate the patient about the binge–purge cycle and its self-perpetuating nature. *The compulsive nature of the binge–purge cycle is maintained by repeated restricting, hunger, binge eatinging, and purging accompanied by feelings of guilt.*

4. Identify triggers that lead to compulsive eating and purging behaviors. *Recognizing triggers helps the patient to substitute healthier coping when they occur.*

5. Explore dysfunctional thoughts that precede the binge–purge cycle. Teach the patient to challenge and reframe these thoughts in healthier ways. *Cognitive behavioral techniques can help combat distorted thinking and promote rational thoughts that lead to healthier behaviors, improved self-esteem, body image, and self-worth.*

6. Encourage the patient to record their thoughts, feelings, and behaviors in a journal and share them with the nurse. *Journaling clarifies thoughts and feelings, and leading to increased self-awareness, problem-solving, and healing. Sharing journal entries allows the patient to receive valuable feedback.*

7. Work with the patient to identify problems and collaboratively establish short- and long-term goals. *The patient needs to develop tools to handle personal problems instead of resorting.*

8. Assess and teach problem-solving skills. *Teaching alternative methods of stress relief and ways to meet needs is crucial in helping individuals replace binge-eating behaviors with healthier alternatives.*

9. Arrange for the patient to learn ways to enhance interpersonal communication, socialization, and assertiveness skills. *Individuals with bulimia often isolated themselves, lack social interaction, and struggle with appropriate communication skills to get their needs met.*

10. Encourage attendance at support groups, recovery groups, or therapy groups with other individuals with bulimia. Provide information for family members as well. *Eating disorders are chronic conditions, and long-term follow-up therapy and support are essential for success.*

Powerlessness

Related to
- Unsatisfying interpersonal interactions
- Lifestyle of helplessness
- Inability to control binge eating
- Distortion of body image
- Feelings of low self-worth
- Impulsivity
- Insufficient coping skills

Desired Outcome By discharge (inpatient) or within 2 weeks (outpatient), the patient will verbalize decreased powerlessness.

Assessment/Interventions and *Rationales*

1. Explore the patient's experience of out-of-control eating behavior. *Listening in an empathetically and without udgment helps the patient feel understood and supported in their experience.*

2. Encourage the patient to keep a journal of thoughts and feelings associated with binge–purge behaviors. *Automatic thoughts and beliefs perpetuate the binge–purge cycle. Journaling is an effective way to identify these dysfunctional thoughts and underlying assumptions.*

3. Teach the patient how to systematically challenge negative and self-defeating thoughts and beliefs. *These automatic dysfunctional thoughts must be addressed and restructured for any meaningful change in the patient thinking and behavior.*

4. Explore cognitive distortions that influence feelings, beliefs, and behaviors. *Cognitive distortions reinforce unrealistic self-perceptions regarding strengths and future potential. Developing a more realistic self-view promotes healing and growth.*

5. Encourage the patient's active participation in decisions and responsibilities related to care and future planning. *Self-advocacy helps the patient regain a sense of control over their life and recognize options for making meaningful changes.*

6. Teach the patient alternative stress-reduction techniques and visualization skills to enhance self-confidence and self-worth. *Visualizing a positive self-image and successful outcomes for life goals stimulates problem-solving and progress toward those goals.*

7. Encourage the patient to role-play new skills in counseling sessions and group therapy, especially regarding communication with others, particularly family. *Role-playing offers a safe environment for the patient to practice new ways of relating and responding to others.*
8. Teach the patient that one lapse does not equate to a relapse. One slip of control does not eliminate all positive accomplishments. *A single slip in control does not negate all positive progress. When a lapse occurs, it is important to examine its causes, knowing that it doesn't invalidate past accomplishments.*

TREATMENT MODALITIES

Biological Treatments

Pharmacotherapy

Fluoxetine (Prozac), an SSRI antidepressant, is the only FDA-approved medication for the treatment of bulimia nervosa in adult patients. This drug can be helpful for people with bulimia even in the absence of depressive symptoms. Other antidepressants have shown efficacy in the treatment of bulimia nervosa at the same dose as used for depression. They include the following:

- SSRIs sertraline (Zoloft), paroxetine (Paxil), and citalopram (Celexa)
- The tricyclic antidepressants imipramine (Tofranil), nortriptyline (Pamelor), and desipramine (Norpramin)
- The monoamine oxidase inhibitor tranylcypromine (Parnate)

Bupropion (Wellbutrin) is contraindicated in patients diagnosed with bulimia due to the increased risk of seizure with this medication. Serotonin-norepinephrine reuptake inhibitors (SNRIs) have not been evaluated through randomized controlled trials in patients with bulimia. Research is exploring the potential for second-generation antipsychotics, antiepileptics, and/or opioid antagonists for decreasing symptoms associated with bulimia.

Psychological Therapies

Advanced practice professionals are qualified to use evidence-based CBT, which is considered a first-line treatment for bulimia. Interpersonal psychotherapy is also recommended. Additional modalities which have been explored and found to be helpful for eating disorders include acceptance and commitment therapy (ACT), integrated cognitive affective therapy (ICAT), dialectical behavior therapy (DBT), exposure and response prevention (ERP), family therapy, and psychodynamic psychotherapy (NEDA, n.d.). Chapter 29 describes these models.

BINGE-EATING DISORDER

Individuals with binge-eating disorder engage in episodes of excessive food intake that go beyond the point of satiety (fullness) and lead to distress afterward. A key difference between this disorder and bulimia nervosa is that compensatory behaviors such as self-induced vomiting and laxatives are typically not present. While some individuals who may begin binge eating at a normal weight, repeated episodes often result in obesity. Binge eating occurs once a week for 3 months.

Epidemiology

Binge eating is the most common eating disorder. The 12-month prevalence for adults is 1.6% in women and 0.8% in men (NIMH, 2024). The lifetime prevalence is 2.8%. All racial and ethnic groups seem to be equally represented.

Risk Factors

Binge-eating disorder tends to run in families, which may be the result of additive genetic influences. As in the case of patients diagnosed with bulimia nervosa, individuals with binge eating also exhibit altered processing in the orbitofrontal cortex (Donnelly et al., 2018). Body dissatisfaction, low self-esteem, and difficulty coping with feelings can contribute to binge-eating disorder. Social pressures to be thin, which are typically influenced by media, can trigger emotional eating. Social weight stigma, which is stereotyping or discrimination based on a person's body, is common in the United States and perpetuates the cycle of binging. A history of trauma, particularly emotional neglect, increases the risk of binge eating.

Assessment

Signs and Symptoms

Psychological

- Feels out of control
- Distress
- Depression
- Grief
- Anxiety
- Shame
- Self-disgust

Behavioral

- Compulsive eating
- Eating rapidly
- Eating until feeling uncomfortably full
- Eating large amounts of food even when not hungry
- Eating alone
- Lack of control
- Isolation
- Stealing or hoarding food
- Creating a lifestyle or rituals to make time for binges
- Withdrawing from others and activities
- Frequent dieting

Physiological

- Normal weight, overweight, or obese
- Obesity may result in:
- Type II diabetes
- High blood pressure
- High cholesterol
- Gallbladder disease/gallstones
- Cardiac disease
- Joint pain
- Sleep apnea
- Cancer (e.g., gallbladder, esophagus)

Nursing Diagnoses

The nursing diagnosis *impaired high nutritional intake* is essential in structuring care for individuals with this disorder. Since binge-eating disorder shares similarities to bulimia nervosa (without the purging behaviors), many of the same nursing diagnoses are relevant. These include *compulsive eating behavior*, *powerlessness*, and *disturbed body image*.

Nursing Care for Binge-Eating Disorder
Impaired High Nutritional Intake
Related to
- Binge eating
- Lack of control over eating
- Eating rapidly
- Eating until uncomfortably full
- Eating when not hungry

Desired Outcome The patient will demonstrate decreased nutritional intake.

Assessment/Interventions and *Rationales*
1. Encourage the patient to keep a journal documenting urges to binge eat, feelings or events immediately before, and responses to these urges. *Understanding the pattern of binge eating can help identify more adaptive ways to respond to these urges.*
2. Identify strategies to challenge irrational thoughts that may arise before binge eating. *Correcting faulty thinking is an evidence-based method for managing this disorder.*
3. Encourage the exploration of alternative, healthy coping strategies. *Since p-atients have been using food to regulate mood, they need to develop new, healthier strategies.*
4. Help the patient set goals for adopting healthy eating patterns and exercise. *Self-care is enhanced when goals are developed collaboratively within the context of the nurse-patient relationship.*
5. Identify social support from friends and community (locally or online). *Social support helps reduce feelings of isolation, making patients feel stronger and more likely to achieve goals.*
6. Identify support groups for eating disorders in general or binge-eating disorder specifically. These groups can be local or available through online forums. *Support groups are a powerful tool for reducing isolation, offering feedback, sharing experiences, helping others, and practicing relational skills.*

TREATMENT MODALITIES

Biological Treatments

Pharmacotherapy

Because of their efficacy in treating bulimia nervosa, researchers have studied the use of SSRIs at or near the high end of the dosage range to treat binge-eating disorder. Although these medications seem to help in the short term, patients regained significant weight after discontinuing them. Some evidence supports the use of SNRIs, including duloxetine (Cymbalta) or venlafaxine (Effexor XR) in the treatment of patients with comorbid binge-eating disorder and major depressive disorder (Brownell & Walsh, 2018). Other medications that are under investigation include the tricyclic antidepressants and antiepileptic agents.

Lisdexamfetamine (Vyvanse), a stimulant used to treat attention-deficit/hyperactivity disorder, also has FDA approval for the treatment of moderate to severe binge-eating disorder in adults. Lisdexamfetamine is correlated with a significantly lower risk of relapse in binge episodes compared with placebo at 6-month follow-up (Brownell & Walsh, 2018). In adults with binge-eating disorder, the most common side effects are dry mouth, insomnia, decreased appetite, increased heart rate, constipation, feeling jittery, and anxiety. The FDA includes a black box warning on the label of lisdexamfetamine due to the potential for misuse.

Popular media sources have recently reported that diabetes medications, such as Ozempic (semaglutide), are being used to treat binge-eating disorder (BED) due to their appetite-suppressing effects. Resarch is just emerging on the effectiveness of these GLP-1 receptor antagonists in binge-eating disorder. Smaller studies indicate they may reduce symptoms. However, larger studies are necessary to determine treatment guidelines, efficacy, and safety data.

Surgical Interventions

Bariatric surgery is a controversial option for the treatment of obesity that is due to binge-eating disorder. Potential complications from this surgery require individuals to consider it carefully (Mitchell et al., 2015). Complications include impaired fasting glucose levels, high triglycerides, and urinary incontinence. Furthermore, surgery does not address psychiatric concerns associated with binge-eating disorder. It is quite common to require psychiatric counseling that addresses food-related thoughts and behaviors as a prerequisite to bariatric surgery.

Psychological Therapies

Advanced practice professionals commonly use IPT to improve relationships, communication, and explore problem areas, which thereby reduces symptoms associated with binge eating (NEDA, n.d.). NEDA also identifies the following therapies as used to treat eating disorders, which can be used for binge eating at the therapist's discretion: acceptance and commitment therapy (ACT), integrated cognitive affective therapy (ICAT), dialectical behavior therapy (DBT), exposure and response prevention (ERP), ramily therapy, and psychodynamic psychotherapy. See Chapter 29 for a description of these models.

👪 Nurse, Patient, and Family Resources

Anorexia Nervosa and Related Eating Disorders (ANRED)
ANRED provides comprehensive information about anorexia nervosa, bulimia, binge eating disorder, and other less well-known eating disorders.
www.anred.com

Center for Discovery Eating Disorder Treatment Support Groups
Offers free online support groups for anyone who has been impacted by an eating disorder or mental health.
https://centerfordiscovery.com/groups/

Families Empowered and Supporting Treatment of Eating Disorders (F.E.A.S.T.)
Feast is a global community offering support, education, and empowerment to families of people affected by eating disorders.
www.feast-ed.org

KidsHealth (Search for Eating Disorders)
The most-viewed site for dependable information on children's health, behavior, and development from before birth through the teen years.
www.kidshealth.org

National Association of Anorexia Nervosa and Associated Disorders (ANAD)
The leading nonprofit in the United States that provides free peer support services to anyone struggling with an eating disorder.
www.anad.org

National Eating Disorders Association (NEDA)
NEDA works to advance research, build community, and raise awareness to support the nearly 30 million Americans who will experience an eating disorder in their lifetimes.
www.nationaleatingdisorders.org

CHAPTER 11

Sleep Disorders

For many, sleep is treated as a dispensable commodity. In our fast-paced society, it is often sacrificed to maintain demanding schedules that disrupt normal sleep patterns. Work, academic pursuits, and commuting are the primary factors influencing total sleep duration. As more time is dedicated to these activities, less time remains for sleep.

Sleep requirements vary from person to person and are likely genetically influenced to some degree. While most adults require 7 to 8 hours of sleep for optimal functioning, a small percentage of individuals are considered to be long sleepers, requiring 10 or more hours per night, or short sleepers needing less than 5 hours per night. The amount of sleep necessary to feel fully awake and able to maintain normal levels of performance is known as the basal sleep requirement.

Nurses frequently work with sleep-deprived patients. Pain, noise, unfamiliar environments, and anxiety disrupt sleep patterns in hospitalized patients. Virtually all psychiatric disorders are associated with sleep disturbance, which can also serve as a precipitating factor for these disorders and increase the risk of relapse. Individuals with major depressive disorder who experience sleep disturbances often show higher levels of suicidal ideation. Long-standing insomnia is common in alcohol use disorder recovery. One of the strongest indicators of recovery from any mental illness is a return to normal sleep patterns, offering hope that with time and proper treatment, restful sleep can be restored.

According to the American Psychiatric Association (APA, 2022), sleep disorders are classified into three specific categories:
1. **Sleep–wake disorders:** Insomnia (insufficient sleep), hypersomnolence (sleeping too much), and narcolepsy (attacks of falling asleep)

185

11. Do you nap? If so, for how long? Do you feel refreshed after napping?
12. Can you identify any stress or problem that may have initially contributed to your sleep difficulties?
13. What are your daily habits, diet, exercise, and medications?
14. What changes, if any, have you made to improve your sleep? What were the results?

Nursing Diagnoses

There are several specific International Classification for Nursing Practice (ICNP) (International Council of Nurses, 2019) nursing diagnoses that address sleep disturbances. The two that will be discussed in this chapter are *insomnia* and *impaired sleep*. Since these diagnoses are closely related with only nuanced differences, students may choose to apply interventions from either diagnosis to create a tailored plan of care based on the individual patient's needs.

Intervention Guidelines

Provide patients with education on the following topics:
A. Reserve the bedroom for sleep and intimacy (i.e., no electronics, reading, or other activities in the bedroom).
B. Avoid clock-watching.
C. Avoid heavy meals before bedtime.
D. Limit alcohol, and avoid its use for several hours before bed.
E. Exercise daily, but not right before bed.
F. Get out of bed if unable to sleep and engage in a quiet activity such as reading or crossword puzzles.
G. Avoid lighted activities, which stimulate the retina in the hour before bed (e.g., no television or computer).
H. Maintain a regular sleep–wake schedule, getting up at the same time each day being the most important factor.
I. Avoid daytime napping. If napping is necessary, limit to 20 to 30 minutes maximum, and set a timer.

Nursing Care for Insomnia

Insomnia

Related to
- Biochemical alterations in the brain

- Anxiety
- Pain
- Grieving
- Daytime napping
- Inadequate physical activity
- Poor sleep hygiene
- Medication
- Caffeine
- Alcohol
- Unsuitable environment

Desired Outcome The patient will report and demonstrate improved sleep.

Assessment/Interventions and *Rationales*
1. Assess the patient's activity pattern and sleep pattern. *Establishing a baseline is crucial for identifying deviations from their norm. This initial assessment provides a foundation for planning interventions and allows for accurate tracking of the patient's progress, whether it reflects improvement or deterioration.*
2. Monitor the effects of sleep medications on the patient's sleep pattern. *If the medication is effective, the patient may need to collaborate with their healthcare provider to gradually withdraw the sleeping medication as more permanent methods [e.g., antidepressants] take effect.*
3. Teach sleep hygiene measures such as limiting daytime naps, avoiding caffeine and nicotine close to bedtime, increasing daytime exercise, establishing a relaxing bedtime routine, and avoiding light-producing electronics 1 hour before sleep. *These simple sleep hygiene measures help patients establish habits that promote a natural sleep-wake cycle and improve sleep quality.*
4. Provide a comfortable, cool, quiet, disturbance free, and dark environment. *Heat, noise, people, and light impair an individual's ability to sleep.*
5. Encourage the use of blackout curtains, eyeshades, earplugs, white noise machines or apps, humidifiers, fans, and other devices. *Nonpharmacological sleep aids are often highly effective in promoting sleep.*
6. Teach relaxation techniques to promote sleep, such as slow, deep breathing; guided imagery; and progressive muscle relaxation. *These methods reduce anxiety and muscle tension, which can interfere with sleep.*

7. Monitor the patient's sleep for physical problems, such as sleep apnea, urinary frequency, or discomfort. *Many physical conditions that interfere with sleep can be effectively treated.*
8. Encourage the patient to keep a sleep diary or use a sleep-tracking device. *Understanding patterns and objectively evaluating sleep practices enhance self-care. Tracking sleep can help correct inaccurate perceptions and improve self-awareness of sleep patterns.*
9. Teach the principles of cognitive behavioral therapy for insomnia (CBT-I), including strategies like sleep restriction, stimulus control, cognitive restructuring, and relaxation techniques. Encourage the patient to practice these strategies consistently and monitor their effectiveness. *These techniques help patients identify and change thoughts and behaviors that contribute to insomnia, improve sleep quality, and establish healthier sleep patterns. Over time, they can enhance overall sleep hygiene and contribute to better long-term sleep health.*

Impaired Sleep

Related to
- Biochemical alterations in the brain
- Physical or psychological pain
- Age-related sleep pattern changes
- Circadian asynchrony
- Restless legs syndrome
- Sleep apnea
- Poor sleep hygiene
- Nightmares, sleepwalking, sleep terrors
- Caffeine
- Sleep interruption for treatments
- Unsuitable environment
- Life demands (e.g., caregiving responsibilities, parental duties, night-shift work)

Desired Outcome The patient will report and demonstrate improved sleep.

Assessment/Interventions (*Rationales*)
1. Assess sleep patterns and document findings. *Accurate baseline data will inform interventions and provide a record for monitoring improvement or lack of improvement.*

2. Provide sedatives or hypnotics, antipsychotics, or other medications prescribed for sleep. *Medication can prevent sustained sleep loss, which, if left unaddressed, could result in a significant decline in overall quality of life and, in severe cases, psychosis (i.e., disturbed thinking, delusions, hallucinations).*

3. Teach the patient that one of the strongest indicators of recovery from any mental illness is the return to normal sleep patterns. In still hope by emphasizing that, with time, medication and other treatments can help restore normal sleep patterns. *Normal sleep patterns are a key indicator of progress in recovery, and with appropriate treatment, restoring sleep can enhance overall mental health and well-being.*

4. If applicable, administer prescribed pain medications as needed and encourage relaxation techniques, such as deep breathing or progressive muscle relaxation, to alleviate discomfort. *Pain, both physical and psychological, can disrupt sleep. Proper pain management and relaxation techniques can help alleviate discomfort and improve sleep quality.*

5. If the patient has restless legs syndrome, collaborate with the healthcare provider to explore treatment options such as medication (e.g., dopaminergic agents) and recommend non-pharmacological approaches like stretching exercises before bed. *Restless legs syndrome can significantly disrupt sleep. Addressing it with medication and lifestyle adjustments can reduce symptoms and improve sleep.*

6. If the patient has sleep apnea, encourage the use of continuous positive airway pressure (CPAP) or biphasic positive airway pressure (BiPAP) therapy if prescribed, and educate on lifestyle changes such as weight management and sleeping on the side to reduce symptoms. *Sleep apnea can lead to fragmented sleep. Using prescribed devices and addressing lifestyle factors can improve sleep quality and prevent health complications.*

7. For patients with parasomnias, assess for underlying psychological issues such as trauma or anxiety, and recommend therapy (e.g., cognitive behavioral therapy) to address them. In the case of sleepwalking or night terrors, ensure a safe environment and consider a referral to a sleep specialist. *Nightmares, sleepwalking, and night terrors disrupt sleep and may indicate underlying psychological or sleep-related issues that require treatment.*

8. Minimize sleep disruption in the hospital whenever possible by medicating before bed and in the morning, and keeping lights dim and voices quiet if medications or treatments must be given at night. *Interruptions for treatments can fragment sleep, and minimizing these disruptions can improve sleep continuity.*

9. Promote a regular bedtime and wake time. *Reestablishing a consistent sleep schedule will help improve functioning and promote better sleep quality.*

10. As sleep normalizes, discourage sleeping during the day. *Initially, patients may be so sleep-deprived that short daytime naps are essential to restoring brain function and body homeostasis. However, after the crisis period, daytime naps can interfere with nighttime sleep.*

11. Limit caffeine-containing drinks and foods such as energy drinks, coffee, tea, colas, and chocolate. *Caffeine is a central nervous system stimulant and can interfere with sleep.*

TREATMENT FOR SLEEP DISORDERS

Biological Treatments

Pharmacotherapy

Long-term use of pharmacotherapy is typically discouraged, as behavioral interventions have shown superior efficacy in reducing insomnia. Medications commonly used for insomnia include benzodiazepines, nonbenzodiazepine receptor agonists, a melatonin receptor agonist, orexin receptor antagonists, and a tricyclic antidepressant. Most of these drugs are classified as schedule IV and have the potential to be habit-forming. Second-generation antipsychotics, including olanzapine (Zyprexa), quetiapine (Seroquel), and risperidone (Risperdal), are used off-label for insomnia, though they lack specific FDA approval for its purpose. Chapter 26 provides a list of FDA-approved drugs for the treatment of insomnia.

Over-the-counter sleeping aids have limited effectiveness. Melatonin, a naturally occurring hormone, is a popular over-the-counter product. While there is partial evidence supporting its use in managing insomnia disorder, new research into prolonged-release forms of melatonin is showing some promise.

Somatic Treatments

Functional magnetic resonance imaging studies indicate that the prefrontal cortex is overly active with insomnia. Racing thoughts interfere with the individual's ability to sleep. The Cerêve Sleep System has FDA approval and significantly reduced sleep latency from stage 1 to stage 2 in clinical trials. This product is a software-controlled bedside device that is placed on the forehead. A fluid-filled pad cools the forehead and reduces activity in the cerebral cortex.

In 2024 another somatic treatment was approved by the FDA. This treatment is the Modius Sleep device that treats chronic insomnia by delivering a small and safe electrical pulse to the head for 30 minutes before bed. Another new somatic treatment is a wellness device not subject to FDA approval. **Elemind** is a wearable headband that provides neurotechnology for sleep and is safe for nightly use. It monitors EEG brain signals to assess and respond to an individual's unique brainwaves, helping to shift the brain from wakeful patterns into deeper sleep on demand.

Psychological Therapies

Effective treatment of insomnia involves incorporating basic sleep hygiene principles, which are practices and conditions that promote continuous, restful sleep. Modifying poor sleep habits and establishing a regular sleep–wake schedule can be achieved using sleep diaries (Fig. 11.1). A 2-week period is typically helpful for identifying overall sleep patterns and assessing sleep efficiency ([time in bed divided by total sleep time] × 100). After reviewing their sleep diaries, patients are often surprised to find that their sleep problems are not as severe as they initially thought.

Sleep restriction, or limiting the total sleep time, creates a temporary mild state of sleep deprivation and strengthens the sleep homeostatic drive. This helps decrease sleep latency and improves sleep continuity and quality. If, for example, a sleep diary indicates that your patient is in bed for 8 hours but sleeping only 6 hours, sleep is restricted to 6 hours, and the bedtime and wake time are adjusted accordingly. Do not reduce the sleep time below 5 hours, regardless of sleep efficiency, and caution patients about the dangers of sleepiness with driving while undergoing a trial of sleep restriction. Once sleep efficiency is improved,

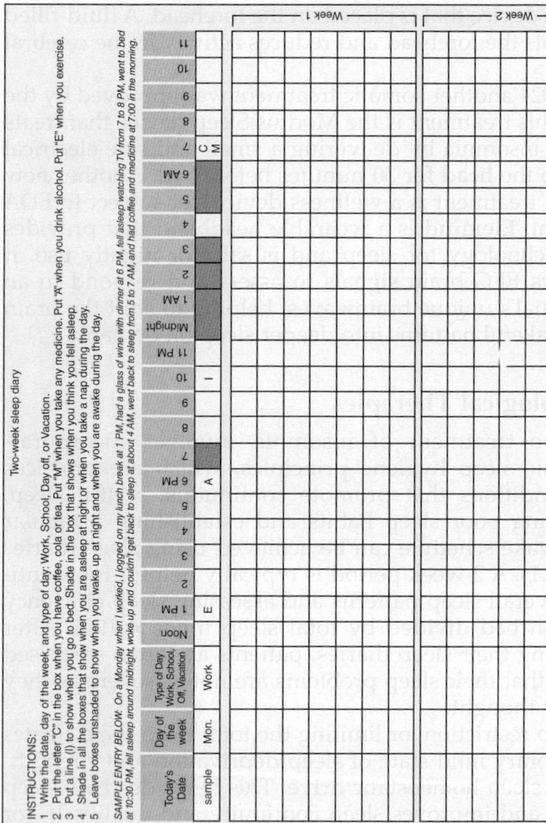

Fig. 11.1 Two-week sleep diary. (Printed with permission from the American Academy of Sleep Medicine. Available from: http://sleepeducation.org/.)

total sleep time is gradually increased by 10- to 20-minute increments.

A specific form of cognitive behavioral therapy (CBT), known asCBT for insomnia (CBT-I), is used to treat insomnia. Patients are encouraged to identify and challenge misperceptions about sleep (e.g., "I must have 9 hours of sleep"). The focus is on improving the quality of sleep rather than the quantity of hours slept. Other goals of CBT-I involve identifying and correcting maladaptive attitudes and beliefs about sleep that contribute to insomnia. For example, patients may justify behaviors like spending excessive time in bed to "catch up" on lost sleep or hold unrealistic expectations about sleep.

The SleepioRx combines psychology and technology to offer CBT-I through a prescription-based mobile app. This software provides a computerized version of CBT-I, enabling clinicians to educate patients about the treatment and track their progress. The program can be tailored to the patient's symptoms and daily sleep tracking, with a duration of 90 days.

NURSE, PATIENT, AND FAMILY RESOURCES

American Academy of Sleep Medicine
The purpose of the American Academy of Sleep Medicine is to advance sleep care and enhance sleep health to improve lives. They emphasize that sleep and circadian care are fundamental to healthcare.
www.aasmnet.org

American Sleep Apnea Association
The American Sleep Apnea Association (ASAA) is a nonprofit organization that works to improve the lives of those affected by sleep apnea and leads the search for the elimination of this syndrome in future generations.
www.sleepapnea.org

American Sleep Medicine
American Sleep Medicine is a provider of sleep diagnostic testing and was established in 2002. Their objective is to provide the highest level of patient care possible in both the diagnosis and treatment of sleep-related disorders.
www.americansleepmedicine.com

Centers for Disease Control and Prevention: Sleep and Sleep Disorders

The Centers for Disease Control and Prevention: Sleep and Sleep Disorders provides information about sleep, sleep facts, and sleep resources for both individuals and healthcare providers.

www.cdc.gov/sleep/resources.html

Narcolepsy Network

Narcolepsy Network assists people with narcolepsy each year through education and information through their website. The Network actively participates in key professional and industry meetings and advocates for our community whenever need and opportunity present.

www.narcolepsynetwork.org

National Sleep Foundation

The National Sleep Foundation is committed to advancing excellence in sleep health theory, research, and practice. They seek to improve health and well-being through sleep education and advocacy.

www.sleepfoundation.org

Restless Legs Syndrome Foundation

The Restless Legs Syndrome Foundation is dedicated to improving the lives of men, women, and children who live with this often devastating disease. The organization's goals are to increase awareness, improve treatments, and advance research to find a cure.

www.rls.org

CHAPTER 12

Substance Use Disorders

Substance use disorders are not illnesses of choice. They are complex diseases of the brain characterized by craving, seeking, and using regardless of consequences. Continuous substance use results in changes in the brain structure and function. Substance use disorders are chronic and relapsing. Deficits in executive functioning that affect self-control and decision-making are both a risk factor for substance use and a consequence of it.

In 2022 about 17.3% (or about 48.7 million people) of the US population aged 12 or older had a substance use disorder (Substance Abuse and Mental Health Services Administration [SAMHSA], 2023). A substance use disorder is a pathological pattern of substance use that leads to dysfunction. Symptoms include:
- Impaired ability to control use
- Social impairment
- Risky use
- Physical effects (i.e., addiction, intoxication, tolerance, withdrawal)

Substance use disorders encompass the use of a broad range of products that individuals take into their bodies through various means such as swallowing, inhaling, and injecting. These disorders span substances ranging from seemingly harmless ones like caffeine to illegal, mind-altering drugs like lysergic acid diethylamide (LSD). No matter the substance, use disorders share many commonalities, intoxication characteristics, and withdrawal attributes.

The American Psychiatric Association (APA, 2022) provides diagnostic criteria for the following psychoactive substances:
- Alcohol
- Caffeine
- Cannabis
- Hallucinogen
- Inhalant

- Opioid
- Sedative, hypnotic, and antianxiety medication
- Stimulant
- Tobacco

In addition to substances, certain behaviors are also recognized as addictive. These behavioral addictions, also called process addictions, do not exhibit the same physical signs as drug addiction. However, the compulsive actions activate the reward or pleasure pathways in the brain similarly to substances. The first process addiction, gambling, was established as a disorder in 2013. Excesses in internet gaming, social media use, shopping, and sexual activity are also process addictions that may be included in future *DSM* editions.

CONCEPTS CENTRAL TO SUBSTANCE USE DISORDERS

Addiction

Addiction is a chronic and progressive medical condition influenced by environmental, genetic, neurotransmission, and life experience factors. It involves a physiological or psychological need for a habit-forming substance, activity, or behavior that results in negative consequences. Like other chronic diseases, addictions involve cycles of relapse and remission. When the addiction substance or behavior is removed, withdrawal symptoms are typically well defined.

Intoxication

Intoxication occurs when a substance is used in excess, inhibiting a person's normal ability to act or reason. The terminology used to describe intoxication may vary depending on the substance. For example, alcohol causes one to be drunk, while marijuana results in being high.

Tolerance

Tolerance develops when a person experiences a diminished physical response to a substance due to repeated use. As tolerance builds, the person may no longer achieve the initial high, leading them to continually "chase" that original sensation. Tolerance does not always equate to addiction. For example, individuals with chronic pain may develop tolerance to prescription medications without being addicted to them.

Withdrawal

Withdrawal refers to a set of symptoms that occur when a person stops using a substance. Withdrawal is specific to the substance being used, and each substance will have its particular syndrome, which may be mild or life-threatening. The more intense symptoms a person has, the more likely the person is to start using the substance again to avoid the withdrawal symptoms.

This chapter focuses on substance use disorders, providing an overview of each major category in the following sections. Nursing care for this population is then discussed.

SUBSTANCE USE DISORDERS

Caffeine

Caffeine is the most widely used psychoactive substance in the world. The typical side effects of caffeine include increased alertness or wakefulness; feeling restless, anxious, or irritable; increased body temperature; dehydration; headache; and increased respirations and pulse. Excessive caffeine use is not an official use disorder. However, caffeine can result in intoxication, withdrawal, and overdose.

Caffeine Intoxication

The stimulatory effects of caffeine may begin as early as 15 minutes after ingestion and last as long as 6 hours. Behavioral symptoms of caffeine intoxication include restlessness, nervousness, excitement, agitation, rambling speech, and inexhaustibility. Physical symptoms of intoxication are flushed face, diuresis, gastrointestinal disturbance, muscle twitching, tachycardia, and cardiac arrhythmia. These symptoms are distressing and impair normal functioning. Individuals with tolerance are less sensitive to intoxication. Conversely, chronic use of high doses of caffeine can cause the body's stress system to produce hormones to counter the stimulation, causing a sedating response.

Caffeine Withdrawal

Removal of caffeine from daily use results in headache, drowsiness, irritability, and poor concentration. Some individuals may experience flu-like symptoms, including nausea, vomiting, and muscle aches. Symptoms occur within 12 to 24 hours after the last dose, peak in 24 to 48 hours, and resolve within 1 week.

Caffeine Overdose

Although caffeine overdoses are rare, extremely high doses of caffeine may lead to death. With the advent of energy drinks, caffeine pills, and caffeinated alcoholic beverages more people are experiencing overdoses. Symptoms of a lethal concentration of caffeine include trouble breathing, vomiting, hallucinations, confusion, chest pain, irregular pulse, uncontrollable muscle movements, and seizures.

Overdose treatment is aimed at managing symptoms while eliminating the caffeine from the body. Activated charcoal, laxatives, or gastric lavage may be used.

Cannabis Use Disorder

Cannabis, or marijuana, is derived from the dried leaves, flowers, stems, and seeds of the cannabis plant. The chemical delta-9-tetrahydrocannabinol (THC) is responsible for its mind-altering effects.

The 12-month prevalence of cannabis use disorder in individuals aged 12 and older was 6.7%, with the highest percentage seen in young adults aged 18 to 25 (16.5%) (SAMHSA, 2023). Males are more likely to be affected.

Cannabis Intoxication

Cannabis intoxication enhances sensory experiences, making colors appear brighter, details in common stimuli seem more vivid, and can make time appear to slow down. At higher doses, individuals may experience depersonalization and derealization. Motor skills are impaired for 8 to 12 hours, and activities such as driving and operating machinery can be hazardous. Physical symptoms of cannabis intoxication include conjunctival injection (red eyes due to vessel dilation), increased appetite, dry mouth, and tachycardia.

Cannabis Withdrawal

Withdrawal occurs within 1 week of cessation. Symptoms include irritability, anger, aggression, anxiety, restlessness, and depressed mood. Since many individuals use marijuana as a sleep aid, insomnia and disturbing dreams may arise during withdrawal. Decreased appetite can lead to weight loss. At least one of the following physical symptoms of withdrawal occurs: abdominal pain, shakiness, sweating, fever, chills, and headache.

Abstinence and support are the main principles of treatment for cannabis use disorder. Hospitalization or outpatient care may be required. Individual, family, and group therapies can provide support. Short-term relief of withdrawal symptoms can be managed with antianxiety medications. Patients with underlying anxiety and major depressive disorder may respond to antidepressant therapy.

Hallucinogen Use Disorder

Hallucinogens cause a profound disturbance in reality and are associated with flashbacks, panic attacks, psychosis, delirium, and mood and anxiety disorders. These substances can be both natural and synthetic substances, with no recognized medical use. They are found in certain plants and mushrooms or can be synthesized. Classic hallucinogens (e.g., LSD) and dissociative hallucinogens (e.g., phencyclidine [PCP] and ketamine) are commonly used. A use disorder leads to significant impairment or distress, causing cravings, difficulty fulfilling role obligations, tolerance, and overall functional impairment, and tolerance.

Hallucinogen Intoxication

Intoxication is characterized by paranoia, impaired judgment, intensification of perceptions, depersonalization, and derealization. Hallucinations, illusions, and synesthesia (e.g., hearing colors or seeing sounds) are prominent. Physical symptoms include pupillary dilation, tachycardia, sweating, palpitations, blurred vision, tremors, and incoordination.

Treatment for hallucinogen intoxication includes reassuring the individual that the symptoms are drug induced and will subside. In severe cases, short-term treatment with antipsychotics such as haloperidol (Haldol) or benzodiazepines such as diazepam (Valium) may be necessary.

Phencyclidine Intoxication

PCP intoxication is a medical emergency. Behavioral symptoms include belligerence, assaultiveness, impulsiveness, and unpredictability. Physical symptoms include nystagmus (involuntary eye movements), hypertension, tachycardia, diminished response to pain, ataxia (loss of voluntary muscle control), dysarthria (unclear speech), muscle rigidity, seizures, coma, and hyperacusis (sensitivity to sound). Hyperthermia and seizure activity may also occur.

Patients who have ingested PCP cannot usually be calmed and may require restraint. Placing the patient in a quiet room with dim lights may help. Mechanical cooling may be needed for severe hyperthermia. Benzodiazepines such as lorazepam (Ativan) or diazepam (Valium) can be administered intramuscularly or intravenously to reduce hypertension, agitation, and control seizures.

Hallucinogen Withdrawal

There is no official withdrawal syndrome for hallucinogens. However, hallucinogen-persisting perception disorder, which may affect about 4% of users, particularly those who have used LSD, can occur. The hallmark of this condition is the re-experiencing of perceptual symptoms that occurred while intoxicated. These symptoms can be distressing and impair the individual's normal functioning for weeks, months, or even years.

Inhalant Use Disorder

Inhalants are toxic gases inhaled through the nose or mouth, entering the bloodstream. Misused household products that contain inhalants include:
- Solvents for glues and adhesives
- Aerosol propellant paint sprays, hair sprays, and shaving cream
- Thinners, such as paint products and correction fluids
- Fuels, including gasoline and propane

Repeated inhalant use leads to increasing use, cravings, and tolerance. Inhalant use impairs an individual's ability to fulfill life roles and causes problems in relationships. This disorder is most common in youth, with 2.7% of adolescents aged 12 and 17 reporting past-year inhalant use (APA, 2022).

Inhalant Intoxication

Small doses of inhalants result in disinhibition and euphoria. Higher doses can lead to fearfulness, illusions, auditory and visual hallucinations, and a distorted body image. Apathy, diminished social and occupational functioning, impaired judgment, impulsive behavior, and aggression often accompany intoxication. Physical symptoms include nausea, anorexia, nystagmus, depressed reflexes, and diplopia. High doses can result in stupor, unconsciousness, and amnesia. In some cases, delirium, dementia, and psychosis are also may occur as outcomes of inhalant use.

Inhalant intoxication usually does not require treatment. However, serious and potentially fatal reactions, such as coma, cardiac arrhythmias, or bronchospasm, may occur and require immediate medical treatment. A psychotic response may also be induced by inhalant intoxication.

Opioid Use Disorder

Opioid misuse, particularly with heroin and prescription drugs, is a chronic relapsing disorder. Cravings and tolerance are significant. The use of this substance results in significant impairment in life roles and interpersonal conflict and puts a person in physically hazardous situations.

In 2022, about 6 million people aged 12 or older misused opioids (SAMHSA, 2023). Specifically, 8.5 million people misused prescription pain relievers, and 900,000 people used heroin.

Opioid use usually begins in the late teens or early 20s. Increasing age is associated with fewer affected individuals, probably due to early mortality and cessation of use after age 40 years.

Opioid Intoxication

Opioid intoxication results in psychomotor retardation, drowsiness, slurred speech, altered mood (ranging from withdrawn to elated), and impaired memory and attention. Physical symptoms include pinpoint pupils (miosis), decreased bowel sounds, a reduced respiratory rate, and normal to low heart rate. Skin disruptions, such as track marks or fresh injection sites, may confirm intravenous drug use.

Opioid Overdose

Death from an opioid overdose usually results from respiratory arrest due to respiratory depression. Symptoms include unresponsiveness, slow respiration, coma, hypothermia, hypotension, and bradycardia. The combination of coma, pinpoint pupils, and respiratory depression strongly suggests an overdose.

Overdose treatment begins with aspirating secretions, inserting an airway, and providing mechanical ventilation. Naloxone, a specific opioid antagonist, can be administered intranasally, intramuscularly, or intravenously. Increased respirations and pupillary dilation occur rapidly. However, excessive naloxone administration may induce withdrawal symptoms. Since naloxone's duration of action is shorter than that of many opioids, repeated doses may be necessary.

Opioid Withdrawal

Withdrawal symptoms occur after a reduction or cessation of heavy opioid use or after the administration of an opioid antagonist. Symptoms include mood dysphoria, nausea, vomiting, diarrhea, muscle aches, fever, and insomnia. Other common symptoms of withdrawal include lacrimation (watery eyes), rhinorrhea (runny nose), pupillary dilation, piloerection (bristling of hairs), and yawning. Males may experience sweating and spontaneous ejaculation.

Morphine, heroin, and methadone withdrawal begins at 6 to 8 hours after use. Symptoms intensify on the second or third day and then subside over the following week. Meperidine (Demerol) withdrawal starts within 8 to 12 hours after abstinence and lasts about 5 days. For information on pharmacotherapy for opioid withdrawal and abstinence, refer to Chapter 27.

Sedative, Hypnotic, and Antianxiety Medication Use Disorder

Sedative, hypnotic, and antianxiety use disorder is applied to the misuse of all prescription sleeping medications and almost all prescription antianxiety drugs. These drugs include benzodiazepines, benzodiazepine-like drugs (e.g., zolpidem, zaleplon), carbamates, barbiturates (e.g., secobarbital), and barbiturate-like hypnotics (e.g., methaqualone). Misuse of these neural depressants negatively affects role performance and relationships. Craving, tolerance, dependence, and withdrawal can develop even when taken for their intended indication. However, a use disorder diagnosis is only given in the presence of clinically significant maladaptive behavior or psychological changes.

The 12-month prevalence of this problem is about 0.2% in adults (APA, 2022). It occurs in males slightly more often than in females. These disorders are highest among 18- to 29-year-olds (0.5%) and lowest among individuals 65 and older (0.04%).

Sedative, Hypnotic, and Antianxiety Medication Intoxication

As depressants, intoxication from these drugs results in slurred speech, incoordination, unsteady gait, nystagmus, and impaired thinking. Inappropriate aggression and sexual behavior, mood fluctuations, and impaired judgment may also occur.

Sedative, Hypnotic, and Antianxiety Medication Overdose

Overdose treatment includes gastric lavage, activated charcoal, and monitoring of vital signs. If the patient is conscious, they are kept awake. If the patient is unconscious, an intravenous line is initiated. Endotracheal intubation may be necessary to ensure a patent airway, and mechanical ventilation may be necessary.

Sedative, Hypnotic, and Antianxiety Medication Withdrawal

Repeated depression of the central nervous system, along with the body's attempts to return to homeostasis, results in rebound hyperactivity when the depressant is removed. As a result, autonomic hyperactivity, tremors, insomnia, psychomotor agitation, anxiety, and grand mal seizures may occur. The drug's half-life is a key predictor of withdrawal duration.

Gradual reduction of benzodiazepines will prevent seizures and other withdrawal symptoms. Barbiturate withdrawal can be managed by using a long-acting barbiturate such as phenobarbital.

Stimulant Use Disorder

Amphetamine-type, cocaine, or other stimulant drugs are the second most widely used illicit substances in the United States, following cannabis (SAMHSA, 2020). These drugs typically produce feelings of euphoria and high energy. Long-distance truckers, students studying for examinations, soldiers in wartime, and athletes in competition may use these substances. As with all use disorders, increased consumption, craving, and tolerance are accompanied by a reduced ability to function in major roles. Stimulant use disorders can develop rapidly, sometimes within just 1 week.

The estimated 12-month prevalence for amphetamine-type stimulant use is about 0.2% in adults (APA, 2022). Both females and males are affected equally, though intravenous stimulant use is more common in males, with a ratio of about around 4:1. Cocaine use disorder is higher at 0.3%, with more male users.

Stimulant Intoxication

Stimulants make individuals feel elated, euphoric, and sociable. They can also increase hypervigilance, anxiety, tension, and anger. Physical symptoms include chest pain, cardiac arrhythmias, high or low blood pressure, tachycardia or bradycardia, and respiratory depression. Other physical signs include dilated pupils, perspiration, chills, nausea or vomiting, weight loss, psychomotor agitation or retardation, weakness, confusion, seizures, and coma.

Stimulant Withdrawal

Withdrawal symptoms can begin within a few hours to several days after cessation. Common symptoms include fatigue, vivid nightmares, increased appetite, insomnia or hypersomnia, and psychomotor retardation or agitation. During this period, functionality is often impaired. The most serious side effects of stimulant withdrawal include depression and suicidal thoughts.

Depending on the stimulant used, specific drugs may help manage withdrawal symptoms in the short term. Antipsychotics may be prescribed for a few days. If no psychosis is present, diazepam (Valium) can be useful in treating agitation and hyperactivity. Once the patient has been withdrawn from the stimulant, antidepressants can be used to manage major depressive symptoms.

For cocaine, the withdrawal period of 1 to 2 weeks generally does not involve physiological disturbances that require inpatient care. However, hospitalization may be helpful to remove the affected individual from their usual social settings and sources of drugs. Some patients experience fatigue, mood changes, disturbed sleep, cravings, and depression. Currently, there are no medications that reliably reduce the intensity of these symptoms.

Tobacco Use Disorder

Craving, persistent use, and tolerance are all symptoms of tobacco use disorder. Dependence develops quickly. The 12-month prevalence of tobacco use disorder is about 13% in adults (APA, 2022). Rates are slightly higher in males compared to females. Most individuals who use tobacco begin before the age of 18 years.

Tobacco Withdrawal

Tobacco withdrawal is distressing and results in irritability, anxiety, depression, difficulty concentrating, restlessness, and insomnia. Within days of smoking cessation, heart rates decrease by 5 to 12 beats per minute. Within the first year of smoking cessation, people typically gain an average of 4 to 7 lbs.

Behavioral therapy helps patients recognize cravings and respond to them effectively. Hypnosis is also used to treat tobacco withdrawal. Nicotine replacement therapies, such as gum, lozenges, nasal sprays, and patches, are effective treatments. The antidepressant bupropion (Zyban) reduces cravings for nicotine. Varenicline (Chantix), a nicotinic receptor partial agonist, provides mild nicotine-like effects and blocks the effects of nicotine from cigarettes if smoking is resumed.

Gambling Disorder

Gambling can become a compulsive activity that leads to severe financial problems and significant disturbances in personal, social, or occupational functioning. Affected individuals are preoccupied with gambling, experience an increasing desire to gamble, and may lie to conceal the extent of the problem. They may attempt to control or reduce their gambling but often fail. Otherwise, honest individuals may commit illegal acts to finance their addiction. They may rely on others to help pay off debts while gambling in an attempt to recoup losses.

The 1-year prevalence rate of gambling disorder is about 0.2% in females and about 0.6% in males (APA, 2022). Early signs of gambling disorder are more common in males, although the progression tends to be more rapid in females. Gambling may be regular or episodic. Heavy gambling may be interspersed with abstinence. Stress and depression may exacerbate this behavior.

Legal problems, family pressure, and other psychiatric illnesses may bring individuals with excessive gambling habits into treatment. Gamblers Anonymous (GA) is a 12-step program modeled after Alcoholics Anonymous (AA). GA involves public confession, peer pressure, and peer counselors who are reformed gamblers. Hospitalization may help by removing patients from gambling environments. Individual, group, and family therapy are also useful in supporting the patient.

Medications are used to decrease either the urge to gamble or the thrill associated with it. Antidepressants such as selective serotonin reuptake inhibitors and bupropion (Wellbutrin), mood stabilizers (e.g., lithium), and anticonvulsants such as topiramate (Topamax) may be beneficial-. Second-generation antipsychotics are also used. Naltrexone, an opioid antagonist, may be prescribed for individuals with the most severe symptoms of gambling disorder.

ALCOHOL USE DISORDER

Although alcohol is a sedative, it initially produces a feeling of euphoria, likely due to decreased inhibitions. Alcohol use disorder is characterized by a cluster of behavioral and physical symptoms. In 2022, the 12-month prevalence rate in individuals aged 12 and older was 10.5%, or 29.5 million people (SAMHSA, 2023).

Types of Problematic Drinking

The US Department of Health and Human Services and US Department of Agriculture (2020–25) have identified dietary guidelines on alcohol consumption that vary based on individual factors such as gender, age, and pregnancy status. Avoiding alcohol is recommended for those who are pregnant, individuals with certain medical conditions, those taking certain medications, and individuals with an alcohol use disorder or those unable to limit their drinking. For those aged 21 and over who choose to drink, the recommendation is to limit alcohol intake to 2 drinks or fewer per day for men and 1 drink or fewer per day for women.

Excessive drinking is categorized into two terms: binge drinking and heavy drinking. Binge drinking refers to consuming large amounts of drinks, defined as four or more drinks for women and five or more drinks for men in about 2 hours. Heavy drinking is characterized by regular excessive consumption—eight or more drinks in a week for women and more than 14 drinks per week for men.

Alcohol Intoxication

In the United States, a standard drink contains about 14 g of pure alcohol (National Institute on Alcohol Abuse and Alcoholism, n.d.). This amount is equivalent to 12 ounces of beer with 5% alcohol content, 5 ounces of wine with 12% alcohol content, and 1.5 ounces of distilled spirits with 40% alcohol content.

The legal definition of intoxication in most states requires a blood concentration of 0.08 to 0.10 g/dL. Blood alcohol levels, the number of drinks, and symptoms of alcohol intoxication are listed in Table 12.1.

Table 12.1 **Blood Alcohol, Drinks, and Symptoms**

Blood Alcohol	Drinks	Symptoms
0.02 g/dL	2	Slower motor performance, decreased thinking ability, altered mood, and reduced ability to multitask
0.05 g/dL	3	Impaired judgment, exaggerated behavior, euphoria, and lower alertness
0.08 g/dL	4	Poor muscle coordination, altered speech and hearing, difficulty detecting danger, impaired judgment, poor self-control, and decreased reasoning
0.10 g/dL	5	Slurred speech, poor coordination, and slowed thinking
0.15 g/dL	6	Vomiting (unless high tolerance) and major loss of balance
0.20 g/dL	8–10	Memory blackouts, nausea, and vomiting
0.30 g/dL	10+	Reduction of body temperature, blood pressure, and respiratory rate; sleepiness; and amnesia
0.40 mg/dL	—	Impaired vital signs and possible death

Excessive amounts of alcohol may result in blackouts, during which new memories cannot be consolidated. During blackouts, a person may actively engage in behaviors, perform complicated tasks, and appear normal, despite having no memory of the events.

Alcohol Withdrawal

Alcohol withdrawal occurs after reducing or quitting alcohol following heavy and prolonged use. A summary of symptoms is provided here, Chapter 27 offers a more thorough discussion of alcohol withdrawal and treatment.

- The classic sign of alcohol withdrawal is tremulousness, commonly called the shakes or jitters, which typically begins 6 to 8 hours after alcohol cessation.
- Mild-to-moderate alcohol withdrawal includes symptoms such as agitation, loss of appetite, nausea, vomiting, insomnia, impaired cognition, and mild perceptual changes. Both systolic and diastolic blood pressure increase, along with pulse and body temperature.
- Psychotic and perceptual symptoms may begin 8 to 10 hours after cessation. Patients progressing to psychosis should receive prompt treatment due to the risks of unconsciousness, seizures, and delirium.
- Withdrawal seizures may occur 12 to 24 hours after alcohol cessation. These seizures are generalized and tonic-clonic in nature.
- Alcohol withdrawal delirium or delirium tremens (DTs) can occur at anytime in the first 72 hours. This is a medical emergency that can be fatal if left untreated patients, often due to complications such as pneumonia, renal disease, hepatic insufficiency, or heart failure. Autonomic hyperactivity is accompanied by delusions and visual and tactile hallucinations.

Cognitive Disturbances

Wernicke–Korsakoff Syndrome Heavy alcohol use can result in a memory-reducing condition called Wernicke's (alcoholic) encephalopathy, an acute and reversible condition. It is characterized by altered gait, vestibular dysfunction, confusion, and several ocular motility abnormalities. Symptoms include sluggish reaction to light and anisocoria (unequal pupil size). Wernicke's encephalopathy responds rapidly to large doses of intravenous thiamine, typically given two to three times daily for 1 to 2 weeks.

Untreated Wernicke's encephalopathy may progress into Korsakoff's syndrome, a more severe and chronic form of the condition. Treatment for Korsakoff's syndrome involves thiamine supplementation for 3 to 12 months. Most patients with Korsakoff's syndrome never fully recover, though cognitive improvement may occur with thiamine and nutritional support.

Fetal Alcohol Syndrome

Alcohol use during pregnancy is the most common cause of intellectual developmental disorder in the United States. The condition in the infant is known as fetal alcohol syndrome. Alcohol during pregnancy inhibits intrauterine growth and postnatal development, resulting in microcephaly, craniofacial malformations, and defects in the limbs and heart. Affected individuals often have short stature as adults. Pregnant women with alcohol-related disorders are at a significant risk of having a child with these defects.

Systemic Effects

Alcohol overuse results in damage to nearly every system in the body. Conditions associated with alcohol use disorder include:

- Peripheral neuropathy
- Alcoholic myopathy
- Alcoholic cardiomyopathy
- Esophagitis
- Gastritis
- Cirrhosis of the liver
- Leukopenia
- Thrombocytopenia
- Cancer
- Pancreatitis
- Alcoholic hepatitis

ASSESSMENT

A substance use assessment is a critical part of a broader, comprehensive evaluation that considers the individual holistically. Ideally, this assessment should be conducted by an addiction professional with specialized knowledge and skills to make an accurate diagnosis.

The Screening, Brief Intervention, and Referral to Treatment (SBIRT) is a comprehensive, integrated, public health approach designed to deliver early intervention and treatment services for individuals with substance use disorders, as well as those at risk of developing them. SBIRT identifies at-risk substance users for early intervention (SAMHSA, 2022) and consists of three major components:

- Screening: A nurse or other healthcare professional in any healthcare setting assesses the severity of substance use and identifies the appropriate level of treatment.
- Brief Intervention: A nurse or other healthcare professional focuses on increasing insight and awareness regarding substance use and motivation toward behavioral change.
- Referral to Treatment: A nurse or other healthcare professional provides those identified as needing more extensive treatment with access to specialty care.

Assessment Tool

A variety of screening tools are available to assist healthcare practitioners in gathering important information to inform plans of care. A simple, crosscutting measure for most misused substances is provided in Table 12.2.

Assessment Guidelines

A. Is immediate medical attention necessary for a severe or major withdrawal syndrome? For example, alcohol and sedative use can be life-threatening during major withdrawal.
B. Is the patient experiencing an overdose of a substance that requires immediate medical attention? For example, opioids or depressants can cause respiratory depression, coma, and death.
C. Does the patient have physical complications related to substance use (e.g., acquired immunodeficiency syndrome [AIDS], abscess, tachycardia, hepatitis)?
D. Does the patient have suicidal thoughts or indicate, through verbal or nonverbal cues, a potential for self-destructive behaviors?
E. Does the patient seem interested in addressing the substance use problem?

Table 12.2 CAGE[a] Questions Adapted to Include Drug Use (CAGE-AID)

Item	0 = No 1 = Yes
1. Have you ever felt you ought to cut down on your drinking or drug use?	
2. Have people annoyed you by criticizing your drinking or drug use?	
3. Have you felt bad or guilty about your drinking or drug use?	
4. Have you ever had a drink or used drugs first thing in the morning to steady your nerves or to get rid of a hangover (eye-opener)?	
Total	

[a]Cut down, annoyed, guilty, and eye-opener.
Scoring: Item responses on the CAGE questions are scored 0 for "no" and 1 for "yes" answers, with a higher score being an indication of alcohol problems. A total score of two or greater is considered clinically significant.

Nursing Diagnoses

Nurses care for patients with substance use disorders in a variety of settings and situations. Some conditions require medical interventions and skilled nursing care, while necessitate the effective use of communication and counseling skills. Substance use can lead to intoxication, overdose, and withdrawal, making *risk for injury* a priority nursing diagnosis (International Council of Nurses, 2019).

Patients often face challenges in managing their health in areas such as finances, nutrition, sleep, and coping skills. The nursing diagnoses *impaired health maintenance* and *impaired coping* are crucial in addressing these issues. Additionally, because individuals with substance use disorders have difficulty acknowledging their use as a problem, the nursing diagnosis *denial* is essential.

Intervention Guidelines

A. Support the patient during detoxification.
B. Assess for feelings of hopelessness, helplessness, and suicidal thinking.
C. Determine whether the patient is being treated for a comorbid physical condition (e.g., liver disease or

infections) or a psychiatric condition (e.g., depression or panic attacks).
D. Intervene with the patient's use of defense mechanisms, such as denial, rationalization, projection, that interfere with motivation for change.
E. Involve family members and provide support to them, while being aware that they may minimize the problem or enable the patient.
F. Emphasize abstinence.
G. Provide referrals to self-help groups (e.g., AA, Narcotics Anonymous [NA], Cocaine Anonymous [CA]) or a recovery program early in treatment.
H. Teach the patient to avoid medications that may be habit-forming, such as antianxiety agents or pain medications.
I. Emphasize personal responsibility, placing control within the patient's grasp.
J. Support residential treatment when appropriate, particularly for patients with multiple relapses.
K. Provide support if the patient relapses.
L. Provide education on the physical and psychological consequences of substance use.
M. Provide both verbal and written education regarding pharmacotherapy for addictions (e.g., naltrexone or methadone) to help prevent relapse in alcohol use disorder and narcotic addiction.

Nursing Care for Substance Use Disorders

Risk for Injury

Related to
- Biochemical alterations in the brain
- Perceptual alteration, loss, or disorientation
- Chemical toxicity (e.g., poisons, drugs, alcohol, nicotine, pharmacological agents)
- Impaired judgment (due to disease, drugs, reality testing, risk-taking behaviors)
- Substance withdrawal
- Severe or panic levels of anxiety and agitation
- Potential for electrolyte imbalance or seizures
- Hallucinations (e.g., bugs, animals, snakes)
- Elevated temperature, pulse, and respirations
- Agitation, attempts to escape, or climbing out of bed
- Combative behaviors
- Misinterpretation of reality (illusions)

Desired Outcome The patient will remain free from injury.

Assessment/Interventions and *Rationales*

1. Monitor vital signs frequently, at least every 15 minutes until stable, and then every hour for 4 to 8 hours, according to hospital protocol or the care provider's order. *Withdrawal from depressants, particularly alcohol, can cause significant and dangerous autonomic hyperactivity. Pulse is a strong indicator of impending delirium tremens (DTs), signaling the need for more intensive sedation.*

2. Provide the patient with a quiet room that has limited environmental stimulation, such as a single room near the nurses' station, if possible. *Reduced stimulation helps decrease irritability and confusion."*

3. Approach the patient calmly and reassuringly. *Patients need to feel that others are in control and that they are safe.*

4. Use simple, direct language and clear instructions. *The patient can follow basic commands but struggles with processing complex or abstract ideas.*

5. Orient the patient to time, place, and person during periods of confusion or disorientation. Highlight the patient's progress during periods of lucidity. *Fluctuating levels of consciousness may occur during intoxication, withdrawal, and overdose from certain drugs. Providing orientation can help reduce anxiety.*

6. Institute seizure precautions according to hospital protocol as needed. *Seizures might occur during intoxication, overdose, and withdrawal, and precautions for patient safety are a priority.*

7. Carefully monitor intake and output, checking for dehydration or overhydration. *Dehydration can aggravate electrolyte imbalance, while overhydration can lead to congestive heart failure.*

8. If hallucinations are present, reassure the patient— that although they seem real, you cannot hear/ see them. Offer to stay with the patient to provide support (e.g., "I don't see rats on the wall. You sound frightened right now. I will stay with you for a few minutes."). *Instilling reasonable doubt as to the reality of the hallucinations is supportive when carefully presented. Staying near a frightened patient provides reassurance.*

9. If the patient is experiencing illusions, gently correct their misinterpretation in a calm and matter-of-fact manner (e.g., "This is not a snake around my neck

ready to bite you; it is my stethoscope. Let me show you."). *Illusions can be explained to a patient who is misinterpreting environmental cues. When the patient recognizes normal objects for what they are, anxiety is reduced.*

10. Administer medications ordered to treat use disorders, intoxication, overdose, and withdrawal. *Medication can reverse uncomfortable responses and prevent mortality when treating responses to use disorders.*

11. Use the least restrictive environment to maintain safety. Restraints and seclusion are used with caution if the patient is combative. Always follow unit protocol. *Myocardial infarction, cardiac collapse, and death have occurred when patients have fought against restraints.*

12. Maintain frequent, accurate documentation of the patient's vital signs, behaviors, medications, interventions, and effects of interventions. *Documentation provides a record of progress, identifies what works best, and alerts for potential complications.*

Impaired Health Maintenance

Related to

- Biochemical alterations in the brain
- Inability to make sound judgments
- Ineffective coping skills
- Perceptual or cognitive impairment
- Preoccupation with obtaining and using the drug
- Depleted finances due to substance use, leaving little or nothing for healthcare, nourishing food, or safe shelter
- Poor nutrition related to prolonged drug binges, taking drugs instead of eating nourishing food, or diminished appetite related to choice of drug (e.g., cocaine)
- Malabsorption of nutrients caused by chronic alcohol use
- Sleep deprivation related to decreased rapid eye movement (REM) sleep as a result of use of stimulants, alcohol, or central nervous system depressants
- Lack of regular health care (e.g., mammograms, dentist, yearly physicals) because of either being intoxicated, being hung-over, or withdrawing from an illicit substance

Desired Outcome The patient will demonstrate improved health maintenance.

Assessment/Interventions and *Rationales*
1. Encourage small feedings and provide bland foods if appropriate. *If the patient has a loss of appetite, small feedings are better tolerated. Bland foods are often more appealing.*
   Assess nutritional status, including conjunctival appearance, body weight, and eating history. *Assessing nutritional status through conjunctival appearance, body weight, and eating history helps identify deficiencies or malnutrition, guiding appropriate interventions to prevent further health complications.*
2. Monitor fluid intake and output and assess skin turgor and ankle edema for signs of fluid imbalance. *Monitoring fluid intake and output, along with assessing skin turgor and ankle edema, helps detect early signs of fluid imbalance, which can indicate dehydration or fluid retention, allowing for timely intervention and prevention of complications.*
3. When skin turgor is poor, encourage fluids containing protein and vitamins (e.g., milk, milkshakes/smoothies, juices), and consider a urine test for specific gravity. *Poor skin turgor may indicate dehydration, and encouraging fluids rich in protein and vitamins helps support hydration and nutritional needs. A urine-specific gravity test can further assess hydration status and guide appropriate intervention.*
4. Promote rest and sleep by providing a quiet environment. *Restorative rest and sleep are disrupted during substance use. Sleep hygiene measures are emphasized during recovery.*
5. Explore the patient's understanding of the detrimental impact of alcohol or substance use (e.g., fetal alcohol syndrome, hepatitis or AIDS, fertility issues). *Before teaching, the nurse must identify what the patient knows about the drugs and evaluate readiness to learn. Patient education allows for personal control over health care.*
6. Review the patient's blood work and physical examination results and discuss these findings with the patient. *Assessment information helps the nurse identify potential causes of symptoms (e.g., infection) and initiate counseling. Sharing this information allows the patient to take an active role in health care.*
7. Set up an appointment for medical follow-up and encourage the patient to record the event on a calendar, cell phone, or appointment book. If possible, follow up reminders through calls, e-mails, and texts. *Follow-up is essential in monitoring physical status. Concrete reminders increase the likelihood of appointments being kept.*

Denial

Related to
- Substance use or process addiction with a need to maintain the status quo
- Fear of acknowledging the destructiveness of the substance or process
- Feelings of hopelessness and helplessness without the substance
- Ineffective coping strategies

Desired Outcome The patient will acknowledge and demonstrate responsibility for behavior.

Assessment/Interventions and *Rationales*
1. Maintain an interested, nonjudgmental, and supportive approach. *A professional and caring approach based on a therapeutic relationship is most effective.*
2. Focus initially on reducing anxiety by addressing the current crisis situation. *Patients are unable to address higher-level needs while experiencing situational anxiety (e.g., practical living problems, family crises).*
3. Avoid criticizing the patient's behaviors. *Disapproval is a nontherapeutic approach to communication with a patient. These reactions will only make the patient more defensive.*
4. Explore the role of denial in continuing addictive behaviors and discuss how it acts as a barrier to seeking treatment. *Addressing denial helps the patient recognize its role in sustaining addictive behaviors, which is crucial for overcoming resistance to treatment and fostering readiness for change.*
5. Explore goals and what the patient wants to change. *Initially, the patient's goal might not be abstinence. Identifying areas the patient wants to change gives the patient a motivation to change.*
6. Use miracle questions to help identify what the patient wants to change. For example, "What if your worst problem were miraculously solved overnight? What would be different about your life the next day?" *Miracle questions help patients perceive their future without some of their problems and give direction to moving forward and identifying long- and short-term goals.*
7. Encourage the patient to evaluate the pros and cons of substance use. *Analyzing the pros and cons helps the patient look at what substances will and will not do for*

them in a clear light. This analysis may help strengthen personal motives for change.

8. Encourage the patient to explore how external problems (e.g., relationships, job-related, legal) relate to substance use. *Denial of the destructive nature of addiction is a major component of addiction. Patients may gradually view external problems as the result of addictive behaviors and not the cause.*

9. Help the patient identify behaviors contributing to problems (e.g., family dysfunction, social difficulties, job-related problems, legal issues). *When individuals take responsibility for maladaptive behaviors, they are more prepared to take responsibility for learning effective and satisfying behaviors.*

10. Encourage the patient to stay in the present moment (e.g., "Let's focus on how you want to respond when criticized by your boss"). *Focusing on past disappointments is not useful for developing new and more adaptive coping methods.*

11. Encourage the patient to find a sponsor within a 12-step program or another therapeutic approach. *Having a sponsor and being a sponsor supports success.*

12. Help the patient identify—vulnerable times for substance use and strategies to cope during those times. *Considering alternative strategies to drinking or taking drugs in vulnerable situations gives the patient a ready choice.*

13. Encourage family and friends to seek support, education, and ways to recognize and stop enabling the patient's substance use. *Enabling behavior supports the patient's use of drugs by taking away the incentive for change.*

14. Educate the patient and family about the physical and neurological effects of the substance or process, potential treatment, and aftercare. *Education allows the patient to take responsibility for personal care. Educating the family provides clarity for them and, ideally, support for the patient.*

15. Acknowledge that treatment is a long process. *Acknowledging that treatment is a long-term process helps set realistic expectations, fosters patience, and supports the patient in maintaining motivation and commitment throughout their recovery journey.*

16. Refer the patient to a 12-step support group, recovery program, or residential program and encourage

attendance. *These referrals can provide essential ongoing support and structure, while encouraging attendance reinforces commitment and accountability in maintaining recovery and preventing relapse.*

17. Attend several open meetings in the local community to better understand the 12-step process. *Attending open meetings helps nursing students and nurses gain insight into the 12-step process, improving their ability to support patients in recovery and foster empathetic, informed care.*

Impaired Coping

Related to
- Biochemical alterations in the brain
- Inadequate resources
- Disturbance in pattern of stress management
- Inadequate level of control or perception of control
- Knowledge deficit
- Coping styles that are no longer adaptive
- Insufficient social support

Desired Outcome The patient will report and demonstrate improved coping.

Assessment/Interventions and *Rationales*

1. Set small, achievable goals at the start of treatment. *Patients with substance use problems often experience cognitive deficits during use, which may persist for months after achieving sobriety.*

2. Encourage the patient to use memory aids, such as writing notes or setting reminders on a smartphone or calendar to help them manage appointments and follow the treatment plan. While *cognition improves with long-term abstinence, memory aids are essential in the early stages of recovery.*

3. Encourage the patient to join relapse prevention groups. *Attending these groups helps the patient anticipate and rehearse healthy responses to stressful situations.*

4. Encourage the patient to identify or seek role models, such as peers in recovery. *Role models can provide motivation and hope by demonstrating successful abstainence from substance use.*

5. Help the patient identify triggers for substance use (e.g., people, feelings, situations) that contribute

to addiction. *Recognizing these triggers for substance use is essential for fostering change and developing new coping skills.*

6. Practice and role-play alternative responses to triggers for substance use. *Increases patient confidence in handling drug triggers effectively.*

7. Give positive feedback when the patient applies new and effective responses to difficult trigger situations. *Validates the patient's positive steps toward growth and change.*

8. Address denial throughout the recovery process. *Addressing denial throughout recovery is essential, as it prevents individuals from acknowledging the impact of their substance use, hindering progress toward sobriety.*

9. Explore coping strategies for personal issues (e.g., relationships), social challenges (e.g., family violence, unemployment), and self-worth. Addressing these areas can foster healing and growth in the absence of substance use. *Exploring coping strategies for personal, social, and self-worth issues helps individuals build healthier ways to manage stress and emotions, promoting healing and growth while reducing reliance on substances.*

10. Recommend family therapy to strengthen strategies for managing family conflict, which is vital to recovery. *Enhanced strategies for dealing with family conflict are essential to recovery. Family therapy also improves the family's sense of empowerment and increases familial support.*

11. Emphasize that substance use affects the entire family, and family members also require support and encouragement. *Helps family members recognize their role in the recovery process and encourages them to seek the support they need, fostering a healthier, more supportive environment for both the patient and their loved ones.*

12. Discuss the potential for relapse and reinforce the patient's ability to achieve and maintain sobriety. This helps reduce feelings of *shame and guilt while rebuilding self-esteem.*

TREATMENT MODALITIES FOR SUBSTANCE USE DISORDERS

Biological Treatment

Pharmacotherapy

Pharmacotherapy for substance use withdrawal and abstinence varies depending on the substance. Pharmacological treatments for substance use disorders are provided in Chapter 27.

Psychological Therapies

Cognitive behavioral therapy (CBT) and motivational interviewing are commonly used evidence-based therapies for substance use disorders. CBT helps patients identify and explore destructive and negative thinking patterns, allowing them to address core beliefs and irrational thoughts. It also involves examining positive and negative consequences of substance use, teaching patients to self-monitor cravings and challenge them realistically. Patients learn to self-monitor their cravings and challenge these cravings realistically. For more detailed information about CBT, refer to Chapter 27.

Motivational interviewing is an approach based on the transtheoretical or stages of change theory. It has gained popularity in its use as a brief, long-term, and supplementary intervention, particularly in the treatment of substance use disorders. It uses a person-centered approach to strengthen motivation for change.

Twelve-Step Programs

Twelve-step programs are peer aid groups for recovery from substance addictions, behavioral addictions, and compulsions. AA, founded in 1930, is the oldest and most well-known of the 12-step programs. Anyone with the desire to quit drinking or using substances is welcome to attend meetings. Individuals learn how to be sober through the support of other members and the 12 steps. In most suburban and urban areas, meetings can be found every day around the clock. Virtual meetings are also available online. All groups are structured for confidentiality and anonymity. Family members and other support are often welcome.

There are also meetings to address the special needs of family and significant others, such as Al-Anon for friends and family members and Alateen for teenage relatives. Other substance-based support groups include Narcotics Anonymous (NA), Pills Anonymous (PA), Cocaine Anonymous (CA), and others.

👥 NURSE, PATIENT, AND FAMILY RESOURCES

Addictions.com
A leading informational resource and web guide for those impacted by substance abuse and co-occurring mental health disorders.
www.addictions.com

Alcoholics Anonymous (A.A.)
A fellowship of individuals who come together to solve their drinking problem. A.A.'s primary purpose is to help alcoholics achieve sobriety.
www.aa.org

Al-Anon
A mutual support group of peers who share their experience in applying the Al-Anon principles to problems related to the effects of a problem drinker in their lives.
www.al-anon.org

Cocaine Anonymous
A fellowship of men and women who share their experience, strength, and hope with each other that they may solve their common problem and help others recover from their addiction.
www.ca.org

Center for Substance Abuse Treatment (CSAT) National Drug Helpline (bilingual)
A free, confidential, 24/7, 365-day-a-year treatment referral and information service for individuals and families facing mental and/or substance use disorders.
1-800-662-HELP (4357)

Marijuana Anonymous
A free, peer-support program focused entirely on the shared problem with marijuana or cannabis addiction.
www.marijuana-anonymous.org

Nar-Anon Family Groups
A worldwide fellowship for those affected by someone else's addiction.
www.nar-anon.org

Narcotics Anonymous
A global, community-based organization with a multilingual and multicultural membership.
www.na.org

National Association for Children of Alcoholics (NACoA)
NACoA is the only national membership organization focusing on the children of parents struggling with alcohol or substance abuse.
www.nacoa.org

National Institute on Drug Abuse (NIDA)
The NIDA is the lead federal agency supporting scientific research on drug use and addiction.
www.drugabuse.gov/

National Mental Health Consumers' Self-Help Clearinghouse
A peer-run national technical assistance and resource center that fosters recovery, self-determination, and community inclusion.
www.mhselfhelp.org/

CHAPTER 13

Neurocognitive Disorders

The ability to reflect on life's meaning and purpose is central to the human experience. This clarity depends on intact cognitive function, which allows individuals to process, interpret, and respond to their surroundings. When cognition is impaired, the ability to navigate life's journey becomes disrupted, leading to challenges in communication, decision-making, and daily functioning.

Cognition operates on two hierarchical levels. Lower-level cognitive functions involve fundamental processes such as attention, orientation, and recognition of previously acquired information. Higher-level cognitive domains are more advanced and include:

- Complex attention—The ability to focus on multiple tasks, filter distractions, and sustain attention
- Executive function—High-level cognitive abilities that enable planning, prioritization, decision-making, task organization, and adaptability
- Learning and memory—The ability to record, store, and retrieve information
- Language—The ability to communicate through writing, reading, and speaking, including naming objects, word retrieval, speech fluency, grammar, syntax, and comprehension
- Perceptual-motor control—The ability to coordinate movement by integrating sensory input (e.g., vision, touch) with motor skills to interact with the environment
- Social cognition—The ability to process and interpret social information, regulate impulses, express empathy, recognize social cues, read facial expressions, and predict behavior.

Psychiatric disorders have a profound impact on cognitive functioning. The American Psychiatric Association

(2022) categorizes neurocognitive disorders into three main classifications: delirium, mild neurocognitive disorder, and major neurocognitive disorder.

In this chapter, delirium, which is an acute and reversible condition affecting lower-level functioning, is discussed and nursing care is addressed. Mild and major neurocognitive disorders, where there is a decline in higher-level cognitive functioning, are then discussed. Mild neurocognitive disorders may or may not progress to the major type. Major neurocognitive disorders, commonly referred to as dementia, are progressive and irreversible.

DELIRIUM

Delirium is an acute cognitive disturbance that is usually reversible. It commonly occurs in hospitalized patients, especially older adults. It is classified as a syndrome, that is, it consists of a constellation of symptoms rather than a distinct disorder. The primary symptoms of delirium include an inability to direct, focus, sustain, and shift attention; an abrupt onset with fluctuating clinical features and periods of lucidity; and disorganized thinking.

Other characteristics include disorientation (often to time and place, but rarely to person), anxiety, agitation, poor memory, and delusional thinking. When hallucinations occur, they are usually visual. These visual hallucinations can be formed (e.g., people, animals) or unformed (e.g., spots, flashes of light).

Epidemiology

Among critically ill adult patients, the incidence is at least 30% (Brennan et al., 2023). The prevalence of delirium in older adults ranges from 30% to 50% (Kim et al., 2023). There is a high degree of variability in the reported incidence and prevalence of delirium, likely due to its under-recognition by healthcare professionals.

Delirium occurs across various healthcare settings, with the highest risk in intensive care units, followed by intermediate care and medical services, and lower rates in surgical services. Patients with delirium tend to be older, have longer hospital stays, and are more likely to have preexisting dementia. They also face a higher risk of in-hospital mortality and are more frequently admitted from and discharged to institutional care.

Box 13.1 **Risk Factors for Delirium**

- Pain
- Infection
- Dehydration
- Hypoxia
- Immobilization
- Poor or inadequate nutrition
- Environmental factors: excessive noise, lack of orienting materials (e.g., calendars, clocks, whiteboards), relocation to a new area
- Sleep deprivation
- Lack of eyeglasses or hearing aids
- Use of restraints

Risk Factors

Delirium is always related to underlying physiological causes. These underlying causes put a patient at risk for developing delirium, and there are immediate factors that precipitate the syndrome. The interaction of the two results in delirium. The risk factors that are modifiable through nursing care are listed in Box 13.1.

Assessment Guidelines

A. Do not assume that acute confusion in an older person is due to dementia.
B. Assess for sudden onset and fluctuating levels of awareness.
C. Evaluate the person's ability to focus on their immediate environment, including responses to nursing care.
D. Determine the person's usual cognition baseline by talking with family or caregivers.
E. Assess for past cognitive impairment—especially an existing dementia diagnosis—and other risk factors.
F. Identify disturbances in physiological status, especially infection, hypoxia, or pain.
G. Review documented physiological abnormalities in the patient's record.
H. Assess vital signs, level of consciousness, and neurological status.
I. Assess the risk of injury, particularly falls and wandering.

J. Maintain comfort measures, especially concerning pain, cold, or positioning.
K. Monitor factors that may worsen or improve symptoms.

Intervention Guidelines

Delirium is reversible with timely treatment
A. Identifying and treating the medical cause of delirium are the first step.
B. Safety becomes a priority since confusion and fear may make patients more prone to accidents.
C. Provide emotional support since delirium is a terrifying experience.
D. Avoid the use of restraints, which are themselves risk factors for developing delirium.

Nursing Care for Delirium

Delirium

Related to
- Biochemical alterations in the brain
- Medical condition (e.g., urinary tract infection, pneumonia)
- Fluid and electrolyte imbalance
- Substance use or intoxication
- Substance withdrawal
- Toxin exposure

Desired Outcomes The patient will be free from symptoms of delirium.

Assessment/Interventions and *Rationales*
1. Introduce yourself and address the patient by name at the beginning of each interaction. *Patients with short-term memory impairment often require frequent reintroductions and orienting.*
2. Maintain face-to-face contact. *If the patient is easily distracted, this helps focus on one stimulus at a time.*
3. Use short, simple, concrete phrases. *The patient may struggle to process complex information.*
4. Briefly explain each action before performing it. *Even if comprehension is unclear, providing explanations reduces misinterpretation and offers reassurance.*

5. Encourage family and friends to visit one at a time. *A familiar presence reduces anxiety and enhances orientation, while multiple visitors can be overwhelming.*

6. Keep the room well lit during the day, preferably with windows, and darken the room at night if possible. *Aligning light exposure with the 24-hour cycle helps regulate circadian rhythms, promote sleep, and improve orientation.*

7. Minimize environmental noise (e.g., television, conversations). *Noise interferes with rest and can be misconstrued as threatening.*

8. Keep the head of the bed elevated whenever possible. *This position can help provide important visual cues and minimize illusions.*

9. Provide clocks, calendars, and whiteboards with caregiver names and scheduled activities. *These visual cues help orient the patient to time, place, and routine.*

10. Encourage and assist the patient in wearing prescribed eyeglasses or hearing aids. *Even if the patient does not express a need for them, sensory aids enhance perception, reducing misinterpretations of visual and auditory stimuli.*

11. When possible, assign the same staff members to care for the patient on each shift. *Consistent caregivers provide familiarity, reduce confusion, and strengthen the nurse–patient relationship, promoting a sense of security and stability.*

12. When hallucinations occur, reassure patients that they are safe (e.g., "I know you are frightened. I'll sit with you a while and make sure you are safe."). *Providing reassurance helps reduce fear and anxiety, promoting a sense of security and emotional comfort.*

13. When illusions occur, gently clarify reality (e.g., "This is a coat rack, not a man with a knife … see?"). *Illusions result from misinterpreted sensory input, and providing clear explanations helps the patient distinguish reality, reducing fear and distress.*

14. During lucid intervals, update and reorient the patient on their progress. *Since consciousness fluctuates in delirium, periodic orientation helps reduce anxiety and provides reassurance.*

15. Ignore insults and name-calling and acknowledge how upset the person might be feeling. For example:
Patient: "You are an incompetent idiot! Get me a real nurse, someone who knows what they are doing."

Nurse: "What you are going through is very difficult. I'll stay with you." *Feelings of fear are often projected onto the environment. Arguing or becoming defensive only increases the patient's anger and aggressive behaviors. Support and reassurance will decrease anxiety.*

16. If the patient's behavior becomes aggressive, follow a structured approach:

    a. Set clear behavioral limits (e.g., "Mr. Jones, you may not hit me or anyone else. Tell me how you feel." "Mr. Jones, if you have difficulty controlling your actions, we will help you gain control.").

    b. Check for prescribed medication to reduce agitation if verbal redirection is ineffective.

    c. As a last resort, consider physical restraints if the patient poses an immediate danger to themselves or others, following proper protocols.

    Establishing clear boundaries ensures safety for the patient, staff, and others. While verbal intervention is preferred, sometime patients may not respond, making medication or, in extreme cases, physical restraints necessary.

17. After the patient regains their premorbid cognitive state, educate and offer counseling for frightening memories and images. *Patients may have fragmented or distorted recollections of their delirium, sometimes believing that illusions or hallucinations were real. Helping them to construct a realistic narrative supports emotional processing and recovery.*

MILD AND MAJOR NEUROCOGNITIVE DISORDERS

Dementia is a broad term describing deterioration and global impairment of cognitive functioning. It does not refer to a specific disease but rather to a collection of symptoms. The *DSM-5* classifies dementia within the diagnostic categories of mild and major neurocognitive disorders. When mild, impairments do not significantly interfere with daily activities, though individuals may need to exert extra effort. These impairments may or may not progress to a major neurocognitive disorder.

While the remainder of this chapter focuses on Alzheimer's disease (AD), nursing care is essentially the same with other dementia disorders. A brief description of the various forms of dementia is listed in Table 13.1.

Table 13.1 **Common Types of Dementia**

Type of Dementia	Symptoms
Alzheimer's disease (60%–70% of dementias)	Early: difficulty remembering recent conversations, names, or events; apathy; and depression Middle: Impaired communication, disorientation, confusion, poor judgment, and behavioral changes Late: Difficulty speaking, swallowing, and walking
Vascular disease (15% of dementias)	One or more documented cerebrovascular events; impaired judgment; difficulties with decision-making, planning and organizing; slow gait; and poor balance
Lewy body disease (10% of dementias)	Same as Alzheimer's disease but includes sleep disturbance, visual hallucinations, movement, and visuospatial impairment
Frontotemporal lobar degeneration (2% of dementias)	Onset is usually between 45 and 64 years old; marked changes in personality, disinhibition, and difficulty with communication
Parkinson's disease dementia (2% of dementias)	Change in memory, cognition, and judgment; visual hallucinations; paranoid delusions; depression; irritability; and rapid eye movement sleep disorder
Mixed dementia (10% of dementias)	Characterized by the presence of more than one type of dementia, which can be more challenging to diagnose and manage.

ALZHEIMER'S DISEASE

AD, the most common cause of dementia, is a devastating disease. It not only impacts the person experiencing it but also results in a tremendous emotional toll and burden for the families and caregivers. AD is classified according to the stage of the degenerative process: mild, moderate, and severe. The first stage roughly corresponds to the *DSM-5* criteria for mild neurocognitive disorders. Stages two and three correspond to the *DSM-5* criteria for major neurocognitive disorder. Table 13.2 describes the stages of AD.

Table 13.2 **Stages of Alzheimer's Disease**

Mild Alzheimer's Disease (Early Stage)

Noticeable memory lapses. May still function independently but will experience:

- Difficulty recalling correct words or names
- Trouble remembering names of newly introduced people
- Challenges in performing tasks in social or work settings
- Forgetting what they have just read
- Losing or misplacing valuable objects
- Difficulty with planning or organizing

Moderate Alzheimer's Disease (Middle Stage)

Confuses words, gets frustrated or angry, or acts in unexpected ways such as refusing to bathe. Symptoms become noticeable to others, and these individuals may:

- Forget events or their personal history
- Become moody or withdrawn, especially in socially or mentally challenging situations
- Be unable to recall their address, phone number, or the school from which they graduated
- Become confused about where they are or what day it is
- Need help choosing appropriate clothing for the season or the occasion
- Change sleep patterns, such as sleeping during the day and becoming restless at night
- Be at risk of wandering and becoming lost
- Become suspicious, delusional, or compulsive

Severe Alzheimer's Disease (Late Stage)

Loses the ability to respond to the environment, to carry on a conversation, and, eventually, to control movement. May still say words or phrases. Personality changes occur. The person may:

- Require full-time, around-the-clock assistance with daily activities and personal care
- Lose awareness of recent experiences and surroundings
- Experience changes in physical abilities, including the ability to walk, sit, and, eventually, swallow
- Have increasing difficulty communicating
- Become vulnerable to infections, especially pneumonia

Adapted from Alzheimer's Association. (2024). *Stages of Alzheimer's.* https://www.alz.org/alzheimers-dementia/stages.

Epidemiology

Although Alzheimer's disease can occur at a younger age (early onset), most of those affected are 65 years of age or older (late onset). In 2021, an estimated 6.2 million in the United States aged 65 and older were living with Alzheimer's dementia. (Alzheimer's Association, 2021). Seventy-two percent are age 75 or older. Women make up two-thirds of individuals with dementia.

Risk Factors

There is an increased risk for individuals with an affected immediate family member. Some rare genetic mutations guarantee that a person will develop AD. Cardiovascular disease and head injury/traumatic brain injury also contribute to the development of AD and other dementias. Modifiable factors that may reduce risk include engaging in mentally stimulating activities, physical exercise, social engagement, a healthy diet, and sufficient sleep.

Assessment

Signs and Symptoms

- Memory impairment, typically beginning with short-term memory loss
- Loss of executive functioning, affecting the ability to organize, plan, and carry out tasks efficiently
- The A's of Alzheimer's:
  Amnesia: Memory loss
  Aphasia: Difficulty with communication, including word loss, language disturbance, and incorrect word usage
  Apraxia: Impaired motor function despite intact physical ability (e.g., difficulty putting on clothes)
  Agnosia: Inability to recognize familiar objects (e.g., a toothbrush) or sounds (e.g., a ringing phone)
  Agraphia: Loss of the ability to write
  Alexia: Loss of the ability to read
  Anomia: Difficulty finding the right word
- Gradual decline in overall functioning
- Poor judgment
- Mood disturbances, including anxiety, hallucinations, and delusions
- Impaired sleep

Assessment Tools

A variety of tools are available to measure mental status in individuals with dementia. The Montreal Cognitive

Intervention Guidelines

1. Educate the patient's family on safety measures for a cognitively impaired family member living at home (see Box 13.3):
   A. Precautions for wandering (e.g., identification bracelet, high-mounted or complex door locks)
   B. Home safety modifications (e.g., removing slippery rugs, labeling rooms and drawers, installing grab bars in showers and bathtubs)
   C. Guidelines for daily care, including maintaining proper nutrition, regular bowel and bladder habits, healthy sleep patterns, and support for activities of daily living
2. Support the family's use of effective communication strategies:
   A. Assist with communication for aphasic patients by allowing time to speak and using alternative methods such as drawings, gestures, writing, and facial expressions. Use yes/no questions to facilitate understanding.
   B. Teach basic communication techniques for confused patients including re-introducing yourself; using simple, short sentences; maintaining eye contact; focusing on one topic at a time; and discussing familiar topics.
3. Family and caregiver support is a priority. Provide information regarding support groups, respite care, adult daycare, protective services, recreational programs, Meals on Wheels, and hospice services.
4. Provide education on medications the patient is taking, including purpose, side effects, and potential adverse effects.

Nursing Diagnoses

Because delirium and major neurocognitive disorders share similar symptoms, the following nursing diagnoses can be individualized and applied to patients with either condition. One of the primary concerns is the patient's safety due to wandering, falls, burns, and accidental ingestion of poisons or medications. *Risk for injury* is always a priority diagnosis.

Patients often struggle with activities of daily living, making *self-care deficit* a key nursing diagnosis. As cognitive decline progresses, difficulties with processing information and communication can result in *impaired verbal communication*.

Box 13.3 Home Safety for Individuals with Cognitive Impairment

Avoid Injury During Daily Activities

Install walk-in showers for easier access.

Add grab bars in showers, bathtubs, and next to toilet to allow for independent, safe movement.

Apply textured stickers to slippery surfaces.

Apply adhesives to keep throw rugs, or remove rugs completely.

Monitor the hot water temperature in the shower or bath. Consider installing an automatic thermometer.

Install locks out of sight. Place a latch or deadbolt either above or below eye level on all doors. Remove locks on interior doors to prevent the person from locking themselves in. Keep an extra set of keys hidden near the door.

Adapt to Vision Limitations

Encourage the use of prescription glasses. Changes in level of lights can be disorienting. Create an even level by adding extra lights in entries, outside landings, and in areas between rooms, stairways, and bathrooms.

Use nightlights in hallways, bedrooms, and bathrooms.

Beware of Dangerous Objects and Substances

Use appliances that have an automatic shut-off feature.

Disconnect the garbage disposal.

Install a hidden gas valve or circuit breaker on the stove so a person with dementia cannot turn it on. Consider removing the knobs.

Store grills, lawnmowers, power tools, knives, and cleaning products in secure places.

Discard toxic plants and decorative fruits that may be mistaken for real food.

Remove vitamins, prescription drugs, sugar substitutes, and seasonings from the kitchen table and counters. Medications should be kept in a locked area.

Remove guns and firearms from the home or lock them up. Firearm accessibility combined with impaired judgment and forgetting who people are could be disastrous.

From Alzheimer's Association.Alz.org. (n.d.). *Home safety and Alzheimer's*. www.alz.org/care/alzheimers-dementia-home-safety.asp.

An important aspect of the patient's care is the support, education, and referrals for the family. *Caregiver stress* is always present, and planning with the family and offering community support are integral parts of appropriate care.

Other nursing diagnoses that may be useful in caring for patients with delirium and dementia include *impaired cognition, acute/chronic confusion, impaired sleep, anxiety, family grief*, and *hopelessness*.

Nursing Care for Major Neurocognitive Disorders

Risk for Injury

Related to
- Biochemical alterations in the brain
- Sensory dysfunction
- Cognitive or emotional impairment
- Confusion and disorientation
- Loss of executive functioning
- Progressive memory loss (initially short-term, eventually long term)

Desired Outcomes Patient will remain free of injury.

Assessment/Interventions and *Rationales*

1. Restrict driving by assessing the patient's ability, involving healthcare providers in discussions, securing car keys if necessary, and providing alternative transportation options to ensure safety. *Cognitive impairment may lead to accidents or result in the individual becoming lost lead to accidents.*
2. Remove area rugs and other objects that could lead to falls. *Removing these hazards minimizes tripping, falling, and serious injury.*
3. Minimize unhelpful sensory stimulation and provide meaningful alternatives. *Minimizing unhelpful and unnecessary sensory stimulation decreases sensory overload, which can increase anxiety and confusion. Providing meaningful verbal stimulation and welcoming background music or other media supports cognitive functioning.*
4. If patients become upset, listen, provide support, and redirect the conversation. *When attention span is short, gentle distraction with a more positive or engaging topic can help de-escalate distress.*
5. Label objects used for activities of daily living with words and pictures. In residential care, label the patients' rooms with their names and photographs. *Labeling objects (e.g., hairbrushes and toothbrushes) supports the patient's functioning. Labeling rooms helps*

prevent wandering into other patients' rooms and increases autonomy.

6. Recommend installing safety bars near the toilet, in the shower, and in the bathtub. *Use of safety bars can prevent falls.*

7. If the patient wanders during the night, consider putting their mattress on the floor. *Putting the mattress on the floor reduces falls when the patient is confused.*

8. Provide an identification bracelet that cannot be easily removed, with the patient's name, address, and phone number. *The patient can be easily identified by police, neighbors, or hospital personnel.*

9. Place locks at the top of the door. *In moderate- tolate-stage neurocognitive disorders, patients often lose the ability to look up or reach high.*

10. Encourage physical activity during the day. *Physical activity during the day helps to decrease nighttime wandering and restlessness.*

11. Explore the possibility of installing sensor devices. *Sensors can provide a warning if the patient wanders.*

12. Enroll the patient in the Alzheimer's Association's MedicAlert Safe Return program (www.alz.org). *This program helps track individuals who wander and are at risk of getting lost or injured.*

Self-Care Deficit

Related to
- Biochemical alterations in the brain
- Perceptual or cognitive impairment
- Neuromuscular impairment
- Decreased strength and endurance
- Confusion
- Apraxia (inability to perform previously routine tasks)
- Agnosia (inability to recognize familiar items)
- Memory impairment

Desired Outcome The patient will demonstrate improved self-care.

Assessment/Interventions and *Rationales*
Dressing and Bathing
1. Encourage patients to perform tasks they are capable of. This helps *maintain self-esteem, engages muscle groups, and minimizes further regression.*

2. Encourage patients to wear their own clothes, even if in the hospital or residential care. *Wearing familiar clothing helps maintain the patient's identity and dignity.*
3. Use clothing with elastic waistbands, and substitute Velcro for buttons and zippers. *Reduces frustration and promotes independence.*
4. Label clothing items with the patient's name and the name of the item. *Helps identify patients if they wander, and gives patients additional cues for patients with agnosia.*
5. Give step-by-step instructions if necessary (e.g., "Take this blouse ... put in one arm ... now the other arm ... pull it together in the front ... now ..."). *Patients can focus on small pieces of information more easily, allowing the patient to perform at an optimal level.*

Eating and Drinking
1. Monitor food and fluid intake. *The patient might have limited appetite or be too confused to eat.*
2. Offer finger foods. *The patient might eat only small amounts while sitting at meals. Offering on-the-go finger foods increases intake throughout the day.*
3. If hyperorality is present, ensure the patient does not ingest nonfood items (e.g., ceramic fruit, food-shaped soaps). *Hyperorality may result in the patients putting inedible objects into their mouths and may result in choking or poisoning.*

Elimination
1. Establish a toileting schedule, directing the patient to the toilet at regular intervals (e.g., early morning, after meals and snacks, before bedtime). *A toileting routine will reduce episodes of incontinence and help to maintain dignity.*
2. Assess the need for adult disposable undergarments. *Disposable undergarments prevent embarrassment and soiling of their surroundings if incontinence occurs.*
3. Label the bathroom door and other key areas with pictures. *Additional environmental clues can maximize independent toileting. Pictures may be more easily interpreted than words.*

Sleep Hygiene
1. Provide dim lighting at night. *Dim lighting reinforces orientation while supporting sleep hygiene through normal light/dark rhythms.*

2. Monitor for side effects of sleep-promoting medications. *Because of metabolic changes, older adults experience more severe side effects including the potential for dangerous falls.*

Impaired Verbal Communication

Related to

- Biochemical alterations in the brain
- Deterioration or damage to neurological centers regulating speech and language
- Decreased cerebral circulation
- Severe memory impairment
- Escalating anxiety

Desired Outcome The patient will demonstrate optimal communication.

Assessment/Interventions and *Rationales*

In addition to the interventions in the first half of this chapter, communication techniques specific to neurocognitive disorders follow.

1. Use a variety of nonverbal techniques to enhance communication:
   a. Point, touch, or demonstrate an action while talking about it.
   b. Ask patients to point to body parts or objects they want to communicate about.
   c. If the patient struggles to find a word, guess their intent and ask for confirmation (e.g., "You are pointing to your mouth, saying pain. Is it your dentures? No. Is your mouth sore? Yes. Okay, let me take a look to see if I can tell what is hurting you."). Always ask the patient to confirm whether your guess is correct.
   d. The use of cue cards, flashcards, alphabet letters, signs, and pictures on doors to various rooms is often helpful for many patients and their families (e.g., bathroom, "Charles's bedroom"). The use of pictures is helpful when the ability to read decreases.
   Both delirium and dementia can cause huge communication problems, and often alternative nonverbal or verbal methods are helpful.

2. Encourage reminiscing about positive life experiences. *Discussing past accomplishments and joyful memories reinforces language use and provides a sense of meaning.*
3. Manage conflicts calmly. If a patient argues with another patient, separate them to prevent escalation. After a brief period (about 5 minutes), explain to each patient, in a respectful and straightforward manner, why intervention was necessary. *Separation prevents escalation to physical acting out and shows respect for the patient's right to know. Explaining in an adult manner helps maintain self-esteem.*
4. Reinforce speech through pictures, nonverbal gestures, and marking days on calendars, to anchor the patient in reality. *Asaphasia progresses, alternative communication methods should be introduced to support continued interaction.*

Caregiver Stress

Related to

- Complexity of activities and severity of the illness
- 24-hour care responsibility
- Lengthy (e.g., years) periods of caregiving
- Lack of support
- Caregiver isolation
- Inadequate use of community support
- Inadequate physical environment (transportation, housing) for providing care

Desired Outcomes Caregivers will demonstrate and verbalize reduced stress.

Assessment/Interventions and *Rationales*

1. Assess what caregivers know about the patient's disorder and provide education. *Empowering caregivers with knowledge of the disorder promotes patience, reduces the tendency to view the patient's actions as bad behavior, and helps them anticipate further deterioration and plan accordingly.*
2. Provide information on community agencies and support groups where the family and primary caregiver can receive support, education, and information regarding respite care. *This support helps diminish a sense of hopelessness, increase a sense of empowerment, and provide a much-needed break from 24-hour care.*

3. Assist the caregiver and family in identifying areas that need intervention. *Healthcare providers are knowledgeable and have experience in the care of individuals with dementia. This makes them able to anticipate specific areas that need assistance and those that may need assistance in the future.*

4. Teach the caregiver and family specific interventions to use in response to behavioral or social problems that result in dementia. *Caregivers are supported by learning new ways to intervene in situations that are common in patients with dementia, such as agitation, sleep–wake disturbances, and wandering.*

5. Safety is a major concern. Box 13.3 identifies some steps the caregiver and family can take to make the home a safer place. *These steps can help make the home safe for individuals with dementia.*

6. Encourage the family to engage in activities with the patient based on the current level of functioning (e.g., watching a favorite movie, reading a simple book with pictures together, performing simple tasks like setting the table, washing dishes, or washing the car). *This promotes participation in family life, reducing feelings of isolation and alienation.*

7. Encourage the caregiver or family to follow family traditions such as church activities, holidays, and vacations as much as is feasible. *Continuing customary activities helps the family transition to and make peace with the eventual loss of a loved one. These experiences also increase the patient's sense of belonging.*

8. Encourage the caregiver or family to use respite care at regular intervals such as every 2 weeks and during vacations. *Regular periods of respite can help prevent burnout, allow caregivers to continue participating in their own lives, and help minimize feelings of resentment.*

9. Identify financial burdens and refer families to available resources. *Any long-term illness can place significant financial strain on families,* so connecting them with community or national assistance programs is essential.

10. Suggest legal and financial planning for future care needs. *Advanced planning for eventual deterioration and death will make these transitions less difficult.*

TREATMENT MODALITIES

Biological Treatment

Pharmacotherapy

Medications with FDA approval for the treatment of AD fall into three categories. These categories include those that inhibit the progression of the disease, treat symptoms related to memory and thinking, and treat non-cognitive symptoms such as insomnia and agitation.

Medications that inhibit disease progression are relatively new and target amyloid plaques, a hallmark of AD pathology. These include lecanemab (Leqembi) and donanemab (Kisunla), which work by reducing amyloid buildup in the brain to slow cognitive decline. While promising, these treatments are most effective in the early stages of AD and require careful patient selection due to potential risks, including brain swelling and bleeding.

T\Medications that target memory and cognitive symptoms are widely used and have shown statistically significant effects compared to placebos. However, their clinical impact on cognition and functioning is modest, and benefits typically diminish after 1–2 years. Given the potential for side effects, patients and families should carefully weigh the risks and benefits before starting treatment.

These medications fall into three categories:

- Cholinesterase inhibitors—used for mild, moderate, and severe AD symptoms. This category includes donepezil (Aricept), rivastigmine (Exelon), and galantamine (Razadyne).
- Glutamate regulators—used for moderate to severe AD symptoms. The primary approved medication in this category is memantine (Namenda).
- Combination therapy (glutamate regulator/cholinesterase inhibitor)—memantine/donepezil (Namzaric) is prescribed for moderate to severe symptoms after a trial of donepezil alone.

For noncognitive symptoms the FDA approved Rexulti (brexpiprazole) as the first atypical antipsychotic specifically indicated for the treatment of agitation in dementia. This approval provides a targeted option for managing agitation, a common and distressing symptom of Alzheimer's disease. However, careful monitoring is required due to potential side effects, including an increased risk of stroke in older patients with dementia.

See Chapter 28 for more information about neurocognitive medications.

Integrative Therapies

Nutrition may play a role in both the prevention and treatment of dementia. Omega-3 fatty acids have been promoted for their potential neuroprotective effects, with some studies suggesting an association between omega-3 fatty acids and a lower incidence of dementia. However, their effectiveness in treating dementia remains controversial, as clinical evidence is inconclusive. See Appendix B for more information on integrative therapies.

Community Resources

The Alzheimer's Association is a national organization that provides support for individuals with Alzheimer's disease and their families. Its Community Resource Finder helps locate local services and assistance.

Some families provide care of their loved one until death. Other families may find it too difficult to manage labile and aggressive behavior, incontinence, wandering, unsafe habits, or disruptive nighttime activity. During this time, families need information, support, and legal and financial guidance. Discussions should include advance directives, durable power of attorney, guardianship, and conservatorship to help them plan for future care needs.

👪 NURSE, PATIENT, AND FAMILY RESOURCES

Alz Connected
ALZ Connected is a free online community designed for people living with dementia and those who care for them. Members can post questions about dementia-related issues, offer support, and create public and private groups around specific topics.
www.alzconnected.org

Alzheimer's Association
The Alzheimer's Association leads the way to end Alzheimer's and all other dementia by accelerating global research, driving risk reduction and early detection, and maximizing quality care and support.
www.alz.org

Alzheimer Society of Canada

The Alzheimer's Society offers programs and support services, develops and pushes forward dementia-focused and dementia-friendly initiatives and campaigns across the country that alleviate the personal and social consequences of dementia, and supports research to improve quality of life.
www.alzheimer.ca

Association for Frontotemporal Degeneration (AFTD)

The AFTD helps to improve the quality of life of people affected by FTD and drive research to a cure.
www.theaftd.org

Lewy Body Dementia Association (LBDA)

The LBDA is dedicated to raising awareness of LBD, supporting people with LBD and their families and caregivers, and promoting scientific advances.
www.lbda.org

National Institute on Aging

The NIA is the primary federal agency supporting and conducting Alzheimer's disease and related dementias research.
www.nia.nih.gov

National Parkinson's Foundation

The Parkinson's Foundation makes life better for people with Parkinson's disease by improving care and advancing research toward a cure.
www.parkinson.org

CHAPTER 14

Personality Disorders

Personality disorders are among the most complex and challenging conditions to treat. Individuals who meet the criteria for these disorders often struggle with self-identity or self-direction, and intimacy in relationships.

Personality is an individual's characteristic and relatively stable pattern of thoughts, feelings, and behaviors that shape their experiences and relationships. A personality is considered unhealthy when it consistently leads to maladaptive or dysfunctional interpersonal patterns. While personality traits can be protective during difficult times, they may also contribute to ongoing relationship conflicts and emotional distress.

People with these disorders often struggle to recognize or acknowledge their personality problems. Some individuals believe the problems originate outside of themselves, while others may be unaware that their behavior is unusual and experience little to no distress. It is uncommon for individuals to seek treatment specifically for a personality disorder, though they may seek treatment for comorbid conditions such as major depressive disorder or generalized anxiety disorder.

TYPES OF PERSONALITY DISORDERS

According to the American Psychiatric Association (APA, 2022), there are 10 personality disorders. They are grouped into clusters of similar behavior patterns and personality traits, as follows:

Cluster A: Behaviors described as odd or eccentric
  Paranoid personality disorder
  Schizoid personality disorder
  Schizotypal personality disorder
Cluster B: Behaviors described as dramatic, emotional, or erratic
  Borderline personality disorder
  Narcissistic personality disorder
  Histrionic personality disorder
  Antisocial personality disorder

Cluster C: Behaviors described as anxious or fearful
  Avoidant
  Dependent
  Obsessive–compulsive

This chapter begins by discussing eight personality disorders, covering their prevalence, characteristics, nursing care guidelines, and treatment modalities. It then provides a more in-depth examination of two of the most common and challenging disorders—antisocial and borderline personality disorders. For each, the application of the nursing process is outlined to guide clinical care.

A short and useful personality disorder questionnaire is provided in Fig. 14.1.

The Personality Inventory for DSM-5—Brief Form (PID-5-BF)—Adult

Name: _____   Age: _____   Sex:☐ Male ☐ Female   Date:_____

Instructions: This is a list of things different people might say about themselves. We are interested in how you would describe yourself. There are no right or wrong answers. So you can describe yourself as honestly as possible, we will keep your responses confidential. We'd like you to take your time and read each statement carefully, selecting the response that best describes you.

		Very False or Often False	Sometimes or Somewhat False	Sometimes or Somewhat True	Very True or Often True	Clinician Use — Item score
1	People would describe me as reckless.	0	1	2	3	
2	I feel like I act totally on impulse.	0	1	2	3	
3	Even though I know better, I can't stop making rash decisions.	0	1	2	3	
4	I often feel like nothing I do really matters.	0	1	2	3	
5	Others see me as irresponsible.	0	1	2	3	
6	I'm not good at planning ahead.	0	1	2	3	
7	My thoughts often don't make sense to others.	0	1	2	3	
8	I worry about almost everything.	0	1	2	3	
9	I get emotional easily, often for very little reason.	0	1	2	3	
10	I fear being alone in life more than anything else.	0	1	2	3	
11	I get stuck on one way of doing things, even when it's clear it won't work.	0	1	2	3	
12	I have seen things that weren't really there.	0	1	2	3	
13	I steer clear of romantic relationships.	0	1	2	3	
14	I'm not interested in making friends.	0	1	2	3	
15	I get irritated easily by all sortsof things.	0	1	2	3	
16	I don't like to get too close to people.	0	1	2	3	
17	It's no big deal if I hurt other peoples'feelings.	0	1	2	3	
18	I rarely get enthusiastic about anything.	0	1	2	3	
19	I crave attention.	0	1	2	3	
20	I often have to deal withpeople who are less important than me.	0	1	2	3	
21	I often have thoughts that make sense to me but that other people say are strange.	0	1	2	3	
22	I use people to get what I want.	0	1	2	3	
23	I often "zone out"and then suddenly come to and realize that a lot of time has passed.	0	1	2	3	
24	Things around me often feel unreal, or more real than usual.	0	1	2	3	
25	It is easy for me to take advantage of others.	0	1	2	3	
					Total/Partial Raw Score:	
				Prorated Total Score: (if 1-6items left unanswered)		
					Average Total Score:	

Krueger RF, Derringer J, Markon KE, Watson D, Skodol AE.
Copyright ©2013American Psychiatric Association. All Rights Reserved.
This material can be reproduced without permission byresearchers and byclinicians for use with their patients.

Fig. 14.1 The Personality Inventory for DSM-5—Brief Form (PID-5-BF)—Adult. (Reprinted with permission from The Personality Inventory for DSM-5, (Copyright ©2013). American Psychiatric Association. All Rights Reserved.)

CLUSTER A PERSONALITY DISORDERS

Paranoid Personality Disorder

Paranoid personality disorder is characterized by pervasive distrust and suspicion of others, driven by unfounded beliefs that others want to exploit, harm, or deceive them. Individuals with this disorder often struggle in relationships due to jealousy, controlling behaviors, and persistent grudge-holding.

The prevalence of paranoid personality disorder is estimated at 2% to 4% (APA, 2022), with slightly higher rates in men. It is more common among relatives of individuals with schizophrenia. Symptoms may emerge in childhood or adolescence.

Nursing Guidelines

- Strictly adhere to all prearranged promises, appointments, and schedules to build trust.
- Avoid being overly friendly, as it may trigger suspicion.
- Provide clear, straight forward explanations of tests and procedures in advance.
- Use simple language and maintain a neutral, yet kind approach.
- Set clear boundaries and enforce limits for any threatening behaviors.

Treatment

Individuals with paranoid personality disorder often resist treatment. If they somehow end up in treatment, they may be suspicious about why this is happening. Their paranoia makes communication challenging, making a professional and trusting therapeutic relationship essential. Although it may be threatening, group therapy is often useful in improving social skills. Role-playing and group feedback can help reduce suspiciousness.

Short-term use of antianxiety agents may help reduce anxiety and agitation. In cases of severe agitation or delusional thinking, low-dose antipsychotic medications may be used temporarily to provide symptom relief.

Schizoid Personality Disorder

Schizoid personality disorder is characterized by a lifelong pattern of social withdrawal and a limited range of emotional expression. Individuals with this disorder are often perceived as odd or eccentric. They neither seek out or enjoy close relationships, and external approval or rejection has little impact on them.

Individuals with schizoid personality disorder may be able to function well in a solitary occupation such as being a security guard on the night shift. They often express feelings of being an observer rather than a participant in life. They may describe feelings of depersonalization or detachment from both themselves and the world.

The prevalence rate for schizoid personality disorder may be as high as 5% (APA, 2022), with males more commonly affected. Symptoms typically emerge before adulthood.

The disorder is more prevalent in families with a history of schizophrenia or schizotypal personality disorder. Abnormalities in the dopaminergic systems may contribute to its development.

Nursing Guidelines

- Maintain a neutral approach and avoid being overly friendly.
- Refrain from pressuring the patient to engage in socialization.
- Patients may be willing to discuss topics such as coping strategies and anxiety.
- Conduct a thorough assessment to uncover symptoms or concerns the patient may be reluctant to share.
- Monitor for potential rejection by group members due to the patient's unusual interests, ideas, and interactions.

Treatment

Individuals with schizoid personality disorder tend to be introspective, making them suitable—though distant—candidates for psychotherapy. As trust develops, they may reveal a rich fantasy life and fears, particularly related to dependence. Group therapy may also be beneficial, even if the patient may be largely silent. Over time, group members may become important to them, serving as their primary source of socialization. Antidepressants may enhance enjoyment in life, while second-generation anti-psychotics can improve emotional expressiveness.

Schizotypal Personality Disorder

Schizotypal (ski·zuh·**tai**·pl) personality disorder is clas-sified as both a personality disorder and the first of the schizophrenia spectrum disorders (APA, 2022). It is char-acteristics by magical thinking, odd beliefs, strange speech patterns, and inappropriate affect (APA, 2022).

These individuals experience severe social and interper-sonal deficits. Their speech often includes lengthy, unclear, and overly detailed and abstract content. As a result of suspiciousness, they tend to misinterpret the motives of others as being out to get them. Odd beliefs (e.g., being overly superstitious) or magical thinking (e.g., "He tripped because I wanted him to") are also common.

Psychotic symptoms such as hallucinations and delu-sions may be present in schizotypal personality disorder, but to a lesser degree with schizophrenia, and only briefly. As opposed to schizophrenia, people with this disorder can often be more easily made aware of their suspiciousness, magical thinking, and odd beliefs.

The prevalence of schizotypal personality disorder ranges from 0.6% to 4.6% (APA, 2022) and is more common in men. Symptoms typically emerge in youth.

Having a first-degree relative with schizophrenia increases the risk. Structural, physiological, and neuro-chemical abnormalities in the brain are similar to those found in schizophrenia.

Nursing Guidelines

- Respect the patient's need for privacy.
- Monitor for increasing suspiciousness.
- Assess for other medical or psychological symptoms that may need intervention (e.g., chest pain, suicidal thoughts).
- Be mindful of and adjust personal responses to the patient's unusual beliefs and activities.

Treatment

Because it is difficult to develop a therapeutic relationship or alliance, the goal should be to provide supportive care.

Helping the patient to identify cognitive distortions may be useful. It is important to be aware that individuals with schizotypal personality disorder may engage in unconventional groups, such as unusual religious sects or occult societies, which can further complicate the clinical picture.

People with schizotypal personality disorder may benefit from low-dose antipsychotic agents such as risperidone (Risperdal) or olanzapine (Zyprexa) to improve functioning, reduce psychotic-like symptoms, and improve day-to-day functioning (Skodol, Bender, & Oldham, 2019). These medications help with such symptoms as ideas of reference or illusions. Antidepressants are used to treat comorbid major depressive disorder and anxiety disorders.

CLUSTER B PERSONALITY DISORDERS

Histrionic Personality Disorder

People with histrionic personality disorder are often high-functioning. They are typically dramatic, extroverted, flamboyant, and colorful. Despite this bold exterior, they tend to have a limited ability to develop meaningful relationships.

Histrionic personality disorder occurs at a rate of nearly 2% (APA, 2022) and is diagnosed more frequently in women than in men. Symptoms typically emerge by early adulthood.

Histrionic personality disorder may stem from childhood experiences, such as a lack of criticism or punishment, receiving parental approval only for specific behaviors, inconsistent attention, and uncertainty about which actions will earn approval. The tendency for histrionic personality disorder to run in families suggests that a genetic cause might exist, although this tendency may also support learned behavior.

Nursing Guidelines

- Encourage and model the use of concrete, descriptive language rather than vague and overly dramatic expression.
- Assist patients in identifying and clarifying their inner feelings, as they often have difficulty identifying them.
- Teach and role model assertiveness to help them express their needs more effectively.

Treatment

Individuals with histrionic personality disorder struggle with regulating and expressing their emotions. Psychotherapy may promote clarification of these feelings and appropriate expression. Both individual and group therapy are useful in this population.

There are no specific pharmacological treatments for people with histrionic personality disorder. Antidepressants can be used for depressive, anxiety, or somatic symptoms. Antipsychotics may be used if the patient exhibits derealization or illusions.

Narcissistic Personality Disorder

Narcissistic personality disorder is characterized by a sense of entitlement, an inflated sense of self-importance, and a lack of empathy. However, beneath this exterior, individuals with this disorder suffer from weak self-esteem and heightened sensitivity to criticism. Compared to other personality disorders, narcissistic personality disorder typically causes less impairment in daily functioning and overall quality of life.

The prevalence of narcissistic personality disorder can be up to 6% of the general population (APA, 2022) and is more common in males. Determining the age of onset is challenging, as narcissistic traits that are commonly found in adolescence.

Genetics is a known risk factor for the development of this personality disorder (Luo & Cai, 2018). This risk may be increased by parents with narcissism who may attribute an unrealistic sense of talent, importance, and beauty to their children, thus putting the children at higher risk.

Nursing Guidelines

- Maintain a neutral and professional tone.
- Avoid power struggles or defensiveness in response to the patient's provocative or controversial remarks.
- Refrain from directly challenging grandiose statements.
- Role model empathy to encourage more meaningful interactions.

Treatment

If a person with narcissistic personality disorder seeks treatment, individual cognitive behavioral therapy (CBT) helps to challenge distorted thinking and encourage more realistic self-perception. Group therapy may also be beneficial by fostering shared experiences, promoting self-awareness, and developing empathy.

There are no FDA-approved medications specifically for narcissistic personality disorder. However, medications such as antidepressants, mood stabilizers, and antipsychotics may be prescribed to alleviate symptoms associated with cooccurring conditions, including anxiety, depression, and other mood disorders.

CLUSTER C PERSONALITY DISORDERS

Avoidant Personality Disorder

People with avoidant personality disorder avoid interpersonal contact due to extreme fears of rejection, criticism, or failure. These individuals are overly sensitive to rejection, feel inadequate, and are socially inhibited. While similar to social anxiety disorder in terms of social avoidance, avoidant personality disorder is primarily driven by low self-esteem rather than anxiety.

Avoidant personality disorder occurs in 2.4% of the population (APA, 2022) and occurs equally in men and women. Early signs include shyness and avoidance in childhood, which tend to intensify during adolescence and early adulthood.

Avoidant personality disorder is influenced by genetics, with studies estimating a 64% heritability rate, as well as temperament traits in infancy, such as hypersensitivity, rigidity, and excessive fear. Additionally, a fearful attachment style and early childhood experiences of rejection or differential treatment may increase the risk of developing AVPD.

Nursing Guidelines

- Approach the patient with warmth, acceptance, and reassurance.
- Recognize that social situations may trigger severe anxiety.

- Validate the patient's fears while maintaining a supportive attitude.
- Provide exercises to enhance new social skills with caution, since failure can increase feelings of poor self-worth.
- Use role playing to help the person develop assertive communication to express needs more effectively.

Treatment

Individuals with avoidant personality disorder are often good candidates for treatment because their distress motivates them to seek help. Individual and group therapy are useful in processing anxiety-provoking symptoms and in planning methods to approach and handle anxiety-provoking situations. Psychotherapy focuses on trust and assertiveness training.

There are no specific medications for avoidant personality disorder (AVPD), but treating cooccurring depression or anxiety can support overall recovery, especially when used alongside psychotherapy. Beta-adrenergic receptor antagonists (e.g., atenolol) can reduce autonomic nervous system hyperactivity. Antidepressants, including selective serotonin reuptake inhibitors (SSRIs) like citalopram (Celexa) and serotonin-norepinephrine reuptake inhibitors (SNRIs) such as venlafaxine (Effexor), may also help alleviate social anxiety.

Dependent Personality Disorder

Dependent personality disorder is characterized by a pattern of submissive and clinging behavior driven by an overwhelming need for care and support. This leads to intense fears of separation and difficulty making decisions without reassurance from others. Individuals with this disorder may experience intense anxiety when left alone, even for short periods, and often go to great lengths to avoid being independent.

A rare condition, the prevalence of dependent personality disorder is estimated at 0.5% (APA, 2022). This disorder is slightly more common among women (0.6%) than men (0.4%).

Dependent personality disorder may develop due to a combination of factors, including a history of abuse, childhood trauma such as neglect or serious illness, and genetic predisposition. Additionally, cultural, religious, or family influences that emphasize reliance on authority may contribute to its development.

Nursing Guidelines

- Encourage the patient to identify and address current stressors while fostering problem-solving skills.
- Monitor for signs of excessive reliance on the nurse.
- Use the therapeutic relationship as a testing ground for increased assertiveness through role-modeling and teaching of assertive skills.
- Support the patient in making independent decisions to reduce reliance on others for validation and guidance.
- Reinforce small steps toward autonomy, providing positive feedback to build confidence in their ability to function independently.

Treatment

Psychotherapy is the preferred treatment modality for dependent personality disorder, with CBT being particularly effective. CBT helps individuals develop healthier perspectives on relationships, build confidence in their ability to function independently, and learn new coping strategies to reduce reliance on others.

For the best results, medication should be used alongside psychotherapy. While no medications are specifically approved for dependent personality disorder, those with the condition may benefit from medications to manage cooccurring depression or anxiety. Addressing these symptoms can help reduce distress and improve overall treatment outcomes.

Obsessive–Compulsive Personality Disorder

Obsessive–compulsive personality disorder is marked by limited emotional expression, stubbornness, perseverance, and indecisiveness. The defining features include a preoccupation with orderliness, perfectionism, and control. Rigidity and inflexible standards of self and others persist even if they are self-defeating or relationship-defeating. Preoccupation with the activity often results in losing the major point of the activity. Projects are often incomplete because of overly strict standards.

Obsessive–compulsive *personality* disorder is distinct from obsessive-compulsive disorder. Obsessive–compulsive personality disorder is characterized by an excessive focus on perfectionism and control, whereas obsessive–compulsive disorder involves intrusive, anxiety-provoking thoughts that lead to compulsive behaviors aimed at relieving distress.

Obsessive–compulsive personality disorder is among the most prevalent personality disorders, with a prevalence ranging from about 2% to 8% (APA, 2022). It is more common in men than women. Risk factors include a background of harsh discipline and having a first-degree relative with the disorder.

Nursing Guidelines

- Avoid power struggles with patients who have a strong need for control.
- Provide structure to help manage difficulties with unexpected changes.
- Allow extra time for patients to complete tasks.
- Assist patients in recognizing ineffective coping and exploring alternatives.

Treatment

Individuals with obsessive–compulsive personality disorder typically seek treatment due to discomfort with their symptoms. Treatment is often lengthy and complex, but group and behavioral therapy can help the person learn new coping skills, manage anxiety, and provide valuable feedback.

While no medications specifically treat obsessive–compulsive personality disorder, individuals with cooccurring depression or anxiety may benefit from medication. Managing these conditions can help reduce distress and support overall treatment effectiveness.

ANTISOCIAL PERSONALITY DISORDER

In this section, we focus on a cluster B personality disorder: antisocial personality disorder. This disorder is characterized by a pattern of disregard for the rights of others, often leading to frequent violations. Key pathological traits include antagonistic behaviors, such as deceitfulness, manipulation for personal gain, or being hostile if needs are blocked. People with this disorder also exhibit disinhibited behaviors, including risk-taking, irresponsibility, and impulsivity. Criminal misconduct and substance use are common.

One of the most disturbing qualities associated with antisocial personality disorder is a lack of empathy, also known as callousness and unemotional traits. This results in a lack of concern about the feelings of others; the absence of remorse or guilt except in the face of punishment; and a disregard for meeting school, family, and other obligations. They may appear concerned and caring if these attributes help them manipulate and exploit others. Wittiness, charm, and flattery may accompany manipulation and exploitation.

Epidemiology

The prevalence of antisocial personality disorder is between 0.2% and 3.3% (APA, 2022), with a prevalence of three times higher among men. The highest prevalence is among males with substance use disorders and in incarcerated individuals.

Risk Factors

Antisocial personality disorder is genetically linked, and twin studies indicate a predisposition to this disorder. An alteration in serotonin transmission, childhood mistreatment, and cultural bias have also been implicated.

ASSESSMENT

Signs and Symptoms

- History of violence
- Violation of others
- Anger and aggression
- Impulsivity
- Substance use
- Illegal and reckless behaviors
- Unstable relationships
- Lacks empathy, callous, and unemotional

Assessment Guidelines

A. Evaluate current life stressors
B. Review criminal history

C. Assess for suicidal, violent, and/or homicidal thoughts
D. Monitor levels of anxiety, aggression, and anger
E. Determine motivation for maintaining control
F. Assess past and present substance use

Nursing Diagnoses

The International Classification for Nursing Practice (International Council for Nurses [ICN], 2019) provides valuable nursing diagnoses for individuals with antisocial personality disorder. Given the disorder's core traits of callous disregard for others and antagonistic behaviors, *risk for violence* is a top priority. Additionally, individuals with antisocial personality disorder demonstrate irresponsibility and fail to maintain work and financial obligations. Therefore, *impaired coping* is a useful nursing diagnosis to address those behaviors.

Intervention Guidelines

A. Recognize attempts to manipulate (e.g., flattery, seductiveness, and instilling guilt).
B. Set clear, realistic limits for specific behaviors.
C. Inform all staff of the treatment plan and discuss the importance of adherence.
D. Help patients to identify feelings of anger, understand their source, and explore healthy coping strategies.
E. Document behaviors objectively, including specific times, dates, and circumstances.
F. Establish and communicate clear boundaries and consequences.

Nursing Care for Antisocial Personality Disorder

Risk for Violence

Related to

- Biochemical alterations in the brain
- Impulsivity
- Inability to control temper
- Emotional dysregulation (e.g., anger, hostility)
- Lack of empathy (callousness)
- Antagonistic behaviors (e.g., deceitfulness, manipulation)

Desired Outcome The patient will refrain from violence.

Assessment/Interventions and *Rationales*

1. Use one-to-one or appropriate level of observation to identify emotional and situational triggers. *Monitoring patients who may exhibit hostility provides external support and reduces the risk of aggression and violence.*

2. Intervene early to calm the patient and defuse potential incidents. *Early intervention facilitates learning before loss of control and offers an opportunity to discuss and role-model new coping strategies.*

3. Set clear, consistent limits in a calm, nonjudgmental manner. *Provides structure, safety, and predictability, which help reduce anxiety and prevent manipulative or aggressive behaviors.*

4. Avoid power struggles and repeated negotiations about rules and limits. *When limits are realistic and enforceable, manipulation is minimized.*

5. Redirect agitation with physical outlets in areas of low stimulation (e.g., punching bag, exercise bike). *Using physical activities to manage anger helps the patient learn to cope constructively and enhances self-control.*

6. Encourage the patient to recognize the impact of their actions on others and explore alternative, prosocial behaviors. *Helps the patient to recognize the consequences of their actions and develop prosocial behaviors, promoting accountability and reducing harmful interactions.*

7. Alert staff if the potential for restraint or seclusion becomes imminent. The priority interventions are (1) setting limits, (2) encouraging time out, (3) offering as-needed medication, and (4) restraint or seclusion. *A team approach to aggression is essential. Always use the least restrictive intervention when managing potentially violent behavior.*

8. Document the patient behaviors, interventions, what seemed to escalate agitation, what helped to calm agitation, if and when as-needed medications were given and their effect, and what proved most helpful. *Documentation provides staff with guidelines for future interventions and legal evidence if necessary.*

Promote problem-solving skills by teaching and reinforcing constructive ways to handle frustration and conflict. *These skills target impulsivity and aggression, equipping the patient with practical strategies to reduce violent behaviors and improve interpersonal interactions.*

Impaired Coping

Related to
- Biochemical alterations in the brain
- Genetic predisposition
- Chaotic childhood environment
- Inadequate coping strategies
- Impulsivity and poor planning
- Irritability and aggressiveness
- Reckless disregard for safety
- Chronic irresponsibility
- Lack of remorse

Desired Outcome Patient will demonstrate improved coping.

Assessment/Interventions and *Rationales*
1. Clearly outline expectations for behavior including unit rules, daily routines, and interactions with others. *Given the patient's history of ineffective and inappropriate coping, a structured understanding of expectations is essential.*
2. Establish consequences with the treatment team for breaking the behavior code and communicate these with the patient. *Undesirable consequences may help to decrease repetition of undesirable behaviors.*
3. Discuss the patient's goals for the hospitalization or treatment period. *Although most people with this disorder do not seek treatment for it, they may seek help for other problems such as major depressive disorder, anxiety, or anger management. Engaging the patient in care by identifying goals is a strong first step.*
4. Encourage the patient to identify usual coping methods such as deceit or aggression. *Identifying coping methods helps to clarify nonproductive responses to stress.*
5. Explore alternate potential coping methods and link these coping methods to their goals. *Understanding that there are choices in the way the patient responds increases motivation for change.*
6. Provide positive reinforcement for the use of new, healthier coping methods. *Positive feedback reinforces learning and* long-term behavior change.
   Teach techniques for emotional regulation such as mindfulness, deep breathing, or grounding exercises to help manage impulsivity and distress. *These techniques help*

to reduce emotional reactivity and promote more constructive responses to stress.

Encourage participation in group therapy. *Group settings can provide peer feedback and reinforcement of healthier coping mechanisms.*

TREATMENT MODALITIES FOR ANTISOCIAL PERSONALITY DISORDER

Biological Therapies

Pharmacotherapy

There are no FDA-approved medications specifically for antisocial personality disorder. However, as with other personality disorders, medications can be used to manage mental health symptoms and co-occurring disorders.

Mood-stabilizers may help reduce aggression, impulsivity, and mood instability. SSRIs can be used to decrease irritability and manage symptoms of anxiety and depression.

Psychological Therapies

Psychological therapies aim to address maladaptive thought patterns, emotional dysregulation, and problematic behaviors associated with antisocial personality disorder. These approaches focus on increasing self-awareness, improving impulse control, and promoting healthier interpersonal interactions.

Behavioral therapy is a basic approach that uses a system of rewards and punishment to promote positive behavior. This approach helps individuals with antisocial personality disorder develop greater impulse control and accountability by linking actions to immediate, tangible outcomes.

CBT helps individuals identify and challenge distorted thinking patterns that contribute to manipulative, deceitful, or aggressive behaviors. It encourages the development of alternative, prosocial coping mechanisms.

Mentalization-based therapy (MBT) aims to improve the ability to reflect on one's thoughts and emotions, as well as those of others. This therapy helps individuals develop empathy and a greater understanding of interpersonal consequences.

Dialectical behavior therapy (DBT) focuses on emotional regulation, distress tolerance, and interpersonal effectiveness to improve impulse control and reduce aggressive behaviors.

Group therapy provides opportunities for individuals to learn from others, practice social skills, and receive peer feedback. Group work also encourages accountability and the development of healthier interpersonal relationships.

BORDERLINE PERSONALITY DISORDER

As previously identified, borderline personality disorder is another cluster B diagnosis. Individuals with borderline personality disorder exhibit marked instability in emotional regulation (dysregulation), impulsivity, self-identity, mood, and interpersonal relationships. Emotional lability—moving from one emotional extreme to another—often occurs in response to a deep fear of separation and heightened sensitivity to rejection.

Another disruptive trait of borderline personality disorder is impulsivity, which leads individuals to act quickly based on emotions without considering the consequences. This impulsivity often damages relationships and can result in suicide attempts or self-destructive behaviors such as cutting, promiscuous sexual behavior, or substance use. Chronic suicidal ideation is common and increases the likelihood of accidental deaths. Additionally, cooccurring mood, anxiety, or substance use disorders complicate both treatment and prognosis. Antagonism is manifested in hostility, anger, and irritability, often leading to violence in relationships and against property.

Splitting, a primitive defense mechanism, is the inability to view both positive and negative aspects of others as part of a whole. As a result, individuals with borderline personality disorder tend to view people as either entirely good or entirely bad, with no middle ground. For example, they may initially idealize a person, such as a nurse, seeing them as exceptional. However, at the first disappointment or frustration, their perception rapidly shifts to devaluation, and the previously admired individual is now despised.

Epidemiology

Borderline personality disorder affects approximately 1.6% of the general population, and up to 20% of the inpatient psychiatric population (Skodol et al., 2019). It is more commonly diagnosed in women, though research suggests that men are underdiagnosed or misdiagnosed, leading to an apparent gender discrepancy. Symptoms often decrease with age, with some individuals experiencing improved emotional stability over time.

Risk Factors

Borderline personality disorder appears to have a genetic component, occurring about five times more often in first-degree biological relatives with the disorder compared with the general population (APA, 2022). Serotonergic dysfunction may contribute to impulsivity, a key trait of this disorder. Additionally, psychological theories, such as those proposed by Mahler and colleagues (1975), suggest that disruptions in the normal separation–individuation-process between a child and their mother may contribute to the development of the disorder.

Assessment

Signs and Symptoms

- Persistent feelings of emptiness
- Engagement in risky behaviors such as reckless driving, unsafe sex, substance use, binge eating, gambling, and overspending
- Intensefear of abandonment, leading to paranoia or dissociation
- Idealization of others with rapid attachment, often followed by devaluation
- A tendency toward anger, sarcasm, and bitterness
- Nonsuicidal self-injury
- Suicidal ideation, behaviors, gestures, or threats
- Sudden shifts in self-identity, causing changes in goals, values, and career focus
- Extreme mood swings occurring within hours or days
- Intense, unstable romantic relationships

Nursing Diagnoses

Individuals with borderline personality disorder are often admitted to psychiatric treatment programs due to comorbid disorders or dangerous behaviors. Common emotional and behavioral challenges include anxiety, rage, depression, withdrawal, paranoia, and manipulation, all require targeted nursing interventions.

The International Classification for Nursing Practice (ICN, 2019) provides the nursing diagnosis *risk for self-mutilation*. This diagnosis is most often associated with borderline personality disorder. Self-mutilation involves deliberate nonsuicidal self-injurious behavior that causes tissue damage. This behavior is used to attain relief from tension and perhaps to enlist the aid and support of others. Other nursing diagnoses directly relevant to borderline personality disorder are *chronic low self-esteem*, *impaired socialization*, and *impaired coping*.

Intervention Guidelines

A. Set realistic goals, using clear action language.
B. Assess for manipulative behaviors (e.g., flattery, seductiveness, guilt instilling).
C. Establish and enforce clear, consistent boundaries and limits.
D. Use clear and straightforward communication.
E. Calmly reinforce therapeutic goals and treatment boundaries when behavioral issues arise.
F. Avoid extremes of rejection or rescue.
G. Regularly assess for suicidal ideation and non-suicidal self-injury, especially during times of stress.

Nursing Care for Borderline Personality Disorder

Risk for Self-Mutilation

Related to
- Biochemical alterations in the brain
- Borderline personality disorder
- History of self-mutilation
- Impulsivity
- Poor self-esteem
- Unstable self-image
- Persistent feelings of emptiness
- Impaired problem-solving abilities
- Social or cultural influences that normalize self-mutilation
- Maladaptive efforts to avoid abandonment
- Intense anger

Desired Outcome Patient will refrain from self-injurious behaviors.

Assessment/Interventions and *Rationales*

1. Assess the patient's history of self-mutilation including:
   a. Types of mutilation
   b. Frequency of self-mutilation
   c. Stressors preceding self-mutilation
   Identifying patterns and circumstances surrounding self-injury helps the nurse plan patient-centered interventions and teach strategies.
2. Identify the patient's emotions around the time of self-mutilation. *Recognizing specific emotional triggers (e.g., rage from feeling abandoned or excluded) helps guide future interventions by addressing the underlying distress and developing healthier coping strategies.*
3. Explore the meaning behind the patient's feelings associated with self-mutilation. *Self-mutilation might be a way to relieve anxiety, feel alive through pain, express guilt, or self-hate, or manipulation.*
4. Help the patient develop a crisis plan by identifying specific steps to take, such as reaching out to a trusted person when feeling the urge to self-mutilate. *Engaging with others during moments of distress can provide emotional support, reduce isolation, and help diminish the frequency and severity of self-injury over time.*
5. Use a matter-of-fact approach when self-mutilation occurs, avoiding criticizing or excessive sympathy. A neutral response helps prevent feelings of shame or increased anxiety while also avoiding reinforcement of the behavior through special attention or emotional reactions.
6. After treatment of the wound, discuss the events, thoughts, and emotions leading up to the self-mutilation episode. Identifying warning signs and triggers helps the patient recognize patterns, develop self-awareness, and learn when to implement coping strategies or seek support before engaging in self-harm.
7. Develop alternatives to self-mutilating behaviors.
   a. Anticipate certain situations that might lead to increased stress (e.g., anger or frustration).
   b. Identify actions that might modify the intensity of such situations.
   c. Identify two or three people whom the patient can contact to discuss and examine intense feelings (e.g., rage, self-hate) when they arise.

Planning for stressful situations provides the patient with increasing self-agency rather than relying on external controls.

8. Set and maintain limits on acceptable behavior and make clear the patient's responsibilities. If the patient is hospitalized, be clear regarding unit rules. *Clear and nonpunitive limit setting is essential for decreasing negative behaviors.*

Chronic Low Self-Esteem

Related to
- Biochemical alterations in the brain
- Borderline personality disorder
- Repeated failures
- Childhood abuse and/or neglect
- Avoidant and dependent behavioral patterns
- Lack of integrated self-identity
- Persistent feelings of shame and guilt
- Inconsistent affection and discipline in family of origin

Desired Outcome The patient will report and demonstrate improved self-esteem.

Assessment/Interventions and *Rationales*

1. Maintain a respectful and empathetic approach to the patient. *This helps feeling respected as a person—even when behavior might not be appropriate—promotes trust and builds on the therapeutic relationship.*

2. Assess for blaming, projection, anger, passivity, and demanding behaviors. *Many behaviors seen in patients with personality disorders cover a fragile sense of self. Often these behaviors are the crux of the patient's interpersonal difficulties in all relationships.*

3. Assess the patient's self-perception across various aspects of life, including strengths and weaknesses in work, school, daily tasks, physical appearance, sexuality, and personality. *A comprehensive assessment helps identify areas of low self-esteem, guiding interventions that promote self-awareness, balanced self-evaluation, and a more positive self-concept.*

4. Review the types of cognitive distortions that affect self-esteem (e.g., self-blame, mind reading, overgeneralization, selective inattention, all-or-none thinking). *These are the most common cognitive distortions.*

Identifying them is the first step to correcting false thoughts.

5. Help the patient to recognize cognitive distortions, their impact on emotion, and their influence on behavior. Encourage the patient to keep a log. *Cognitive distortions are automatic. Keeping a log helps make automatic, unconscious thinking clear.*

6. Teach the patient to reframe and dispute cognitive distortions. Disputes need to be strong, specific, and nonjudgmental. *Practice and belief in the disputes over time help patients gain a more realistic appraisal of events, the world, and themselves.*

7. Discourage the patient from dwelling on and reliving past mistakes. *The past cannot be changed. Dwelling on past mistakes prevents the patient from appraising the present and planning for the future.*

8. Discourage the patient from making self-blaming and negative remarks. *Words become feelings, thoughts, and beliefs that result in a negative cycle of more negative verbalizations. Stopping negative is a step in breaking the cycle.*

9. Use positively framed, action-oriented questions to help the patient shift focus to the present and future. For example: "What could you do differently now?" or "What have you learned from that experience?" *Encouraging reflection in a constructive and solution-focused manner helps the patient reframe past behaviors, fostering a sense of control and empowerment over future choices.*

10. Provide honest and genuine feedback regarding your observations as to strengths and areas that could use additional skills. *Feedback helps give the patient a more accurate view of self, strengths, and areas to work on, as well as a sense that someone understands.*

11. Set goals realistically, and revise goals as needed in small steps. *The patient's negative self-view and distrust of the world took years to develop. Unrealistic goals can set up hopelessness in patients and frustration in staff.*

12. Help the patient to set realistic short-term goals for the future. Identify skills the patient will need to reach these goals. *Focusing on the future reduces negative self-rumination. Meeting realistic goals fosters a sense of accomplishment, direction, and control, enhancing self-perception.*

Impaired Socialization

Related to
- Biochemical alterations in the brain
- Inability to engage in mature, reciprocal interactions
- Manipulative behaviors
- Self-concept disturbance
- Unacceptable or maladaptive social behavior or values
- Disruptive or abusive early family background

Desired Outcome The patient will demonstrate improved socialization.

Assessment/Interventions and *Rationales*

1. Assist the patient in recognizing maladaptive patterns of social interaction. *The patient does not recognize patterns of maladaptive behaviors. Change cannot happen until this recognition occurs.*
2. Identify alternative social interaction methods. *Once maladaptive behavior is eliminated, new methods of social interaction must be identified and adopted.*
3. Role-play and practice successful social interaction. *The nurse–patient relationship is an ideal testing ground for developing relationship skills.*
4. Encourage attendance at group therapy and group work. *Group member influence, confrontation, altruistic learning, and recognition of own behaviors in others are often more valuable than one-to-one encounters.*

Teach emotional regulation strategies. *Since intense emotional reactions often disrupt relationships, helping the patient manage emotions through mindfulness, distress tolerance, and grounding techniques improves social stability.*

Encourage self-reflection after social interactions by the patient evaluating their interactions, identifying what went well and what could be improved. *This intervention promotes self-awareness and behavioral adjustments.*

Assist in developing healthy boundaries. *Teaching the patient to set and respect boundaries prevents unstable, overly intense, or conflict-ridden relationships, a common issue in borderline personality disorder.*

Address fear of abandonment in relationships. *Helping the patient recognize and challenge irrational fears of rejection reduces clinginess, manipulative behaviors, and social withdrawal, fostering healthier interactions.*

Impaired Coping

Related to
- Biochemical alterations in the brain
- Maladaptive tension relief patterns
- Intense and unstable emotional states
- Lack of intent to change behavior
- Lack of motivation for behavioral change
- Negative attitudes toward health-promoting behavior

Desired Outcome The patient will report and demonstrate improved coping.

Assessment/Interventions and *Rationales*

1. Assess for suicidal ideation and non-suicidal self-injury. *Maintaining safety by monitoring for urges or acts of self-mutilation and suicidal thoughts is a priority.*
2. Intervene in times of intense and labile mood swings, anxiety, depression, and irritability. *Many dysfunctional behaviors of patients (e.g., parasuicidal, anger, manipulation, substance use) are used as behavioral solutions to intense pain.*
   a. Anxiety: Teach stress-reduction techniques such as deep breathing, relaxation, meditation, and exercise. *Patients experience intense anxiety and fear of abandonment. Stress-reduction techniques help the patient focus more clearly.*
   b. Depression: The patient might need medications to improve mood. Assess for side effects. *Medication combined with talk therapy and exercise is effective in decreasing depression. Side effects should be managed or medication changed to promote adherence.*
   c. Irritability, anger: Use interventions early before irritability and anger escalate.
   Intervening early can help reduce or eliminate escalation.
3. Reduce manipulation through consistency, limit setting, and unit or community rules. *External structure will decrease negative behaviors, while patients develop internal control.*
4. Set firm, clear, and nonjudgmental limits on the patient's demands for time and attention. *Assertive limit-setting provides necessary structure, helping the patient develop appropriate boundaries and reducing manipulative or attention-seeking behaviors.*

5. Be nonjudgmental and respectful when listening to the patient's thoughts, feelings, or complaints. *Developing a trusting relationship with the nurse lays the groundwork for future relationships.*

6. Encourage the patient to explore feelings and concerns (e.g., identify fears, loneliness, self-hate). *The patient is used to acting out feelings rather than expressing them verbally. Appropriate self-expression is an essential new skill.*

7. When the patient is ready and interested, teach coping skills to help diffuse tension and troubling feelings (e.g., anxiety reduction, assertiveness skills). *Increasing skills helps the patient to use healthier ways to diffuse tensions and get needs met.* Developing these skills provides healthier alternatives for tension relief, reducing reliance on maladaptive behaviors to cope with emotional pain and meet personal needs.

8. Provide referrals or involve professional experts for advanced training (e.g., dialectical behavioral therapy [DBT], interpersonal skills, anger management skills, emotional regulation skills). *Training teaches the patient to refine skills in changing behaviors, emotions, and thinking patterns associated with problems in living that are causing misery and distress.*

9. Treatment of substance use is best handled by well-organized treatment professionals. *Keeping detailed records and having a team involved with each patient can minimize manipulation.*

10. Provide and encourage the patient to use professionals in other disciplines such as social services, vocational rehabilitation, social work, or the law. *Patients with borderline personality disorder often have multiple social problems and do not know how to obtain these services.*

Encourage the use of distress tolerance techniques (e.g., distraction, grounding exercises, sensory-based strategies). *Distress tolerance skills—such as engaging in distracting activities, using grounding techniques (e.g., focusing on the five senses), or employing sensory-based strategies (e.g., holding an ice cube or practicing deep breathing)—help patients manage overwhelming emotions in the moment without resorting to maladaptive behaviors like self-harm or impulsivity.*

TREATMENT FOR BORDERLINE PERSONALITY DISORDER

Biological Treatments

Pharmacotherapy

There are no FDA-approved medications specifically for borderline personality disorder. However, medication may be used to manage cooccurring symptoms such as severe depression, anxiety, psychosis, or crisis-related distress.

- SSRIs are commonly prescribed to address mood instability and emotional dysregulation.
- Mood stabilizers may help regulate impulsivity and mood swings.
- Naltrexone (Revia, Vivitrol), an opioid receptor antagonist, has emerging evidence supporting its use in reducing self-injurious behaviors (Karakula-Juchnowicz et al., 2023).
- Second-generation antipsychotics can be used to manage brief psychotic episodes or severe emotional dysregulation.

While medication does not directly treat BPD, it can play a supportive role in managing distressing symptoms and improving overall functioning when combined with psychotherapy. Chapters 22–24 and 27 discuss the medications mentioned in this paragraph.

Psychological Therapies

Three essential therapies for borderline personality disorder are cognitive-behavioral therapy, dialectical behavior therapy, and schema-focused therapy.

- CBT helps individuals identify and modify distorted core beliefs about themselves and others, improving social interactions and emotional regulation.
- DBT integrates cognitive and behavioral techniques with mindfulness, encouraging individuals to be aware of their thoughts and actively reshape them to manage emotional distress.
- Schema-focused therapy blends elements of CBT with psychodynamic approaches, targeting deeply ingrained self-perceptions and maladaptive coping patterns. These therapies help individuals with borderline personality disorder develop healthier thought patterns, improve emotional regulation, and enhance interpersonal relationships.

These psychological therapies are discussed further in Chapter 29.

NURSE, PATIENT, AND FAMILY RESOURCES

Internet Mental Health
A health technology company guiding people towards self-understanding and connection. The platform offers reliable resources, accessible services, and nurturing communities.
www.mentalhealth.com

MedlinePlus
A service of the National Library of Medicine that presents high-quality, relevant health and wellness information that is trusted, easy to understand, and free of advertising, in both English and Spanish.
www.medlineplus.gov/personalitydisorders.html

National Alliance on Mentally Illness (NAMI)
NAMI is the National Alliance on Mental Illness, the nation's largest grassroots mental health organization dedicated to building better lives for the millions of Americans affected by mental illness. Educational materials and support for individuals with mental illness and their families.
www.nami.org

Self-Injury Outreach and Support
A nonprofit outreach initiative providing information and resources about self-injury to those who self-injure, those who have recovered, and those who want help.
sioutreach.org

Stop Walking on Eggshells
Includes information on Borderline Personality Disorder and Narcissistic Personality Disorder for patients and family members.
https://stopwalkingoneggshells.com

CHAPTER 15

Suicide

Suicide has profound and lasting effects on family, friends, and communities. Yet, it is largely preventable. A 2018 study (Stone et al.) found that 83% of individuals who died by suicide had used healthcare services in the year before their deaths, yet more than half (54%) had no documented mental health diagnosis. These findings underscore the need for broader mental health screening all healthcare settings-not just in psychiatric care.

Given the critical need for early identification and intervention, this chapter focuses on suicide and strategies to keep individuals safe. Suicide risk involves a range of behaviors and warning signs that require careful assessment and support. Terms associated with suicide include:

- *Suicidal ideation* refers to thoughts about wanting to be dead or actively thinking about killing oneself, without engaging in preparatory behavior.
- A *suicide attempt* is self-injurious behavior carried out with the intention of dying, also called a nonfatal suicide attempt or suicidal act.
- *Suicide* is death resulting from self-directed injurious behavior undertaken with the intent to die.
- *Suicidality* is a broad term encompassing suicidal ideation, planning, suicide attempts, and suicide.
- *Suicide survivors* are family members, significant others, or acquaintances who have lost someone to suicide. This term may also refer to individuals who have survived suicide attempt.

Some words used to describe suicide concepts are problematic and are avoided. One familiar term is to commit suicide. However, using the word "commit" is discouraged due to its association with criminal activity. Historically, suicide was illegal, and this language reinforces outdated stigma. Other problematic terms imply a judgmental or misleading tone. For example, *completed suicide* and *successful suicide* suggest a positive outcome, while *failed suicide attempt* implies a negative one. Instead, neutral and accurate terms such as *died by suicide* or *suicide attempt* are preferred.

EPIDEMIOLOGY

According to the Centers for Disease Control and Prevention ([CDC]; 2022), nearly 50,000 people died by suicide in 2022. Since 2020 COVID-19 replaced suicide as one of the top 10 leading causes of death (CDC, 2024).

This entirely preventable cause of death is especially prominent in younger people. In 2022 suicide was the second leading cause of death for people ages 10 to 14 and 25 to 34, and among the 9 leading causes of death for ages 10 to 64.

Men died by suicide about 4 times more often than women, while over a lifetime, women attempted suicide almost 1.5 times more often than men. White males accounted for almost 70% of all suicide deaths. Non-Hispanic American, Indian, or Alaskan Natives had the highest suicide rates for both males and females in all age groups in 2022.

RISK FACTORS

Twin and adoption studies suggest genetic factors in suicide, as concordance rates are higher among monozygotic (identical) twins than dizygotic (fraternal) twins. Biological factors also play a role, particularly serotonin levels. Low serotonin is associated with depressed mood, and postmortem examinations of individuals who died by suicide reveal low levels of serotonin in the brainstem and/or the frontal cortex.

Hopelessness is the central emotional factor underlying suicide intent. Certain cognitive styles also increase risk including all-or-nothing thinking, difficulty considering alternative solutions, and perfectionism. Adolescents are particularly vulnerable due to immaturity of their prefrontal cortex, the portion of the brain that controls the executive functions involving judgment, frustration tolerance, and impulse control.

Assessment

- History of suicide attempts or self-mutilation
- Family history of suicide attempts or death by suicide
- History of bullying and/or victimization
- History of a mood disorder, schizophrenia, or drug or alcohol use
- History of chronic pain, recent surgery, or chronic physical illness
- History of personality disorder (e.g., borderline, paranoid, antisocial)
- Bereavement or another significant trauma (e.g., divorce, loss of job or home)
- Legal or disciplinary problems

Signs and Symptoms

- Talking or writing about death, dying, or suicide
- Making comments about being hopeless, helpless, or worthless
- Expressions of having no reason to live; no sense of purpose in life; saying things like "It would be better if I wasn't here"
- Increased alcohol and/or substance use
- Withdrawal from friends, family, and community
- Reckless behavior or more risky, impulsive activities
- Dramatic mood changes
- Talking about being a burden to others

Assessment Tools

A variety of assessment tools measure suicide risk. The Columbia-Suicide Severity Rating Scale (C-SSRS) assesses patients through a series of simple questions. Responses to these questions can help to identify suicide risk, assess the severity and immediacy of that risk, and determine the necessary level of support. The C-SSRS is in Box 15.1.

Box 15.1 **Columbia-Suicide Severity Rating Scale (C-SSRS)**

Suicide Ideation Definitions and Prompts	Past Month	
Ask Questions That Are Bolded and Underlined	Yes	No

Ask Questions 1 and 2

1). Wish to be Dead:

Have you wished you were dead or wished
  you could go to sleep and not wake up?

1). Suicidal Thoughts:

Have you actually had any thoughts of killing
  yourself?

**If YES to 2, Ask Questions 3, 4, 5, and 6. If NO to 2, go
directly to Question 6**

1). Suicidal Thoughts with Method (Without
  Specific Plan or Intent to Act):

*E.g. "I thought about taking an overdose, but I
  never made a specific plan as to when, where, or
  how I would actually do it….and I would never
  go through with it."*

Have you been thinking about how you
  might do this?

1). Suicidal Intent (Without Specific Plan): As
  opposed to *"I have the thoughts, but I definitely
  will not do anything about them."*

Have you had these thoughts and had some
  intention of acting on them?

1). Suicide Intent With Specific Plan:

Have you started to work out or worked out
  the details of how to kill yourself? Do you
  intend to carry out this plan?

1). Suicide Behavior Question:

Have you ever done anything, started to do
  anything, or prepared to do anything to end
  your life?

Examples: Collected pills, obtained a gun,
  gave away valuables, wrote a will or suicide
  note, took out pills but didn't swallow any,
  held a gun but changed your mind or it was
  grabbed from your hand, went to the roof
  but didn't jump; or actually took pills, tried
  to shoot yourself, cut yourself, tried to hang
  yourself, etc.

If YES, ask: Was this within the past 3 months?

Box 15.1 Columbia-Suicide Severity Rating Scale (C-SSRS)—cont'd

Suicide Ideation Definitions and Prompts	Past Month	
Ask Questions That Are Bolded and <u>Underlined</u>	Yes	No

Response Protocol to C-SSRS Screening (linked to last item marked Yes)

Item 1: Behavioral health referral

Item 2: Behavioral health referral

Item 3: Behavioral health consult and consider patient safety precautions

Item 4: Immediate notification of physician and/or behavioral health and safety precautions

Item 5: Immediate notification of physician and/or behavioral health and safety precautions

Item 6 (over 3 months ago): Behavior health consult and consider patient safety precautions

Item 6 (3 months ago or less): Immediate notification of physician and/or behavioral health and safety precautions

---

From Posner, K., Brent, D., Lucas, C., Gould, M., Stanley, B., Brown, G. et al. (2009). Columbia-Suicide Severity Rating Scale. Retrieved from https://www.thenationalcouncil.org/about/contact/.

Assessment Guidelines

Suicide

1. Assess risk factors (Box 15.2).
2. Assess protective factors (see Box 15.2).
3. Determine the level of suicide precautions for the patient based on the following questions:
   a. Are you thinking of killing/hurting yourself?
   b. How long have you been thinking about suicide (i.e., frequency, intensity, duration)?
   c. Do you have a plan? Obtain specific information if there is a plan.
   d. Do you have the means to carry out the plan (e.g., accessibility of a weapon, medications, drugs)?
   e. Have you attempted suicide in the past? If yes, how?
   f. Has someone in your family died by suicide? If yes, how?
   g. Is there anything or anyone to stop you such as religious beliefs, children left behind, or pets?

Box 15.2 Risk and Protective Factors for Suicide

Risk Factors
- Previous suicide attempt
- A history of suicide in the family
- Substance use
- Mood disorders (depression, bipolar disorder)
- Access to lethal means (e.g., keeping firearms in the home)
- Losses and other events (e.g., breakup of a relationship or a death, academic failure, legal difficulty, financial problems, bullying)
- History of trauma or abuse
- Chronic physical illness including chronic pain
- Exposure to the suicidal behavior of others

Protective Factors
- Effective and accessible mental healthcare clinical interventions
- Strong connections to individuals, family, community, and social institutions
- Significant other
- Having children
- Problem-solving skills

---

4. Assess for a sudden mood improvement. Often a decision to die by suicide provides a way out of severe emotional pain.
5. Assess social supports and helpfulness of significant other(s).

NURSING DIAGNOSES

A thorough assessment provides the framework for determining the level of protection the patient requires. Therefore, *risk for suicide* is the first area of concern (International Council of Nurses, 2019). Believing that one's situation or problem is intolerable, inescapable, and interminable leads to feelings of hopelessness. *Hopelessness* is often associated with suicide and is a priority nursing diagnosis.

Reinforcing the patient's problem-solving skills and helping to reframe life difficulties as events that can be controlled are strategic parts of the counseling process. Therefore, *impaired coping* is the third point of intervention. Other potential nursing diagnoses include *low self-esteem, impaired socialization, spiritual distress, and impaired family process.*

Nursing Care for Patients With Suicidality

Risk for Suicide

Related to
- History of prior suicide attempt
- Family history of suicide
- Suicidal ideation
- Suicide plan
- Alcohol and substance use
- Adverse childhood experiences
- At-risk demographics (e.g., older adult, young adult male, adolescent, widowed, white, American Indian)
- Physical illness, chronic pain, terminal illness
- Grief, bereavement, loss of important relationship, job, home
- Psychiatric disorder (e.g., major depressive disorder, schizophrenia, bipolar disorder)
- Poor support system, loneliness
- Legal or disciplinary problems
- Hopelessness or helplessness

Desired Outcome The patient will be free from suicidal risk.

Assessment/Interventions and *Rationales*
Hospitalized
1. Follow agency protocol to ensure a safe environment, such as removing potential weapons (e.g., belts and sharp objects) and monitoring visitor belongings. *While having suicidal ideation, the access to the means of self-harm increases the risk of death.*
2. Suicide precautions range from one-on-one with a staff member at arm's length at all times to less frequent checks. *Close contact with healthcare workers not only provides safety for a patient with suicidal ideation but also fosters socialization and self-esteem.*
3. If there is an imminent risk of self-harm, seclusion or restraint may be required. *For patients with the most*

severe suicidal ideation, temporary seclusion or restraint may be the safest option.

4. Follow unit protocol and document the patient's behavior and statements along with nursing interventions. *Documentation supports for continuity of care with other healthcare workers, tracks progress, and provides a legal record of nursing care.*

5. Encourage the patient to discuss stressors, responses to stressors, and alternative responses to stressors. *Talking about feelings, responses to stressors, and looking at alternatives can help reduce suicidal thoughts.*

Outside the Hospital

1. If an individual is managed outside the hospital, notify the family, significant other, or friends of the risk and treatment plan. Provide education about signs of worsening depression such as hopelessness. *Family and friends can support the individual and also facilitate access to healthcare if suicidal ideation continues or increases.*

2. Provide education or referral for medication, counseling (a general nursing intervention), and/or psychotherapy (advanced practice interventions). *Antidepressants are initiated quickly due to the significant lag time before they take effect, while counseling and psychotherapy will provide immediate support.*

3. Provide the patient, family, and friends with the number for the emergency department, crisis care facilities, or an emergency hotline (i.e., 988 for the US mental health hotline). *Patients, family, and friends need access to 24/7 support.*

4. Schedule a follow-up visit as early as the next day if decisions concerning hospitalization need to be reconsidered. *During a crisis period, individuals are monitored carefully for increasing suicidal ideation.*

5. Educate friends and family regarding signs of increased suicidal ideation. These signs include withdrawal, preoccupation, silence, remorse, and sudden mood changes from sad to happy and carefree. *Friends and family can intervene and facilitate the patient receiving more acute care.*

6. Identify social supports and encourage the patient to initiate contact. *Social connections reduce self-absorption and hopelessness. Talking with other people is one of the best activities for improving mood and reducing suicidal thoughts.*

7. List support people and agencies to use as outpatient and crisis hotline numbers. Significant others. *Suicide attempts are often impulsive. Immediate access to another person can be lifesaving.*
8. Work with the patient and fa*mily to limit access to lethal means,* such as firearms and medications, in the home. *Limiting access to lethal means, such as firearms and medications, reduces the risk of suicide by preventing impulsive attempts, increasing safety, and involving family in supportive prevention efforts.*

Hopelessness

Related to
- Deteriorating physical or psychiatric condition
- Social isolation
- Long-term stress
- Spiritual distress
- Severe loss (financial hardship, termination of a relationship, loss of job)
- Chronic pain
- Negative perception of the future

Desired Outcome The patient will demonstrate and verbalize hopefulness for the future.

Assessment/Interventions and *Rationales*
1. Encourage the patient to reframe negative thoughts into neutral or balanced perspectives. *Cognitive reframing helps individuals view situations more objectively, reducing feelings of hopelessness and promoting problem-solving, which can lower suicide risk.*
2. Identify and challenge unrealistic and perfectionistic thinking. *Constructive interpretations of events and behaviors promote realistic thinking, expand problem-solving options, and foster hope for the future, reducing suicide risk.*
3. Work with the patient to identify strengths. *When people are feeling overwhelmed, they no longer view their lives or behavior objectively and dismiss their strengths.*
4. Spend time discussing the patient's dreams and hopes for the future. Identify short-term goals for the future. *Renewing realistic dreams and hopes can give promise to the future and meaning to life.*
5. Help the patient to identify past sources of life that have given meaning and joy and explore ways to

reintegrate them into their life (e.g., religious or spiritual beliefs, group activities, creative endeavors). *Reawakens the patient's abilities and experiences that tap areas of strength and creativity. Creative activities give people intrinsic pleasure, joy, and life satisfaction.*

6. Encourage contact with religious or spiritual individuals or groups that have supplied comfort and support in the patient's past. *During times of hopelessness, people might feel abandoned and too paralyzed to reach out to caring people or groups.*

Impaired Coping

Related to
- Situational or maturational crises
- Disturbance in pattern of tension release
- Inadequate social support
- Inadequate coping skills
- Impulsive use of extreme solutions
- Inadequate resources

Desired Outcome The patient will demonstrate improved coping.

Assessment/Interventions and *Rationales*

1. Identify situations that trigger suicidal thoughts. *Identifying triggers for suicidal thoughts helps to identify targets for learning more adaptive coping skills.*

2. Assess the patient's strengths and positive coping skills (e.g., talking to others, creative outlets, social activities, problem-solving abilities). *Use these strengths and skills when planning alternatives to self-defeating behaviors.*

3. Assess the patient's ineffective coping behaviors (e.g., drinking, angry outbursts, withdrawal, denial, procrastination) that result in negative emotions. *This helps to identify areas to target for teaching and planning strategies for more effective and self-enhancing behaviors.*

4. Role-play adaptive coping strategies that can be used when suicidal thinking begins to emerge. *Practice helps the patient use skills when/if suicidal thoughts occur.*

5. Assess the need for assertiveness training. *Assertiveness skills can help the patient develop a sense of control and balance.*

6. Clarify aspects of life that are not under the patient's control such as other's actions, likes, choices, or health

status. *Recognizing one's limitations in controlling others is, paradoxically, a beginning to finding one's strength.*

7. Assess the patient's support system. *Social supports improve coping by reducing isolation, thereby lowering the risk of suicide attempts.*

8. Encourage the patient to identify two potential social activities with others who share mutual interests such as walking, books, or dining, which can be easily found online. *Involvement in outside activities with others reduces introspection and self-absorption.*

Nurse, Patient, and Family Resources

Alliance of Hope for Suicide Survivors
Created by survivors for survivors to provide online healing support and other services for people who are coping with devastating loss to suicide.
www.allianceofhope.org

American Association of Suicidology (AAS)
The AAS promotes the research of suicide and its prevention, public awareness programs, public education, and training for professionals and volunteers.
www.suicidology.org

American Foundation for Suicide Prevention (AFSP)
AFSD is a voluntary health organization that gives those affected by suicide a nationwide community empowered by research, education, and advocacy to take action against this leading cause of death.
www.afsp.org

Crisis Text Line
Crisis text line provides free, 24/7 mental health support via text message.
www.crisistextline.org

Friends for Survival, Inc
Friends for Survival is not just a support group, but a "suicide bereavement support program" that offers a variety of services on a long-term basis to meet the complicated needs of families.
www.friendsforsurvival.org

(If You Are Thinking About) Suicide… Read This First
An online letter with resources for individuals who are thinking about suicide.
www.metanoia.org/suicide

National Suicide Prevention Lifeline
1-800-273-8255
Samaritans
Samaritans is a unique charity dedicated to reducing feelings of isolation and disconnection that can lead to suicide.
www.samaritans.org

Suicide Awareness Voices of Education (SAVE)
SAVE is a national nonprofit working to end the tragedy of suicide through education, training, advocacy, and supporting suicide loss survivors.
www.save.org

CHAPTER 16

Crisis Intervention

The previous edition of the *Clinical Companion, Varcarolis' Psychiatric Nursing Care* was revised in the midst of a global pandemic. Any nursing student reading this chapter experienced this crisis/disaster situation firsthand. Most of us were afraid, if not for ourselves, for loved ones who were older or had preexisting conditions. Anxiety levels ran high as the country and states wrestled with the accompanying economic disaster. People were isolated and cut off from their usual support and social outlets. For some vulnerable individuals, the stress of the coronavirus pandemic caused an emergence or exacerbation (i.e., worsening) of psychiatric symptoms. Even now, years later, most remember that period vividly.

This shared experience of collective stress highlights the importance of understanding how the human body and mind respond to challenges. Despite stress, the human organism's internal environment maintains a relatively stable state while interacting with external forces. This stable state is referred to as *homeostasis* or *equilibrium*. A crisis, which is a major disturbance caused by a stressful event or threat, disrupts this homeostasis. In a crisis, normal coping mechanisms fail, resulting in an inability to function as usual. Equilibrium is replaced by disequilibrium. Crisis intervention efforts are aimed at promoting (1) a realistic perception of the event, (2) adequate situational support, and (3) adequate coping skills.

PERCEPTION OF THE EVENT

A person's perception of a crisis can range from realistic to distorted. Individuals vary in how they absorb, process, and use information from the environment. Some may respond to a minor event as if it were life-threatening, while others may remain calm and rational even during a genuinely life-threatening situation.

SITUATIONAL SUPPORT

Situational support includes all the people who are available and who can be depended upon to help during the time of a crisis. This includes family, friends, and healthcare professionals who provide emotional or practical assistance. Nurses and other healthcare professionals who use crisis intervention are providing situational support.

COPING SKILLS

The quality and quantity of a person's usual coping skills affect a person's ability to cope with a crisis situation. Other factors may compromise a person's ability to cope with a crisis event. These factors include the number of other stressful life events with which the person is coping, other unresolved losses, the presence of psychiatric disorders or other medical problems, and excessive fatigue or pain.

Crisis, by definition, is self-limiting and typically resolves within 4 to 6 weeks. The overall goal of crisis intervention is to regain the pre-crisis level of functioning. However, an individual can emerge from the crisis at a lower or higher level of functioning. This variability highlights the critical importance of crisis intervention and community services.

TYPES OF CRISES

Crises can be classified using various frameworks. Three primary types: (1) maturational (or developmental) crises, (2) situational crises, and (3) adventitious crises. Identifying which type of crisis the individual is experiencing or has experienced helps in the development of a patient-centered plan of care in childhood, adolescence, and adulthood.

Maturational

Erikson (1963) identified eight stages of growth and development, each defined by two opposing psychological tendencies—one positive and one negative—with specific tasks that must be mastered to progress through the growth process. Former coping styles may no longer be age-appropriate, and new coping mechanisms have yet to be developed.

A maturational crisis occurs when former coping mechanisms are inadequate to handle the stress common to a particular stage in the life cycle. Temporary disequilibrium might impact interpersonal relationships, body image, and social or work roles. Examples of triggers to a maturational crisis include leaving home for the first time, marriage, the birth of a child, retirement, and the death of a parent.

Situational

A situational crisis arises from events that are unusually distressing and often unexpected. Examples of triggers to a situational crisis include a job loss or change, the death of a loved one, a change in financial status, divorce, or the onset of psychiatric or physical illness. These situations are often referred to as life events or crucial life problems because most people encounter some of these challenges during the course of their lives.

Adventitious

An adventitious crisis is a traumatic, external event that occurs unexpectedly. These rare crises can be natural, human-caused, or accidental. Natural disasters include pandemics, epidemics, floods, fires, and earthquakes. Human-caused adventitious crises may involve one-on-one violence—such as rape and murder—as well as acts of terrorism, wars, riots, shootings, and bombings. Accidents, such as airline crashes, structural collapses, or nuclear power plant failures, are another source of adventitious crisis. In addition to injury and loss of life, adventitious crises may result in long-term psychological trauma.

PHASES OF CRISIS

Through extensive study of individuals experiencing crisis, Caplan (1964) identified behaviors that follow a fairly predictable path. He categorized these behaviors into four distinct phases of a crisis.

Phase 1

When a person is exposed to a serious stressor or problem, they experience increased anxiety. This heightened anxiety triggers the use of familiar coping methods in an effort to resolve the problem and reduce discomfort.

Phase 2

If the usual coping methods fail and the threat persists, anxiety continues to rise, causing greater distress. As anxiety intensifies, individual functioning becomes disorganized. Trial-and-error attempts to solve the problem and restore balance begin.

Phase 3

If the trial-and-error attempts are unsuccessful, anxiety may escalate to severe and even panic levels. At this stage, the person may resort to automatic relief behaviors, such as withdrawal and flight. Resolution—such as compromising needs or redefining the situation to reach an acceptable solution—can sometimes occur during this stage.

Phase 4

If the problem remains unresolved and new coping skills prove ineffective, anxiety may overwhelm the person. These powerful feelings can lead to serious consequences, including personality disorganization, depression, confusion, violence against others, or suicidal behavior.

ASSESSMENT

Assessing History

A history of potential crises may include:
- An overwhelming life event (maturational, situational, or adventitious)
- Previous violent behavior
- Previous suicidal behavior
- A psychiatric disorder (e.g., major depressive disorder, personality disorder, bipolar disorder, schizophrenia, anxiety disorder)
- A significant physical condition (e.g., cancer, cardiac disease, uncontrolled diabetes, lupus, multiple sclerosis)

Signs and Symptoms

Individuals in crisis may exhibit a range of behaviors, including:
- Confusion, disorganized thinking

- Immobilization, social withdrawal
- Violence against others, suicidal thoughts, or attempts
- Agitation, increased psychomotor activity
- Crying and feelings of sadness
- Flashbacks, intrusive thoughts, nightmares
- Forgetfulness, poor concentration

Sample Questions

Three main areas are assessed during a crisis: (1) perception of the event, (2) support system, and (3) coping skills. Nurses use a variety of therapeutic techniques to gather information by asking the following questions:

1. **Perception of the Event**
   "What happened in your life before you started to feel this way?"
   "What does this event or problem mean to you?"
   "How is this event or problem affecting your life?"
   "How do you see this event or problem affecting your future?"

2. **Support System**
   "Is there anyone—family or friends—you would like to have involved in your care?"
   "Are these people available now?"
   "Do you have a religious affiliation?"
   "Where do you go to school? Are you involved in any community-based activities?"

3. **Coping Skills**
   "What do you usually do when you feel stressed or overwhelmed?"
   "What has helped you get through difficult times in the past?"
   "What have you done so far to cope with this situation?"
   "Do you have any thoughts of killing yourself?"
   "Do you have any thoughts of killing or hurting someone else?"

Assessment Guidelines

- Determine whether the patient can identify the precipitating event.
- Assess the patient's situational support system.

- Identify the patient's usual coping styles, and evaluate which coping mechanisms may be helpful in the present situation.
- Consider any religious or cultural beliefs that may influence assessment and intervention.
- Assess whether the patient requires health promotion (e.g., education, environmental manipulation, or new coping skills), crisis intervention, or rehabilitation.

Nursing Diagnoses

When anxiety levels escalate to moderate, severe, or panic levels, problem-solving ability becomes impaired. In an acute crisis, an individual's usual coping skills may no longer be effective. For individuals with already compromised coping abilities, this challenge is even greater. The International Council Nurses (2019) provides useful and logical nursing diagnoses. One key diagnosis is impaired coping, evidenced by an inability to meet basic needs, reliance on inappropriate defense mechanisms, or alterated social participation. This chapter addresses *impaired coping* both in the context of acute crisis intervention and separately during the rehabilitation phase.

Another essential nursing diagnosis focuses on anxiety. *Anxiety (moderate, severe, panic)* is always present in various levels during crisis situations. Reducing anxiety so that individuals can begin problem-solving on their own is central to crisis management.

Because a crisis in one family member affects the entire family, *impaired family processes* must also be addressed. Family members may struggle to support one another, leading to disorganized communication and difficulty expressing emotions appropriately. Interventions support the individual and family to engage in healthy interactions.

Intervention Guidelines

Levels of Crisis Intervention

Crisis intervention levels correlate with the public health levels of prevention model. The levels are health promotion (primary prevention), acute crisis intervention (secondary prevention), and stabilization and rehabilitation (tertiary prevention).

Health Promotion

The goal of health promotion is to prevent crisis responses from occurring. Nurses help to promote mental health with the following interventions:

- Evaluate the patient's experience of stressful life events.
- Provide education on specific coping skills, such as decision-making, problem-solving, assertiveness, meditation, and relaxation techniques.
- Encourage the patient to reduce or eliminate stress by postponing major life changes such as moving to a new residence or changing jobs.

Acute Crisis Intervention

Acute crisis intervention focuses on identifing and reducing prolonged crisis responses once they occur. This care is provided in hospital units, emergency departments, clinics, or mental health centers.

Essential nursing interventions for acute crisis intervention include:

- Conducting regular screening to detect psychiatric symptoms that may lead to crisis responses. Key symptoms include depressive, anxious, obsessive–compulsive, psychosis, and suicidality.
- Prioritizing safety by addressing harmful thoughts and impulses.
- Assessing the patient's problems, support systems, and coping styles.
- Promoting a realistic perception of events, strengthening social support, and exploring alternate coping methods.
- Taking an active and directive approach to care.

Crisis Stabilization and Rehabilitation (Tertiary Prevention)

Crisis stabilization and rehabilitation programs provide long-term support for individuals who have experienced a crisis. The primary goals are to facilitate optimal levels of functioning and prevent further emotional disruptions. This care is delivered in rehabilitation clinics, day hospitals, sheltered workshops, and outpatient settings. Individuals with serious mental illness are more susceptible to crises, and community facilities offer a structured, supportive environment that helps reduce stress and promote stability.

Nurses support crisis stabilizaon and rehabilitaon through the following interventions.

- Assess and address the educational needs of the patient and family.
- Assess and provide for social skills training as needed.
- Assess and refer paents to vocaonal rehabilitaon programs when appropriate.
- Evaluate and refer patients to supportive group therapy.
- Teach cognive techniques and/or refer paents to cognive behavioral therapy programs.

Table 16.1 describes the impact of stress based on mental health and mental illness.

Acute Crisis

- Assess for suicidal or homicidal thoughts or plans.
- Prioritize safety and work to reduce anxiety.
- Take an active, directive approach (e.g., make phone calls, arrange social support).
- Continuously monitor the patient's progress.

Table 16.1 **Responses to Stress in Mental Health and Mental Illness**

Mental Health	Mental Illness
Adapts to day-to-day disappointments and changes	May perceive even mild disruptions as crises (e.g., a cancelation of a healthcare provider appointment)
Maintains a healthy sense of self, place, and purpose in life with strong problem-solving abilities	Has an inadequate sense of self, purpose, or abilities, along with poor problem-solving skills
Typically has adequate situational support and can activate is them during stressful times	May lack family or friends, live in isolation, or experience homelessness
Possesses effective coping skills and a variety of techniques to reduce anxiety and adjust to challenges	Coping ability is often compromised, requiring additional support

Crisis Stabilization and Rehabilitation

- Individuals with serious mental illness are more vulnerable to crises.
- Adapting the crisis model for this group involves emphasizing the patient's strengths, setting realistic goals, and taking a more active role in their care.

After Crisis Stabilization

- Assess and address the educational needs of the patient and family.
- Evaluate the needs for social skills training and provide support as needed.
- Assess and refer to vocational rehabilitation programs when appropriate.
- Evaluate and refer patients to supportive group therapy.
- Teach cognitive techniques and/or refer patients to cognitive behavioral therapy programs.

Acute Crisis Intervention

Impaired Coping

Related to
- Maturational crisis
- Situational crisis
- Adventitious crisis
- Inadequate social support
- Inadequate level of perceived control
- Inadequate resources available
- High degree of threat
- Lack of opportunity to prepare for stressors
- Disturbance in pattern of appraisal of threat
- Disturbance in pattern of tension release

Desired Outcome The patient will demonstrate improved coping.

Assessment/Interventions and *Rationales*
1. Provide a liaison such as a social worker who has expertise in community resources to link the patient to emergency support. *The patient's physical needs (e.g., shelter, food, protection from abuser) are the initial priority.*

2. Facilitate making appointments for medical or other healthcare providers. *During an acute crisis, patients' attention may be limited. Making sure that healthcare appointments are made reduces the potential for missing other health problems.*

3. Document the date and time of appointments, their purpose, and location. *A written reminder for follow-up is essential because anxiety reduces the capacity for attention and memory formation.*

4. Assess for patient safety. Examples of questions to ask include: Do you have suicidal thoughts? Is there child or spouse abuse? Are you living in unsafe living conditions? *The patient's physical safety is the priority. Identifying immediate risks allows for timely intervention and the implementation of appropriate protective measures.*

5. Identify the patient's perception of the event. Help the patient to reframe this perception of the event if memories of the event seem to be unrealistic or distorted. *The patient's distorted perception increases anxiety.*

6. Assess whether helplessness or hopelessness has interfered with the patient's usual coping skills. *Help the patient to view the event as a problem that can be solved.*

7. Assess stressors and the precipitating cause of the crisis. *Assessing for these stressors helps identify areas for change and intervention.*

8. Identify the patient's current skills, resources, and knowledge to deal with problems. *This reminder supports the patient's self-esteem while encouraging the patient to use strengths and usual coping skills.*

9. Identify other skills that may be helpful (e.g., decision-making skills, problem-solving skills, communication skills, relaxation techniques) and support the patient's use of these skills through patient education. *Teaching the patient additional skills helps to regain more control over the present situation and helps minimize crisis situations in the future.*

10. Assess the patient's support systems. Encourage the patient to contact these supports or, with the patient's consent, make the contact yourself if the patient is overwhelmed. *Engaging a support system often reduces anxiety. Helping the patient to make contact if the patient is initially immobilized is a useful intervention.*

11. Identify and arrange for external support such as self-help groups. These groups are especially important if

the patient's current support system is unavailable or insufficient. *The patient might have lost important support because of death, divorce, or distance, for example, or the patient may simply not have sufficient support in place.*

12. Take an active role in crisis intervention (e.g., make telephone calls; arrange temporary child care; arrange for shelters, emergency food, or first aid). *Patients in crisis are often incapacitated by anxiety and unable to problem-solve. The nurse can provide much-needed organization so the patient views the situation as solvable and controllable.*

13. Provide small amounts of information at a time. *Only small pieces of information can be understood when a person's anxiety level is high.*

14. Encourage the patient to stay in the present to deal with the immediate situation. *Crisis intervention deals with the immediate problem disrupting the patient's present situation.*

15. Listen to the patient's story. Avoid interrupting. *Telling the story can be healing in itself.* Allowing the patient to set the pace is important in processing facts and feelings.

16. Help the patient set achievable goals. *Working in small, achievable steps helps the patient gain a sense of control and mastery.*

17. Work with the patient on devising a plan to meet goals. *A realistic and specific plan helps decrease anxiety and promote hopefulness.*

18. Identify and contact other members of the healthcare team who can support the patient in addressing specific concerns after a crisis event. *Other members of the healthcare team with specific expertise broaden the base of support and increase the patient's network for future problems.*

19. Provide debriefing for patients and family members after a crisis and for staff after a serious unit event such as a suicide attempt. *Survivors, family members, and staff all need to discuss the effects of a crisis, and debriefing provides the structure in which to do so.*

Crisis Stabilization and Rehabilitation

Crisis stabilization and rehabilitation addresses long-term needs of individuals with limited resources or support. This care may address deficits that result in a lower level of functioning after the crisis than before the crisis. This may happen to veterans who return from war after prolonged exposure to traumatic events. At other times, individuals with limited coping skills are faced with overwhelming situations, which for many people would not result in a crisis. For example, individuals with serious mental illnesses such as schizophrenia may experience a situational crisis based on seemingly trivial events such as a canceled therapist appointment.

The nursing diagnosis *impaired coping* applies to people with serious mental illness. These disorders usually impact multiple areas of functioning including activities of daily living (e.g., cooking, hygiene), health maintenance, relationships, leisure activities, safe movement within the community, finances, vocational and academic activities, and coping with stressors.

Impaired Coping

Related to

- Situational crisis
- Maturational crisis
- Adventitious crisis
- Serious mental illness
- Inadequate social supports
- Impaired ability to reduce anxiety
- Impaired ability to accurately appraise threat
- Poor coping skills
- Inability to problem-solve
- Inadequate level of personal resources

Desired Outcome The patient will demonstrate improved coping.

Assessment/Interventions and *Rationales*

1. Nurses and trained mental healthcare workers meet with the patient and family to assess the patient's various needs. *Patients with psychiatric problems have a wide range of needs that are best addressed in the context of the healthcare team.*
2. Identify the patient's highest level of functioning in terms of living skills, learning skills, and working skills. *Identifying the highest level of functioning provides*

a baseline evaluation of whether interventions help maintain or improve the patient's level of functioning.

3. Identify the social supports available to the family such as community support to help the patient function optimally through support groups and education. *Family members need a variety of supports to prevent family deterioration.*

4. Identify community support that can promote continuity of care, such as:
   a. Residential services
   b. Transportation services
   c. Outpatient services
   d. Case management
   e. Peer support and peer-led services
   f. 24/7 emergency and crisis stabilization services
   g. Crisis lines and text services
   h. Homeless and crisis hotlines
   Comprehensive community support services are available to help individuals function at optimal levels and slow their rate of relapse.

5. Obtain a referral for social skills training, especially if the patient is living with family. *Social skills training is an evidence-based practice that helps individuals understand and improve social behavior. This training is associated with decreased relapses and improved interactions with others, including families.*

6. Work with the patient and family to identify the patient's prodromal (early) signs of impending relapse. *The patient and family can access professional services before a full exacerbation of the illness occurs.*

7. Assist patient and family in identifying a vocational rehabilitation service for the patient. *Vocational rehabilitation prepares individuals with serious mental illness for work. Employment makes a significant contribution to relapse prevention, improved clinical outcomes, and enhanced self-image.*

8. Teach the patient and family about psychiatric medications, including their purpose, benefits, potential side effects, adverse effects, and who to contact with questions or concerns. *Providing education on medications empowers the patient to engage in self-care, reduces relapse rates, and helps prevent or delay future episodes by promoting adherence and early recognition of concerns.*

👪 NURSE, PATIENT, AND FAMILY RESOURCES

Crisis Text Line
A 24/7, free, confidential line where a live, trained volunteer Crisis Counselor receives the text and responds from a secure, online platform.
www.crisistextline.org

Emotions Anonymous
Follows the Twelve-Step program of Alcoholics Anonymous, as adapted for people with emotional problems.
www.emotionsanonymous.org

988 Lifeline Chat and Text
Provides emotional support from caring crisis counselors, 24/7/365.
https://suicidepreventionlifeline.org/chat/

Mental Help Net
Mentalhelp.net provides accurate and up-to-date information available in the field of addiction medicine and behavioral health and has enlisted an acclaimed team of authors, treatment professionals, and editorial experts to write, review, and update content to check that it meets our high editorial standards.
www.mentalhelp.net

NAMI (National Alliance on Mental Illness)
NAMI is the National Alliance on Mental Illness, the nation's largest grassroots mental health organization dedicated to building better lives for the millions of Americans affected by mental illness. Educational materials and support for individuals with mental illness and their families.
www.nami.org

Red Cross Disaster Mental Health Services (DMHS)
Red Cross volunteers and staff work to deliver vital services—from providing relief and support to those in crisis, to helping individuals be better prepared to respond in emergencies.
www.redcross.org

Teenline Online
Teenline provides support, resources, and hope to any teen through a hotline of professionally trained teen counselors, and outreach programs that de-stigmatize and normalize mental health.
www.teenlineonline.org/talk-now

CHAPTER 17

Anger, Aggression, and Violence

Anger, aggression, and violence are complex emotional and behavioral responses that can strain the skills and resources of healthcare providers and society. Distinguishing between these terms provides a starting point for intervening and preventing potentially damaging outcomes and society.

- Anger is a primal and natural human emotion that can motivate and energize individuals to take productive action. However, when anger becomes overwhelming or uncontrollable and lead to aggressive or violent behavior.

- Aggression is the behavioral expression of anger, characterized by directing angry or hostile feelings toward others.

- Violence is an extreme form of aggression, involving the intentional physical manifestation of anger and aggression—whether threatened or actual—that can result in psychological harm, physical injury, or death.

Some individuals are more prone to angry, aggression, and violent behaviors than others. Those at higher risk include individuals who misuse substances, have poor coping skills, experience psychosis, or exhibit antisocial, borderline, or narcissistic traits. Additionally, cognitive disorders, paranoia, or mania can contribute to increased aggression.

Managing anger, aggression, and violence in healthcare settings is critical, as safety is always a top priority. Fortunately, most patients demonstrate signs of increasing anxiety before escalating to dangerous levels. The most effective nursing interventions occur early, before anger spirals out of control. However, when anger has already escalated, aggression is evident, and the risk of violence is imminent, different intervention strategies are necessary.

RISK FACTORS

Anger, aggression, and even violence were once necessary for survival—early humans relied on these responses to defend themselves against predators, secure resources, and project their communities. For instance, hunter-gatherers who lack the instinct to fight off a threat might not have lived long enough to pass on their genes. As a result, some individuals may be more biologically predisposed to respond to life events with irritability, frustration, and anger.

Anger, frustration, and impulsive reactions may also be influenced by underlying neurological or psychiatric conditions. Conditions such as brain tumors, Alzheimer's disease, temporal lobe epilepsy, and traumatic brain injuries can lead to disinhibition, increasing the likelihood of violence. Additionally, abnormalities in the amygdala, hippocampus, hypothalamus, and prefrontal cortex are linked toh anger and aggression. Altered levels of neurotransmitters—especially serotonin, dopamine, and gamma-aminobutyric acid (GABA)—may play a role in regulating these responses.

Nursing Care for Anger, Aggression, and Violence

The following sections provide nursing guidelines for (1) assessing anger and potential the potential for aggression when a patient's behavior escalates and (2) implementing interventions, including the use of restraints or seclusion when a patient's anger has escalated to physical violence. All interventions follow hospital protocols that adhere to legal and ethical standards for safety and patient care.

Assessment

- History of violence (the strongest predictor of future behavior)
- Paranoia
- Alcohol or drug use
- Mania or agitated depression
- Personality disorders (e.g., antisocial, borderline, or narcissistic)
- Oppositional defiant disorder or conduct disorder
- Psychosis (i.e., hallucinations, delusions, and disorganized thought)
- Command hallucinations
- Neurocognitive disorder

- Intermittent explosive disorder
- Physical conditions (e.g., chronic illness, pain, or loss of body function)

Important questions:

- Have you thought of harming someone else?
- Have you ever seriously injured another person?
- What is the most violent thing you have ever done?

Assessment Guidelines: Violence and Aggression

- A history of violence is the strongest predictor of violence.
- Does the patient express a desire or intent to harm another?
- Does the patient have a specific plan?
- Does the patient have the means or access to carry out the plan?
- Consider demographic risk factors, including sex (male), age (14–24 years), low socioeconomic status, and limited support systems

Self-Assessment

Evaluate your own responses to the patient's anger, as reacting defensively or taking it personally can escalate the situation. Consider whether you are:

- Responding aggressively toward the patient
- Avoiding the patient
- Suppressing or denying either your own feeling of anger or the patient's anger

Additionally, assess your level of comfort in managing the situation and determine whether you need support from other staff to help de-escalate a potentially volatile encounter.

Interventions for Anger, Aggression, and Violent Behavior

When managing angry, aggressive, or potentially violent patients, interventions should follow a least restrictive approach to help them gain control. This typically begins with verbal and nonverbal de-escalation techniques, progresses to pharmacological interventions if needed, and only as a last resort, involves seclusion and physical restraints to ensure safety.

Verbal and Nonverbal Interventions

Begin by telling the patient that you are concerned and want to listen. It is important to clearly state your expectations for the patient's behavior: "I expect that you will stay in control."

Approach the patient in a controlled, nonthreatening, and caring manner. Allow enough personal space so that you are not perceived as threatening. Stay about 1 foot farther than the patient can reach with arms or legs. Make sure that the patient is not between you and the door. Choose a quiet place to talk to the patient but one that is visible to other staff. Inform the staff about the situation so they can be prepared to intervene if the situation escalates.

When anger escalates, a patient's ability to mentally process information decreases. It is important to speak to the patient slowly and in short sentences, using a low and calm voice. Use open-ended statements and questions such as "You think people are treating you unfairly?" Ask what is behind the angry feelings and behaviors. You may want to give two options such as, "Do you want to take a break in your room or the quiet room for a while?" This approach decreases the sense of powerlessness that often precipitates violence while also providing external boundaries.

Pharmacological Interventions

When a patient is showing increased signs (e.g., pacing, hitting the wall, or yelling) or symptoms (e.g., "I'm so angry!") of anxiety or agitation, it is appropriate to offer the patient an as-needed medication, as ordered, to relieve symptoms. When used in conjunction with psychosocial interventions and de-escalation techniques, medication can prevent an aggressive or violent incident.

Inhaled loxapine (Adasuve), a first-generation antipsychotic, has FDA approval for the acute treatment of agitation associated with schizophrenia or bipolar I disorder in adults. This medication is rapidly absorbed in the lungs. However, its use is restricted due to the risk of fatal bronchospasm and must be administered only in a certified healthcare setting.

Second-generation injectable antipsychotics, such as olanzapine (Zyprexa) and ziprasidone (Geodon), are useful in reducing agitation. An orally disintegrating tablet version of olanzapine (Zyprexa Zydis) is an alternative

Table 17.1 Drugs Used for Acute Management of Violent Behavior

Generic (Trade)	Forms	Considerations
Antianxiety Agents (Benzodiazepines)		
Lorazepam (Ativan)	PO, SL, IM, IV	Drug of choice in this class. Short half-life and less hepatic metabolism relative to most other agents in class.
Alprazolam (Xanax)	PO	Paradoxical (opposite response) with personality disorders and older adults.
Diazepam (Valium)	PO, IM, IV	FDA approved for alcohol withdrawal agitation. Rapid onset of calming and sedating. Long half-life; use with caution in older adults.
First-Generation Antipsychotics		
Haloperidol (Haldol)	PO, IM, IV	Favorable side effect profile. IV administration requires ECG monitoring. Due to risk of neuroleptic malignant syndrome, keep hydrated, check vital signs, and test for muscle rigidity.
Loxapine (Adasuve)	Inhalation	Rapid systemic delivery. Available only through a restricted program. Risk for fatal bronchospasm—contraindicated for individuals with breathing disorders.
Perphenazine	PO	Risk of neuroleptic malignant syndrome increases; keep hydrated. Frequent vital sign checks and testing for muscular rigidity are recommended.
Chlorpromazine (Thorazine)	PO, PR, IM	Very sedating. Injections can cause pain; watch for hypotension.

Second-Generation Antipsychotics

Drug	Route	Comments
Risperidone (Risperdal)	PO, disintegrating tablet	Calms while treating the underlying condition. Watch for hypotension with reflex tachycardia. Increased risk of stroke in older adults.
Olanzapine (Zyprexa, Zyprexa Zydis)	PO, IM, disintegrating tablet	IM is FDA-approved for agitation with schizophrenia or bipolar I in adults. Useful in patients unresponsive to haloperidol. Calms while treating the underlying condition. Avoid IM combination with lorazepam. Increased risk of stroke in older adults.
Ziprasidone (Geodon)	PO, IM	IM is FDA-approved for agitation with schizophrenia in adults. Use cautiously with QT prolongation. Less sedating.
Combinations		
Haloperidol (Haldol), lorazepam (Ativan), and diphenhydramine (Benadryl) or benztropine (Cogentin)	IM	Commonly used in the acute setting. Men who are young and athletic are at increased risk of dystonia. Consider akathisia if agitation increases.

FDA, Food and Drug Administration; *IM*, intramuscularly; *IV*, intravenously; *PO*, orally; *PR*, per rectum (rectally); *SL*, sublingually. From U.S. Food and Drug Administration (various dates). Online label repository. https://labels.fda.gov/ .

to injectable medication. The tablets disintegrate in saliva almost immediately, and the effects occur rapidly.

A combination of an antipsychotic and a benzodiazepine can be administered intramuscularly. Diphenhydramine or benztropine added to the injection reduces extrapyramidal side effects. Table 17.1 lists medications that have been found useful in managing aggression.

Seclusion or Restraints

In some cases, aggression and the risk for violence necessitate the use of seclusion or restraints to ensure the safety of the patient and others. Seclusion involves confining a patient to a room they cannot leave at will. Restraint refers to any method that restricts the movement of arms, legs, body, or head. These interventions require an order from a licensed provider, though in emergency situations, the order may be obtained retroactively. Licensing and accreditation agencies regulate the frequency of observation and assessment.

All team members are trained in the proper use of seclusion and physical restraint. A designated leader communicates clearly with the patient, explains the necessity of the intervention, and directs the team's actions. The leader informs the patient of the team's intent to either seclude or restrain and the reason for the actions. Once the patient is secluded or restrained, the nurse may obtain an order for medication and administer it if needed. Box 17.1 provides guidelines for the use of seclusion and restraints.

Signs and Symptoms

Violence is usually preceded by the following:
- Hyperactivity is the most significant predictor of imminent violence (e.g., pacing, restlessness)
- Increasing anxiety and tension: clenched jaw or fists, rigid posture, fixed or tense facial expression, mumbling, shortness of breath, sweating, rapid pulse
- Verbal aggression such asusing profanity, argumentativeness, intrusive demands
- Voice changes—loud or high-pitched voice, or unusually soft voice, requiring others to strain to hear
- Altered level of consciousness—confusion, disorientation, memory impairment

Box 17.1 **Guidelines for the Use of Seclusion and Restraint**

Indications for Use
- To protect the patient from self-harm
- To prevent the patient from harming others

Legal Requirements
- Multidisciplinary involvement
- Signed order from an appropriate health care provider per state law
- Notification of a patient advocate or relative
- Discontinuation of restraint or seclusion as soon as it is no longer necessary

Documentation
- Behaviors that led to restraint or seclusion
- Least restrictive interventions attempted prior to restraint
- Patient's response to interventions
- Plan of care for seclusion or restraint use implementation
- Ongoing evaluations by appropriate healthcare providers

Clinical Assessments
- Patient's mental status at time of restraint
- Physical examination to identify medical conditions contributing to behaviors
- Evaluation of the necessity of restraints

Observation
- Continuous 1:1 staff observation
- Document patient status every 15 minutes
- Assess range of motion
- Monitor vital signs regularly
- If restrained, observe circulation in hands and feet and check for chafing
- Ensure adequate nutrition, hydration, and elimination

Release Procedure
- Ensure that the patient can follow instructions and maintain control
- Safely discontinue seclusion or restraints
- Conduct a debriefing with the patient

Other Tips
- Physically holding a patient constitutes a restraint
- Raising all four side rails is considered a restraint unless for seizure precautions
- Tucking sheets too tightly, restricting movement, is a form of a restraint
- Orders for seclusion or restraint are never written on an as-needed basis

- Abnormal eye contact—either intense or avoidance of eye contact
- Recent violent acts, including property violence
- Verbal silence with a sudden refusal to speak
- Alcohol or substance intoxication
- Possession of a weapon or object that might be used as a weapon such as a fork, knife, meal tray
- Conditions conducive to violence:
  - Overcrowding
  - Inexperienced staff
  - Confrontational/controlling staff
  - Poor limit setting
  - Arbitrary revocation of privileges

Nursing Diagnoses

Impaired coping is an appropriate nursing diagnosis for patients who exhibit angry and aggressive responses to stressful, frustrating, or threatening situations (International Council of Nurses, 2019). When a patient's anxiety and anger escalate to a level where there is a potential for harm to self and others, *risk for violence* becomes the priority. During this time, talking-down skills are used first. Offering as-needed medication is the next step. If pharmacotherapy is ineffective, restraint or seclusion of an aggressive patient may be necessary.

Patients Who are Angry and Hostile

Impaired Coping

Related to
- Biochemical alterations in the brain
- Inadequate perception of control
- Perception of being threatened
- Impaired tension management
- Misperception of others' motives
- Knowledge deficit
- Overwhelming crisis situations
- Impaired reality testing
- Severe anxiety
- Substance use, intoxication, or withdrawal
- Ineffective problem-solving strategies or skills
- Personal vulnerability

Desired Outcome The patient will demonstrate improved coping.

Assessment/Interventions and *Rationales*

1. Assess your own feelings in the situation. Do not take the patient's abusive statements personally or become defensive. *Although patients are often skillful at making personal and pointed statements, they do not know nurses personally and have no basis on which to make accurate judgments.*

2. Avoid angry responses, no matter how threatened or angry you feel. *Confrontational responses by an authority figure will increase hostility.*

3. Monitor anger and aggressive behavior. Do not minimize such behavior in the hope that it will go away. *Ignoring or downplaying aggressive behavior can delay necessary interventions and increase the risk of escalation.*

4. Set clear, consistent, and enforceable limits on behavior, and stress the consequences of not adhering to those behaviors. *Behavioral limits provide structure for the patient and promote consistent responses from the staff.*

5. Emphasize that cognitively aware patients are responsible for the consequences of their aggressive behavior, including legal charges. *Some patients may mistakenly believe that aggressive behavior in a hospital setting carries no legal consequences, but most states classify assaults on healthcare providers as a felony.*

6. Emphasize that you are setting limits on specific behaviors, not feelings (e.g., "It is okay to be angry with Dennis, but it is not okay to threaten him or yell at him"). *Patients can learn to express feelings safely while recognizing that acting on feelings is not acceptable.*

7. Use a matter-of-fact, neutral approach. Remain calm using a moderate, firm voice and calming hand gestures. *A matter-of-fact approach can help interrupt the cycle of escalating anger.*

8. If anger escalates and the situation becomes unsafe, inform the patient that you will step away briefly and return at a specified time. Always follow through to reinforce consistency and prevent reinforcing aggression. *When this response is given in a neutral, matter-of-fact manner, the patient's anger is not rewarded.*

9. Provide positive feedback for interactive communication, such as non–illness-related topics, by responding to requests and providing emotional support. *This reinforces appropriate communication and behaviors and gives the patient and nurse time to share healthier communication and increase rapport.*

10. Avoid power struggles. *Power struggles are perceived as a challenge and generally lead to escalation of the conflict.*

11. Respond to feelings of anxiety or anger with active listening and validation of distress. *Active listening and validation build trust and allow the patient to feel heard and understood.*

12. Work with the patient to identify triggers for anger. *Recognizing triggers is an important step in a structured violence-prevention strategy.*

13. Identify factors that contribute to violence, such as family dysfunction, psychiatric conditions, or environmental stressors. *Treating the risk factors (e.g., getting family counseling, finding a job) reduces the family cycle of violence.*

14. Work with the patient to identify what supports are lacking, and problem-solve ways to attain support. *Feeling alone feeds into a sense of powerlessness and anger. Gaining external support promotes a sense of safety.*

15. Teach the patient, and if possible, the family or significant others, the steps in the problem-solving process.
    a. Define the problem
    b. Generate alternative solutions
    c. Select an alternative solution
    d. Implement the solution
    e. Evaluate the results of the solution
    Many people have never learned a systematic and effective approach to dealing with and mastering tough life situations or problems. A concrete method for problem solving empowers the patient.

16. Role-play alternative behaviors that can be used in stressful and overwhelming situations when becoming angry. *Role-playing allows the patient to rehearse alternative ways of handling stressful and angry feelings in a safe environment.*

17. Work with the patient to set behavioral goals. Give positive feedback when goals are reached. *Setting goals and giving positive feedback allow the patient a sense of control while learning goal-setting skills. Achieving self-set goals can enhance a person's sense of self and support new and more effective approaches to feelings of frustration.*

18. Explore outlets for stress and anxiety such as exercising, listening to music, reading, talking to others, attending support groups, and participating in a sport. *Alternative means of channeling emotions may help patients decrease anxiety and stress and allow for*

more cognitive approaches to their situation (e.g., using a problem-solving approach).

19. Provide the patient and family with community resources that teach assertiveness training, anger management, and stress-reduction techniques. *Goal-directed and structured activities provide patients and families with continued support in the community.*

Patients With Potential to Harm Self or Others

Risk for Violence

Related to
- Biochemical alterations in the brain
- History of violent behavior
- History of childhood abuse or witnessing family violence
- History of violence against others
- Psychosis (i.e., hallucinations, delusions, disorganized thought)
- Impulsivity
- Rage
- Mania
- Cognitive impairment
- Substance use, intoxication, or withdrawal
- Excitement, irritability, agitation

Desired Outcome The patient will be free from violence.

Assessment/Interventions and *Rationales*

1. Keep environmental stimulation at a minimum during periods of anger and aggressive behavior (e.g., lower lights, keep levels of noise down, ask patients and visitors to leave the area, or have staff take the patient to another area). *Overstimulation can increase the patient's anxiety level, leading to increased agitation or aggressive behaviors.*

2. Keep your voice calm and speak in a low, steady tone. A high-pitched or rapid voice can escalate anxiety, whereas a calm, slow-paced tone promotes de-escalation. *A calm, steady tone of voice helps regulate emotional responses by signaling safety and stability to the patient. Speaking slowly and evenly can have a soothing effect, promoting de-escalation by reducing the patient's physiological arousal and helping them process information more effectively.*

3. Call the patient by name and, if necessary, introduce yourself. Orient the patient as needed and explain what you are going to do. *Calling the patient by name helps to establish contact. Orienting and giving information can minimize misrepresentation of nurses' intentions.*

4. Use personal safety precautions:
   a. When you are in the patient's room, leave the door open.
   b. If you sense a potential for violence, alert other staff to stay nearby.
   c. Never turn your back on an angry patient.
   d. Have an exit available.
   e. For home visits: (1) Visit the patient with a colleague if there is concern regarding aggression, and (2) leave the home immediately if there are signs that the patient's behavior is escalating.
   Your safety is always the first priority. Always call in colleagues or other staff if you feel threatened or in physical danger.

5. Nursing and security staff require initial and ongoing training in managing disruptive behavior, including anger de-escalation and seclusion and restraint procedures. *Professional training increases safe responses and reduces negative outcomes such as injury.*

6. Document the patient's behaviors and staff interventions during each level of intervention. *Documentation provides direction for future episodes and is essential from a legal standpoint.*

7. When addressing escalating anger, start with the least restrictive intervention first and progress to more restrictive methods only if necessary:
   a. Verbal intervention
   b. Decrease environmental stimulation or suggest a quiet area
   c. Pharmacological interventions
   d. Physical seclusion or restraint
   Human dignity and autonomy are supported through the least restrictive approach. Use seclusion or restraint only when there is no less restrictive alternative.

8. Encourage the patient to talk about angry feelings and find ways to tolerate or reduce angry and aggressive feelings. *When the patient feels heard and understood and has help with problem-solving alternative options, de-escalation of anger and aggression is often possible.*

9. Use empathetic verbal interventions (e.g., "It must be frightening to be here and to be feeling out of control"). *Empathetic verbal intervention is the most effective method of calming an agitated, fearful, anxious patient.*
10. When interpersonal interventions fail to decrease the patient's anger, consider the need for medication. Assessment includes determining whether aggression is acute or chronic. *Often pharmacological interventions can help patients gain control of their behavior and prevent continued escalation of anger and hostile impulses.*
11. Alert other staff and hospital security if anger and aggressive responses are evident and ask for their presence at a distance. *Having staff present at a distance can provide support and encourage the patient to regain control without direct confrontation.*
12. When interpersonal interventions and pharmacological interventions fail, physical intervention (i.e., seclusion or restraint) is the final resort. Follow organization protocol. Refer to Box 17.1 for guidelines for the use of restraints. *Protocol tells staff when to restrain, how to restrain, how long before a provider's order is needed, nursing interventions for the patient during the period of restraint or seclusion, how often to check restraints or the patient in seclusion, whom to call, and how often the need for restraints or seclusion must be reevaluated by a physician.*

NURSE, PATIENT, AND FAMILY RESOURCES

The Center for Anger Resolution
The Center provides counseling, education, and training on anger management.
www.angerbusters.com

Anger Management
Mentalhelp.net provides accurate and up-to-date information available in the field of addiction medicine and behavioral health and has enlisted an acclaimed team of authors, treatment professionals, and editorial experts to write, review, and update content to check that it meets our high editorial standards.
www.mentalhelp.net
Search for "anger management."

Centers for Disease Control and Prevention
CDC is the nation's leading science-based, data-driven, service organization that protects public health.
www.cdc.gov
Search for "anger" to find multiple articles.

Centers for Medicare and Medicaid Services
CMS is the federal agency that provides health coverage and works in partnership with the entire healthcare community to improve quality, equity, and outcomes in the healthcare system.
www.cms.gov
Search for "seclusion and restraint" for national guidelines

National Anger Management Association (NAMA)
NAMA is the international professional association for the fields of anger management, crisis intervention, domestic violence, and parent training.
https://namass.org/index.html

CHAPTER 18

Family Violence

This chapter provides a comprehensive overview of the various forms of violence and abuse, emphasizing that abuse is not limited to physical harm but extends into emotional, sexual, neglectful, and economic domains. Family violence can take the form of emotional, physical, or sexual abuse, neglect, or economic abuse.

- Emotional abuse undermines self-worth and can leave lasting scars on one's ability to connect, feel deeply, and succeed later in life.
- Physical abuse encompasses not only emotional harm but also the risk of enduring physical injuries—including scarring, chronic pain, and, in severe cases, death.
- Sexual abuse of children can inflict deep psychological harm, leading to low self-esteem, self-hatred, emotional instability, and increased anger or aggression. This trauma often undermines the ability to trust others, making it difficult to form healthy relationships and protect oneself.
- Neglect can have equally devastating effects, resulting in malnutrition, insufficient supervision, failure to thrive, and a lack of basic necessities such as adequate clothing, shelter, and medical care. In response, children may exhibit apathy, heightened fearfulness, and even destructive behavior.
- Economic abuse is controlling a person's access to economic resources, making an individual financially dependent. This financial abuse is the greatest barrier to partners leaving abusive situations. Older adults may lose assets, property, and self-agency.

In this chapter, we discuss abuse as it occurs in the lifespan. Family violence includes child abuse, intimate partner violence, and older adult abuse.

Box 18.1 Interview Guidelines

- Conduct the interview in a private setting.
- Be direct, honest, and professional.
- Use language that the patient easily understands.
- Ask the patient to clarify any words or terms that are unclear.
- Demonstrate empathy and understanding.
- Remain fully attentive.
- Inform the patient if a referral to child or adult protective services is necessary, and clearly explain the process.
- Assess the patient's safety, and take steps to reduce danger.
- Avoid suggesting that the patient was at fault.

ASSESSMENT

Sensitivity is required of a nurse who suspects family violence. A person who feels judged or accused of wrongdoing is likely to become defensive. This defensiveness will undermine attempts to modify family coping strategies. The nurse should ask about ways of solving disagreements or methods of disciplining children rather than using the word abuse or violence, which appears judgmental and therefore is threatening to the family. It is also important not to assume a person's sexual orientation. Use the term partner when asking about the relationship. Interview guidelines are suggested in Box 18.1.

Signs and Symptoms

- Feelings of helplessness or powerlessness
- Repeated visits to the emergency room or hospital
- Vague complaints such as insomnia, abdominal pain, hyperventilation, headache, or menstrual problems
- Unexplained bruises at various stages of healing
- Injuries (e.g., bruises, fractures, scrapes, lacerations) that do not match the reported accident
- A frightened, withdrawn, depressed, or despondent appearance

Assessment Questions

The nurse uses therapeutic communication techniques to gather detailed information. Using your discretion, decide which questions are appropriate to complete your assessment. A general question that can be posed to any victim of family violence is "Tell me about what happened to you." Other questions are based on the relationship between the abused and the perpetrators of violence.

For Children

"Who takes care of you?"

"Have you been taken to the hospital for accidents or injuries?"

For Parents

"What arrangements do you make when you have to leave your child alone?"

"How do you discipline your child?"

"When your infant cries for a long time, how do you get your infant to stop?"

"What about your child's behavior bothers you the most?"

"Who helps you care for your children?"

"How much time do you have for yourself?"

For Intimate Partners

"How do you and your partner resolve disagreements?"

"Have you been hit, kicked, or otherwise hurt by someone in the past year? By whom?"

"Do you feel safe in your current relationship?"

"Is there a partner from a previous relationship who is making you feel unsafe now?"

For Older Adults

"Do you feel safe at home?"

"Has anyone limited your daily activities?"

"Does anyone speak to you in a threatening way?"

"Does anyone hit you?"

"Has anyone asked you for money or asked you to sign contracts you didn't recognize?"

Assessment Guidelines

During your assessment and counseling, maintain an interested and empathetic manner. Retain self-awareness and avoid expressions of anger, shock, or disapproval of the perpetrator or the situation. Assess for the following:

A. Signs and symptoms of family violence
B. Qualities of individuals who are vulnerable to abusing children are listed in Box 18.2
C. Physical, sexual, or emotional abuse and neglect and economic maltreatment in the case of older adults
D. Family coping patterns
E. Patient's support system
F. Substance use
G. Suicidal or homicidal ideation
H. Posttrauma syndrome

If the patient is a child or an older adult, identify the protection agency in your state that will need to be notified.

SELF-ASSESSMENT

Working with individuals who experience violence can evoke intense and overwhelming feelings, particularly in new nurses. Strong negative feelings regarding abuse may cloud your judgment, potentially interfering with objective assessment and intervention. Additionally, a personal history of abuse may lead to excessive identification with the victim. Sharing your experiences and emotions with trusted colleagues can manage these reactions, easing anger and frustration while preventing the impulse to overstep professional boundaries.

Box 18.2 Assessing Vulnerability for Child Abuse

- New parents who display rejecting, hostile, or indifferent behavior toward their infant.
- Teenage parents, many of whom are still minors, may require additional support and guidance in infant care, managing expectations, and establishing a reliable support system.
- Parents with intellectual disabilities benefit from careful, explicit, and repeated instructions on child care and recognizing the infant's needs.
- Parents who grew up in abusive homes, which is the strongest risk factor for perpetuating family violence.

Nursing Diagnoses

Violence inflicts pain, psychological anguish, and physical injury and can even result in death. Therefore *risk for violence* is a major concern for nurses and other healthcare professionals (International Council of Nurses, 2019). This chapter discusses *risk for violence* among children, intimate partners, and older adults.

Although survivors of family violence clearly require intervention, a second level of nursing care is also directed toward the perpetrators. In this chapter, we use *impaired family coping* to address the support needed to break the cycle of violence. Perpetrators may include parents, intimate partners, and older adult caregivers.

There are many other nursing diagnoses the nurse can address in caring for children and adults who are suffering from abuse at the hands of others. These include *anxiety, fear, impaired family role performance, posttrauma response, powerlessness, caregiver stress, disturbed body image, chronic low and situational low self-esteem*, and impaired *parenting*.

Intervention Guidelines

Child, Intimate Partner, and Older Adult

A. Establish rapport before focusing on the details of the violent experience.
B. Provide reassurance that the patient is not to blame for the abuse.
C. Allow the patient to share their experience without interruptions.
D. If the patient is an adult, assure confidentiality.
E. If the patient is a child, report abuse to the appropriate state-designated authorities.
F. If the patient is an older adult, consult state laws to determine the correct reporting procedures.
G. Develop a comprehensive safety plan in situations of partner abuse.

Nursing Care for Family Violence

Survivors of Abuse

Risk for Violence

Related to
- A history of rage reactions
- Inadequate coping skills

- Current or past substance use
- Limited impulse control
- Pathological family dynamics
- Experiences of violence, neglect, or emotional deprivation during childhood
- Psychiatric disorders

Abused Child

Desired Outcome The child will be free from violence.

Assessment/Interventions and *Rationales*

1. Use a nonthreatening, nonjudgmental relationship with the parents. *If the parents feel judged or blamed, they may become defensive, potentially withdrawing support, seeking help elsewhere or not seeking help at all.*
2. Understand that children often avoid betraying their parents. *Even in an intolerable situation, the parents are the most important security the child knows.*
3. Perform a complete physical assessment of the child. *A complete physical assessment will support essential care and substantiate reporting to the child welfare agency if required.*
4. Use dolls to help tell the child's story. The child might not know how to articulate what happened or might be afraid of punishment. *Using dolls can be a more comfortable, less direct way for the child to express themselves.*

Forensic Issues With an Abused Child

1. Identify your agency and state policies on reporting child abuse. Contact the supervisor or social worker to implement appropriate reporting. *Healthcare workers are mandated to report cases of suspected or actual child abuse.*
2. Ensure that proper procedures are followed, and evidence is collected. *If the child is temporarily taken to a safe environment, appropriate evidence helps protect the child's future welfare.*
3. Keep accurate and detailed records of the incident:
   a. Verbatim statements of who caused the injury and when it occurred
   b. Body map to indicate size, color, shape, areas, and types of injuries, along with an explanation
   c. Physical evidence, when possible, of sexual abuse
   d. Photographs (check hospital policy regarding permissions)

*Accurate records can help ensure the child's future safety
and court presentation.*

4. Conduct a forensic examination of a sexually assaulted
   child according to specific protocols provided by law
   enforcement agencies and particular medical facilities.
   Ideally, SANE nurses, or nurses who have advanced
   training, will conduct the examination. *The proper
   collection, handling, and storage of forensic specimens are
   crucial to the court presentation.*

Abused Partner

Desired Outcome The abused partner will be free from
violence.

Assessment/Interventions and *Rationales*

1. Ensure that medical attention is provided to the
   patient. Ask permission to take photographs. *If the
   patient wants to file charges, photographs will support the
   case.*
2. Set up an interview in private and ensure confidentiality. *The patient might be terrified of retribution and further
   attacks from the partner for telling someone about the abuse.*
3. In a non-threatening manner, assess the following
   areas:
   a. Sexual abuse
   b. Physical abuse
   c. Economic abuse
   d. Suicidal or homicidal thoughts
   *These are all vital issues in planning care. Sexual abuse
   often accompanies physical abuse. Economic abuse may deter
   the individual from leaving. Self-directed or other-directed
   violence may seem like the only way out.*
4. Encourage the patient to talk about the incident
   without interruptions. *Listening, along with attending
   behaviors, will facilitate full sharing.*
5. Assess for the level of violence in the home (Box 18.3).
   *Each cycle of violence may intensify over time, increasingly
   endangering the lives of survivors and their children. For
   instance, when a perpetrator resorts to choking, it signifies
   an immediate and heightened risk to the individual's life.*
6. Ask about the welfare of the children in the home.
   Intimate partner abuse is often accompanied by child abuse.
7. Assess whether the patient has a safe place to retreat
   when violence is escalating. Provide a list of shelters

> ### Box 18.3 Partner Abuse—Assessing the Level of Violence in the Home
>
> Does the patient feel safe?
> Has there been a recent increase in violence?
> Has the patient been choked?
> Is there a weapon in the house?
> Has the perpetrator used or threatened to use a weapon?
> Has the perpetrator threatened to harm the children?
> Has the perpetrator threatened to kill the patient?

or safe houses with other written information. *When an abused partner decides to leave, the risk of homicide can dramatically increase. Access to an emergency shelter may be the critical factor between life and death.*

Forensic Issues With an Abused Partner

1. Identify whether the patient is interested in pressing charges. If yes, give information on:
   a. Attorneys who specialize in abuse
   b. Nonprofit law firms for low-income individuals and families
   c. Community advocates
   Legal support and advocates who can direct the abused partner to community resources are essential in helping to establish independence.
2. Identify your state laws for documenting and reporting suspected partner abuse. *State laws vary on the process for documenting and reporting domestic violence.*
3. Provide a written plan that includes shelter and referral numbers that can be used during the escalation of anxiety, before actual violence erupts. *A sense of emergency may be the motivation to leave, and a plan must be in place to keep the patient safe.*
4. Emphasize the following messages:
   a. "No one deserves to be beaten."
   b. "You cannot make anyone hurt you."
   c. "It is not your fault."
   When self-esteem is eroded, people often buy into the myth that they deserved the abuse because they did something wrong, and if they had not done it, then it would not have happened.

5. Encourage patients to reach out to family and friends whom they might have been avoiding or isolated from. *Often survivors of violence are isolated from family and friends due to shame and/or control on the part of their partners who want to isolate them. Rallying support will strengthen the patient's resolve.*

6. Become familiar with therapists in your community with experience working with battered partners. *Psychotherapy with survivors of trauma requires special skills on the part of even an experienced therapist.*

7. If the patient is not ready to act at this time, provide a list of community resources available:
   a. Hotlines
   b. Shelters
   c. Support groups
   d. Community advocates
   e. Social services
   It can take time for patients to make decisions to change their life situation. Survivors of abuse need appropriate information.

   See Box 18.4 for a personalized safety plan for when the abused partner is in a relationship and when the relationship is over.

Abused Older Adult

Desired Outcome The older adult will be free from violence.

Assessment/Interventions and *Rationales*

1. Conduct weekly assessments to evaluate the signs and symptoms of abuse, as well as the potential for further abuse. *This regular monitoring is essential for determining the need for further intervention.*

2. Evaluate the environmental conditions contributing to abuse or neglect (Box 18.5). *This assessment will pinpoint areas requiring intervention and determine the extent and severity of the abuse or neglect.*

3. If abuse is suspected, it is advisable to speak with the older adult and caregiver separately. *This approach can provide clearer insights into the situation, while reducing potential friction between the parties involved.*

4. Discuss with the older adult the factors leading to abuse. *Discussing these factors identifies triggers to abusive behaviors and areas for teaching for the perpetrator.*

Box 18.4 **Personalized Safety Plan**

Suggestions for Increasing Safety—In the Relationship

I will have important phone numbers available to my children and myself.

I can tell_____ and_____ about the violence and ask them to call the police if they hear suspicious noises coming from my home.

If I leave my home, I can go (list four places)____,____,____, or_____.

I can leave extra money, car keys, clothes, and copies of documents with_____.

If I leave, I will bring_____ (see checklist below).

To ensure safety and independence, I can: keep change for phone calls with me at all times; open my own savings account; rehearse my escape route with a support person; and review my safety plan on_____ (date).

Suggestions for Increasing Safety—When the Relationship Is Over

I can change the locks. I can install steel or metal doors, a security system, smoke detectors, and an outside lighting system.

I will inform_____ and_____ that my partner no longer lives with me and ask them to call the police if my former partner is observed near my home or my children.

I will tell people who take care of my children the names of those who have permission to pick them up. The people who have permission are:_____,_____, and_____.

I can tell_____ at work about my situation and ask_____ to screen my calls.

I can avoid stores, banks, and_____ that I used when I lived with my abusive partner.

I can obtain a protective order from_____. I can keep it on or near me at all times, as well as have a copy with_____.

If I feel down and ready to return to a potentially abusive situation, I can call_____ for support or attend workshops and support groups to gain support and strengthen my relationships with other people.

Important Phone Numbers

Police_____

Hotline_____

Friends_____

Shelter_____

Box 18.4 Personalized Safety Plan—cont'd

Items to Take Checklist
Identification
Mobile phones and chargers
Birth certificates for me and my children
Social Security cards
School and medical records
Money, bankbooks, credit cards
Keys (house/car/office)
Driver's license and registration
Medications
Change of clothes
Welfare identification
Passports, Green Cards, work permits
Divorce papers
Lease/rental agreement, house deed
Mortgage payment book, current unpaid bills
Insurance papers
Address book
Pictures, jewelry, items of sentimental value
Children's favorite toys and/or blankets

Box 18.5 Older Adult Abuse/Neglect—Home Assessment

- House in poor repair
- Inadequate heat, lighting, furniture, cooking utensils
- Presence of garbage, rodents, or old food in the kitchen
- Lack of assistive devices
- Locks on refrigerator
- Blocked stairways
- Older adult lying in urine, feces, or food
- Unpleasant odors that may signal unsanitary conditions

---

5. Stress concern for physical safety. *Stressing concern validates that the situation is serious.*

Forensic Issues With An Abused Older Adult

1. Know your state laws regarding older adult abuse. Notify your supervisor, healthcare providers, and

social services when a suspected abuse is reported. *Knowing the laws keeps the channels of communication open and emphasizes the need for accurate and detailed records.*

2. If undue influence is suspected, consult with an expert who is experienced in geriatric or forensic psychiatry. *Consulting with an expert can help determine whether the older adult is making medical, legal, or financial decisions based on coercion and manipulations of others to gain control of the older adult's finances, home, or decision-making.*

3. Stress that no one has the right to abuse another person. *Often individuals who have been abused begin to believe they deserve the abuse.*

4. Discuss the following with the patient:
   a. Hotline
   b. Crisis unit
   c. Emergency numbers
   Discussing these options with the patient maximizes older adult safety through the use of support systems.

5. Explore with the older adult ways to make changes. *Exploring the various ways to make changes directs the assessment to positive areas.*

6. Empower the older adult to make informed decisions about their future. *By actively involving them in planning the next steps, you can help reduce feelings of helplessness and facilitate the identification of realistic options for addressing the abusive situation.*

7. Engage community agencies to help monitor and provide resources for the older adult. *It is best to involve as many agencies as can take a legitimate role in maintaining the older adult's safety.*

Perpetrators of Abuse

Impaired Family Coping

Related to
- Domestic violence
- Inadequate support system
- Family conflict
- Young age, developmental level
- Low socioeconomic status
- Substance or alcohol use
- Psychiatric disorders

- Lack of resources
- Lack of knowledge about role skills

Parents Who Abuse

Desired Outcome Parents will demonstrate improved family coping.

Assessment/Interventions and *Rationales*
1. Identify whether the child needs the following:
   a. Hospitalization for treatment and observation
   b. Referral to child protective services
   Immediate safety of the child is foremost. Temporary removal of the child in a volatile situation gives the nurse or counselor time to assess the family situation and coping skills and to rally community resources to decrease family stress.
2. Discuss with parents the stresses the family unit is currently facing. Contact the appropriate agencies to help reduce stress:
   a. Economic aid
   b. Job opportunities
   c. Social services
   d. Family service agencies
   e. Social supports
   f. Public health nurse
   g. Daycare teacher
   h. School teacher
   i. Social worker
   j. Respite worker
   k. Anger management therapy
   l. Encourage and give referrals for a specialist in family therapy. Family therapy is complex—it teaches family members how to develop new strategies,
   With the help of outside resources, family stress can be reduced, leading to an improved ability to problem solve.
3. Reinforce the parents' strengths and acknowledge the importance of continued medical care for the child. *Giving parents credit and support for positive parenting skills will encourage growth.*
4. Work with the parents to try safe methods to effectively discipline the child. *Understanding alternatives to abuse increases healthy family functioning while minimizing feelings of frustration and helplessness.*

5. Encourage parents to join a self-help group (e.g., Parents Anonymous, family counseling, group counseling). *Learning new ways of dealing with stress takes time, and support from others acts as an important incentive to change.*
6. Provide comprehensive, written information that includes hotline numbers, community support groups, and agency contacts. *External resources not only reduce isolation but also increase support during crisis periods.*

Partners Who Abuse

Desired Outcome The partner who abuses will demonstrate improved family coping.

Assessment/Interventions and *Rationales*
1. If the partner who abuses is motivated, arrange for participation in an anger management program. *Some evidence suggests that a 6- to 8-week structural program that trains patients with anger issues may help to deactivate angry emotional states.*
2. Work with the perpetrator to recognize signs of escalating anger. *Often the perpetrator is unaware of the process leading up to the rage reaction.*
3. Work with the perpetrator to learn ways of channeling anger nonviolently. *Violence is often a learned coping skill. Adaptive skills for dealing with anger must be learned.*
4. Encourage the perpetrator to discuss thoughts and feelings with others who have similar problems. *Discussing these thoughts and feelings minimizes isolation and encourages problem-solving.*
5. Refer to self-help groups that are available virtually or in the community (e.g., Batterers Anonymous). *These groups offer a supportive environment where individuals can reflect on their behaviors alongside peers facing similar challenges.*

Provide the number of the National Domestic Violence Hotline, which is 1-800-799-SAFE (7233). *Hotlines provide immediate support for individuals who are beginning to escalate or want to stop the cycle of abuse.*

Older Adult Caregivers Who Abuse

Desired Outcome The perpetrator of older adult abuse will demonstrate improved family coping.

Assessment/Interventions and *Rationales*

1. Research your state laws regarding older adult abuse. *State laws vary regarding documenting and reporting abuse of older adults.*
2. Encourage the perpetrator to verbalize feelings about the older adult and the abusive situation. *The abuser might feel overwhelmed, isolated, and unsupported.*
3. Encourage problem-solving when identifying stressful areas. *Encouragement assesses the perpetrator's approach to problem-solving skills and explores alternatives.*
4. Meet with the entire family and identify stressors and problem areas. *Other family members might not be aware of the strain the perpetrator is under or the lack of safety for the abused family member.*
5. If there are no other family members, notify other community agencies that might help stabilize the situation:
   a. Meals on Wheels
   b. Daycare for seniors
   c. Respite services
   d. Visiting nurse service
   Support minimizes family stress and isolation and increases safety.
6. Initiate referrals for education, psychotherapy, group therapy, and support groups for the older adults and the perpetrator. *Education and therapy for an abusive caregiver may provide tools to deal with stress, develop coping skills, gain social support, and treat underlying mental health conditions such as major depressive disorder and anxiety.*
7. Suggest that family members meet together on a regular basis for problem-solving and support. *Meeting will encourage the family to learn to solve problems together.*

👪 NURSE, PATIENT, AND FAMILY RESOURCES

Adult Survivors of Child Abuse

A private Meetup group with weekly meetings based on the principles and resources of the ASCA (Adults Survivors of Child Abuse) Program, a Morris Center program for healing from the trauma of childhood abuse.
http://www.survivorsanonymousgroup.com

Child Abuse Prevention—KidsPeace

A private charity dedicated to serving the behavioral and mental health needs of children, families, and communities. (800) 334-4KID.
www.kidspeace.org

Childhelp USA

Exists to meet the physical, emotional, educational, and spiritual needs of abused, neglected, and at-risk children.
(800) 4-A-CHILD—(800) 422-4453 (hotline)
www.childhelp.org

Institute on Violence, Abuse, and Trauma (IVAT)

IVAT is a leading international resource and training center that shares and disseminates vital information, improves cross-discipline collaborations, conducts research and training, and provides direct professional services, program evaluation, and consulting.
https://www.ivatcenters.org

National Coalition Against Domestic Violence

NCADV is dedicated to supporting survivors, holding offenders accountable, and supporting advocates.
www.ncadv.org

National Domestic Violence Hotline

Provides essential tools and support to help survivors of domestic violence so they can live their lives free of abuse. Available 24 hours a day, seven days a week, 365 days a year.
www.thehotline.org
(800) 799-SAFE (hotline)

Rape, Abuse, and Incest National Network (RAINN)
The nation's largest anti-sexual violence organization that
created and operates the National Sexual Assault Hotline
(800-656-HOPE). The organization carries out programs to
prevent sexual violence, help survivors, and ensure that
perpetrators are brought to justice.
www.rainn.org

Survivors of Incest Anonymous
A 12-step, self-help recovery program, modeled after
Alcoholics Anonymous, for men and women aged 18 years
and older who were sexually abused as children.
www.siawso.org

Teen Line
Provides personal, teen-to-teen education and support
before problems become a crisis, using a national hotline,
current technologies, and community outreach.
www.teenlineonline.org
(800) TLC-TEEN

CHAPTER 19

Sexual Assault

Sexual assault is a violent crime driven by power, control, and hate, with sex used as a weapon by the perpetrator. Sexual assault includes fondling, unwanted sexual touch, and forced sexual acts. This form of violence encompasses child sexual abuse, incest, intimate partner sexual violence, sexual assault of men and boys, and drug-facilitated sexual assault.

Sexual violence often results in severe and long-term trauma. Psychological effects of include major depressive disorder, anxiety, fear, **posttraumatic stress disorder (PTSD)**, and, in some cases, suicide. Victims of incest may experience a negative self-image, major depressive disorder, eating disorders, personality disorders, self-destructive behavior, and substance use disorders.

Rape is an extreme form of sexual assault. According to the Federal Bureau of Investigation (FBI) (U.S. Department of Justice, 2013, para 1), rape is defined as, "Penetration, no matter how slight, of the vagina or anus with any body part or object, or oral penetration by a sex organ of another person, without the consent of the victim."

Although men are more often the perpetrators and women the victims, sexual assault is not gender exclusive. Women can sexually assault other women, and male-on-male sexual assault is more prevalent in prisons and the military than in the general population. Male survivors are more likely to experience physical trauma and multiple assailants compared to female survivors. However, both men and women experience **long-lasting** psychological effects.

The International Council of Nurses (ICNP, 2019) provides the nursing diagnosis of rape-trauma, defined as the physical and psychological condition that follows forced participation in sexual relations or intercourse. However, nursing care focuses on the victim's response to the rape rather than the event itself.

The ICNP defines rape-trauma response as a maladaptive reaction that disrupts a survivor's lifestyle and results in a long-term process of reorganization. This nursing diagnosis closely aligns with two DSM-5-TR disorders: acute stress disorder (ASD) and posttraumatic stress disorder (PTSD). Similar to these conditions, rape-trauma response consists of two distinct phases:

1. Acute Phase (0–2 weeks)
2. Long-term reorganization phase (2 weeks or more)

Nurses may encounter a patient right after the sexual assault or weeks, months, or even years later. In either case, the individual will benefit from compassionate and effective nursing interventions.

When available, special care for this population is provided by sexual assault nurse examiners (SANEs). They are forensic nurses who have been certified to work with victims of sexual assault. The functions of the SANE are to perform a physical examination of the survivor, collect forensic evidence, provide expert testimony regarding forensic evidence collected, and support the psychological needs of the survivor.

ASSESSMENT

Signs and Symptoms

Acute Phase (0–2 Weeks)

- Shock, numbness, and disbelief
- Appearing calm and composed
- Severe anxiety
- Tearfulness, sobbing
- Smiling or laughing inappropriately
- Disorganization and confusion
- Somatic symptoms (e.g., headaches, nausea, fatigue)

Long-Term Reorganization Phase (2 Weeks or More)

- Intrusive thoughts of the rape (daytime and nighttime)
- Flashbacks (reexperiencing the trauma)
- Violent dreams
- Insomnia
- Increased motor activity (e.g., excessive travel, changing phone numbers, avoiding certain locations)

- Mood swings, crying spells, depression
- Fears of:
  - The indoors (if the assault occurred indoors)
  - Being outdoors (if the assault occurred outdoors)
  - Being alone
  - Crowds
  - Sexual encounters

Assessment Guidelines

Assessment should be conducted in a nonthreatening, supportive manner. Use open-ended questions, broad openings, and general leads, such as "It must have been very frightening to feel like that you had no control over what was happening."

A. Assess:
  1. Physical trauma: Document using a body map, and ask permission to take photographs.
  2. Emotional trauma: Document verbatim statements of the patient.
  3. Level of anxiety: If patients are in severe-to-panic levels of anxiety, they will not be able to problem-solve or process information.
  4. Support system: Often partners or family members do not understand rape and might not be the best support at this time.
  5. Community supports (e.g., attorneys, support groups, therapists) who work in the area of sexual assault.
B. Encourage patients to tell their story, but do not pressure them to do so.

Intervention Guidelines

A. Follow institutional protocol for sexual assault cases.
B. Never leave the patient alone—continuous support is essential.
C. Maintain an accepting attitude.
D. Ensure confidentiality.
E. Encourage the patient to talk, but never pressure them to disclose details. Listen empathetically.
F. Emphasize that the survivor is not responsible for the rape.

Nursing Care for Sexual Assault

Rape-Trauma Response

Related to
• Sexual assault

Desired Outcome The patient will return to pre-crisis level of functioning.

Assessment/Interventions and *Rationales*

1. Arrange for a trusted individual to stay with the patient (e.g., friend, neighbor, or staff member) while the patient is waiting to be treated in the emergency department. *Individuals who are experiencing high levels of anxiety need someone with them until the anxiety level is reduced to moderate or mild.*

2. Approach the patient in a nonjudgmental manner. *A nurse's attitude significantly impacts the patient's emotional well-being and can enhance the therapeutic relationship.*

3. The patient's situation should not be discussed with anyone other than medical personnel involved, unless the patient gives explicit consent. *Confidentiality is crucial from a moral and ethical standpoint, as well as a legal right.*

4. Provide support and anticipate acute symptoms such as shock, numbness, disbelief, anxiety, tearfulness, disorganization, and somatic symptoms. *Patients need external support and direction during the acute phase of the rape-trauma response when anxiety levels are high.*

5. Listen and let the patient talk, but do not pressure the patient to talk. *When the patient feels understood and sets the pace of the conversation, the patient feels more in control of the situation. Allowing the patient to set the pace.*

6. If the patient expresses guilt or shame about the rape, stress that the patient did nothing wrong. *Individuals who are raped might feel guilt or shame. Reaffirming that they did nothing wrong can reduce guilt and maintain self-esteem.*

7. Ensure patient safety and assess for risk of self-harm or suicidal ideation. *Sexual assault survivors are at increased risk for depression, PTSD, and suicidal thoughts, making safety assessment essential.*

8. Avoid judgmental language. For example, consider the difference between the following words: reported rather than alleged, declined rather than refused,

penetration rather than intercourse. *Sensitive word choices support the patient during the crisis phase and as the patient recovers.*

9. Provide written information on available resources, including crisis hotlines, legal aid, and counseling services. *Survivors may have difficulty processing verbal information in crisis and benefit from written materials for later reference.*

10. Arrange for follow-up support:
    a. Rape counselor
    b. Support group
    c. Group therapy
    d. Individual therapy
    e. Crisis counseling
    Ongoing support through counseling and peer groups helps survivors process trauma, reduce isolation, and decrease the risk of long-term psychological effects such as PTSD, depression, and anxiety.

11. As anxiety resolves, identify the symptoms that patients may experience during the long-term reorganization phase, such as nightmares, phobias anxiety, depression, insomnia, and somatic symptoms. *Identifying symptoms of the long-term reorganization phase helps patients understand their experiences, reducing fear and reinforcing that these reactions are a normal part of the healing process.*

Forensic Issues for Sexual Assault Survivors

1. Assess the patient for signs and symptoms of physical trauma, with a focus on common injury sites such as the face, head, neck, and extremities. *Patients may be unaware of the extent of their injuries, and identifying trauma early ensures that immediate medical needs are prioritized.*

2. Assess for signs of drug-facilitated sexual assault (e.g., memory loss, confusion, physical symptoms). *Some survivors may not realize they were drugged, and early detection ensures appropriate medical and forensic testing.*

3. Make a body map to identify the size, color, and location of injuries. *A body map provides essential guidance for the treatment team and serves as critical legal documentation.*

4. Obtain the patient's consent before taking photographs to document injuries. *Photographic evidence provides accurate medico-legal documentation that may support future medical care and legal proceedings.*

5. Clearly explain all procedures before performing them, using a calm, matter-of-fact approach (e.g., "We would like to perform a vaginal (or rectal) examination to obtain evidence. Have you had this type of examination before?"). *Providing clear explanations helps reduce fear and anxiety in patients experiencing high levels of distress, fostering a sense of control and cooperation.*

6. Explain the forensic specimens to be collected. Inform the patient of their use in identifying and prosecuting the perpetrator:
   a. Pubic hair
   b. Skin from underneath nails
   c. Semen samples
   d. Blood
   Clear communication about forensic evidence collection helps the patient make informed decisions, reducing uncertainty and emphasizing the role of evidence in seeking justice.

7. Encourage the patient to undergo evaluation and treatment for sexually transmitted infections (STIs) before leaving the emergency department. *Many survivors do not seek follow-up care, and immediate treatment ensures timely protection against potential infections.*

8. Ensure that emergency contraception is offered and provided to women survivors of sexual assault. *Immediate access to emergency contraception reduces the risk of unintended pregnancy, addressing a critical concern for survivors.*

9. Carefully document all data:
   a. Verbatim statements
   b. Detailed observations of physical trauma
   c. Detailed observations of emotional status
   d. Physical examination findings
   e. Laboratory test results
   Accurate and thorough documentation provides essential legal evidence and supports the patient's medical and forensic needs.

🚶 NURSE, PATIENT, AND FAMILY RESOURCES

Institute on Violence, Abuse, and Trauma (IVAT)
IVAT is an organization that condemns violence and oppression in all its forms. They host two international summits annually, house three academic journals, maintain several research databases, and provide program evaluation, consultation, and a wide array of trainings addressing violence, abuse, and trauma.
www.ivatcenters.org

Rape, Abuse, and Incest National Network (RAINN)
RAINN is the nation's largest antisexual violence organization, and created and operates the National Sexual Assault Hotline.
(800) 656-HOPE (4673)
www.rainn.org
Online chat: online.rainn.org

Survivors of Incest Anonymous (SIA)
SIA is a 12-step, self-recovery program modeled after Alcoholics Anonymous, and is for men and women, 18 years and older, who were sexually abused as children.
www.siawso.org

David Baldwin's Trauma Information Pages
This site provides information for clinicians and researchers in the traumatic stress field.
www.trauma-pages.com
Focuses on emotional trauma and traumatic stress

Male Survivor
Male Survivor is a nonprofit, public benefit organization committed to preventing, healing, and eliminating all forms of sexual victimization of boys and men through support, treatment, research, education, advocacy, and activism.
www.malesurvivor.org

CHAPTER 20

Grieving

Loss is an inevitable part of life, and grieving is the response that allows individuals to accept, reconcile with, and adapt to change. Losing a significant other by death is a major life crisis, as long-term relationships deeply shape our world and sense of identity. The loss of a loved one can profoundly impact our own self-concept and sense of identity.

Other types of loss include the loss of a valued possession, job, status, home, and functions of one's body. Grief is experienced holistically, affecting us emotionally, cognitively, physically, and spiritually.

A couple of terms related to the timing of grief are bereavement and mourning. Bereavement, derived from the Old English word *berafian*, poignantly meaning "to rob," refers to the period of grieving after a death. Mourning encompasses the actions and rituals people engage in to cope with grief, including shared social expressions such as calling hours, funerals, and bereavement groups. The length of time, degree, and specific mourning rituals are often shaped by cultural, religious, and familial influences.

Grieving is a complex, personal, and culturally influenced process of accepting death. It involves experiencing the pain of loss, reconstructing identity, and adapting to a transformed environment. The process varies widely and can take months to several years, depending on individual and situational factors.

Losses fundamentally reshape lives, leaving individuals forever changed. However, over time, most people move from grief that defines them to living with residual pain while integrating the memory of their loved ones into their future.

Successful grieving is evidenced by the following attributes:
- Accepting the death of a loved one.
- Fewer distressing memories of the deceased.
- Resolution of anger related to the loss.
- No longer avoiding of reminders of the deceased.

- Feeling that life is worth living without the deceased.
- A strengthened sense of identity apart from the lost relationship.
- Reengagement in life, including activities, relationships, or planning for the future.

GRIEF VERSUS MAJOR DEPRESSIVE DISORDER

Symptoms of grieving may mirror those of major depressive disorder. Feelings of intense sadness, constant thinking about the loss, insomnia, lack of appetite, and weight loss may be understandable. However, in grief, the predominant feelings are emptiness and loss that occur in waves, sometimes alternating with feelings of acceptance. The depression experienced in major depressive disorder, on the other hand, results in a global inability to experience joy and feelings of guilt and self-loathing.

Previously, the bereavement exclusion in the *Diagnostic and Statistical Manual of Mental Disorders (DSM)*, discouraged clinicians from diagnosing major depressive disorder within 2 months of a loved one's death. However, this exclusion was removed from the *DSM-5*, recognizing that grief can be complicated by major depressive disorder. This change has led to more individuals receiving treatment, helping to alleviate painful depressive symptoms.

PROLONGED GRIEF DISORDER

In the text revision of the American Psychiatric Association (APA, 2022), *prolonged grief disorder* was officially recognized. This diagnosis applies to individuals whose bereavement persists beyond 12 months in adults and 6 months in children. The defining characteristic of this disorder is its significant interference with normal functioning, distinguishing it from the typical grieving process. Suicidal ideation and disinterest in living make this condition particularly dangerous.

Symptoms of this complicated grieving include intense yearning/longing for the deceased person, preoccupation with thoughts of the deceased person, feelings of emptiness, anger, depression, disbelief, detachment, and rumination. Self-blame may be a prominent symptom. For example, a widow may obsessively blame herself for her spouse not seeking help for chest pain.

THEORY

Kübler-Ross's (1973) groundbreaking work provides a framework for understanding individuals' reactions to dying. Over time, her stage theory was eventually applied to the grieving process as well. The five stages—denial, anger, bargaining, depression, and acceptance—describe common emotional responses to loss.

Although viewing the grieving process as linear—from denial to eventual acceptance—is appealing, grieving is not that simple. In reality, these stages overlap and may be nonsequential. Stroebe and Schut (1999) incorporated the stage–phase models of loss-oriented processes with the restoration of a new lifestyle. This process involves coping with everyday life, building a new identity, and developing new relationships. Table 20.1 summarizes the dual process model.

Assessment

Signs and Symptoms of Anticipatory Grief and Grief

- Anger
- Blame
- Despair
- Preoccupation with the deceased
- Crying
- Detachment
- Disorganization
- Altered activity level
- Disturbed sleep pattern
- Pain
- Panic behavior
- Vegetative signs (e.g., anorexia, insomnia, bowel dysfunction, immobility)

Table 20.1 **Dual Process Model of Coping**

Loss-Oriented Processes	Restoration-Oriented Process
Grief work	Attending to life changes
Intrusion of grief	Distraction from grief
Denial or avoidance of restoration changes	Doing new things
Breaking bonds or ties	Establishing new roles, identities, and relationships

Additional Signs and Symptoms of Dysfunctional Grief

- Prolonged, severe symptoms beyond 12 months in adults and 6 months in children
- Limited response to support
- Profound feelings of hopelessness
- Excessive withdrawal
- Fears of being alone
- Inability to work
- Inability to feel emotion
- Feeling dead or unreal
- Panic attacks
- Self-neglect
- Suicidal ideation
- Maladaptive behaviors: alcohol or substance use, indiscriminate sexual activity, compulsive spending, fugue states, and aggression
- Recurrent nightmares, night terrors, and compulsive reenactments
- Other common expressions of grieving are found in Table 20.2

Assessment Guidelines

A. Identify the patient's perception of the loss.
B. Identify the stage of grieving that the patient is experiencing or has experienced (i.e., denial, anger, bargaining, depression, or acceptance).
C. Evaluate whether the individual is at risk for complicated grieving.
D. Evaluate for psychotic symptoms, agitation, increased activity, alcohol or substance use, and extreme vegetative symptoms (e.g., anorexia, insomnia, weight loss, bowel dysfunction, immobility).
E. Consider individuals who do not express significant grief in the context of a major loss as at risk for dysfunctional grief.
F. Always assess for suicide with signs and symptoms of depression.
G. Assess for significant anger and the potential for violence.
H. Assess social support and support available in the community.
I. Determine whether religious or spiritual counseling would be useful.

Table 20.2 **Common Expressions of Grieving**

Yearnings	Survivors often long to reunite with their deceased loved one and may even experience thoughts of dying to be with them.
Deep sadness	Waves of deep sadness and regret about the loved one; crying is common.
Other negative emotions	Anger, remorse, and guilt.
Somatic disturbances	Grief commonly results in sleep problems, changes in appetite, digestive difficulties, dry mouth, or fatigue after a loss. Restlessness and agitation may also occur.
Disbelief	It takes people a long time to accept that a loved one has died. People may forget the loved one is gone until some reminder brings the reality back.
Apathy	People often withdraw or disengage when grieving. People may become irritable toward others.
Emotional surges	Although the worst emotions and disturbances diminish with time, the grieving process also involves surges of emotions. Holidays, anniversaries, birthdays, and other significant events can trigger grief reactions.
Vivid memories	Recalling vivid memories of the deceased is common. Images of the deceased—or even the sound of a loved one's voice—may emerge without warning. Vivid dreams of the loved one may occur.

Nursing Diagnoses

Four nursing diagnoses are applicable to grief: *anticipatory grief, grief, risk for dysfunctional grief,* and *dysfunctional grief* (International Council of Nurses, 2019). This chapter presents nursing care separately for *anticipatory grief, grief,* and then *dysfunctional grief.* Interventions for *risk for dysfunctional grief* may be drawn from both the *grief* and *dysfunctional grief* sections.

Because nurses frequently care for individuals and families experiencing painful losses, additional responses may be the focus of care. Nurse may need to address *impaired coping, impaired family coping, powerlessness, risk for spiritual distress,* or *spiritual distress.* Additionally, nursing diagnoses related to major depressive disorder may be relevant when caring for individuals experiencing grief (see Chapter 7).

Intervention Guidelines

A. Listening is the most effective nursing intervention that a nurse can use. People need to tell their stories, usually over and over, and move through the storyline in their own time.

B. Express sincere sympathy such as "I am so sorry for the death of your wife. You must be devastated" demonstrates engagement, interest, and empathy.

C. Avoid clichés and minimizing statements such as "She is no longer suffering" or "Will you have another child?" These comments can be emotionally painful and are not helpful.

D. Incorporate spiritual and religious support. For individuals with spiritual convictions and religious beliefs, offer spiritual support and referrals to pastoral counseling (when available) or community resources.

E. Grief support groups are available in the community and virtual settings for every type of loss (e.g., spouse, child, pet), age group, and special conditions (e.g., disease, suicide, casualty of war).

Nursing Care for Anticipatory Grief, Grief, and Dysfunctional Grief

Anticipatory Grief

Related to

- Impending loss of significant object (e.g., possession, job, status, home, parts and processes of body)
- Anticipated death of a loved one

Desired Outcome The patient will express feelings about the imminent loss and express feeling supported during the process.

Assessment/Interventions and *Rationales*
At the imminent death of a family member:

1. Inform the family of the imminent death of the family member in a private place. *Family members can support each other in an atmosphere in which they can respond and behave naturally.*

2. Provide support, answers to questions, and guidance regarding immediate tasks and information. *Nurses are*

the constant members of the healthcare team who have the experience and expertise to provide support during this difficult period.

Acknowledge and validate the patient's emotions. *Recognizing feelings of sadness, fear, or anger helps individuals process grief and feel supported.*

3. If only one family member is available, stay with that member until a family member, a friend, or another supportive professional (e.g., hospice worker, clergy) arrives. *The presence and comfort of the nurse during the initial stage of shock can help minimize feelings of acute isolation and anxiety.*

If the family requests to see the dying person:

1. Prepare the family before the visit. Explain the patient's condition, including physical deterioration, medical equipment, and visible marks from medical interventions to help set expectations.: *Providing clear information helps reduce shock and emotional distress, allowing loved ones to focus on their time with the patient.*

2. Support the request to see the dying person. **Acknowledge their need** to say goodbye, ask for forgiveness, or collect a keepsake, such as a lock of hair. *These actions help family members process grief and accept the reality of death.*

3. Remain physically available and reasonably close while the family is with the dying person. *Witnessing a loved one's death is a profound experience, and a nurse's presence offers comfort, reassurance, and guidance if needed.*

If angry family members suggest that healthcare professionals have mismanaged the care of the dying:

1. Continue providing the highest quality care possible for the dying patient. Avoid involvement in angry and painful arguments and power struggles. *Anger is a common initial response to a painful loss. Ensuring compassionate, competent care remains the priority, regardless of family emotions.*

2. Show patience and tact and offer sympathy and warmth. *Shock and disbelief are the first responses to anticipatory grief, and grieving individuals need ways to protect themselves from the overwhelming reality of loss.*

3. Allow the grieving individual to cry. *Crying helps provide relief from feelings of acute pain and tension.*

4. Offer a private place for grieving. *Privacy allows for the unrestricted expression of grief and provides an opportunity to regain composure.*

Grief

Related to
- Death of a loved one
- Loss of a significant object (e.g., possession, job, status, home, or bodily function)

Desired Outcome The patient will express positive expectations for the future and report a successful life reorganization.

Assessment/Interventions and *Rationales*
1. Provide your full presence: use appropriate eye contact, listen attentively, and use appropriate touch. *Appropriate eye contact helps the patient know you are there. Listening supports the patient's processing of the loss. Suitable touch can express warmth and nurturance.*
2. Be patient with the grieving individual during times of silence. Do not fill the silence. *Sharing painful feelings followed by periods of silence allows the patient to process thoughts and feelings without being rushed. Listening patiently helps the patient express feelings, even those that are negative.*
3. Avoid euphemisms (i.e., replacing direct words with less direct words) such as, "I am sorry to tell you this, but James is *declining*. or "You *lost* your husband." The words *death, dead,* and *dying* should be used when it's important to be clear about what is happening.
4. Avoid trite and philosophical statements such as "He's no longer suffering" "You can always have another child" or "It's better this way." Table 20.3 provides recommendations for communicating with grieving individuals. *Making these statements gives the grieving individual the impression that the experience is not understood and that you are minimizing the feelings and pain.*
5. It is helpful to acknowledge the individual's painful feelings:
   a. "His death will be a terrible loss."
   b. "No one can replace her."
   c. "He will be missed for a long time."
   d. "Your relationship was complicated."
   Verbalizing painful feelings reduces feelings of isolation.
6. Instead of asking what you can do to help, encourage the support of family and friends for the following:
   a. Getting food to the house

Table 20.3 Communication and Grief

What Not to Say	What to Say	Rationale
"I know how you feel."	"Your loss must be devastating. I can't imagine how you must be feeling right now."	No one can truly know another person's grief experience. Acknowledging their pain without assuming their emotions shows empathy and respect.
"When my mother died, I cried for months and could hardly eat... [*and proceed with long story*]."	"When I lost my mother, I was in a fog for days. This must be difficult for you right now."	Although it is helpful to know that others have experienced loss, during the acute grief period, the focus should be on the griever. Sharing lengthy stories is not helpful.
After a sudden and unexpected death: "At least he didn't suffer."	"It must have been so shocking to lose your husband so suddenly. Did he have any symptoms?"	While avoiding suffering is a comfort to some, sudden deaths can be deeply traumatic due to the lack of preparation and opportunity for closure. Acknowledging the shock validates the griever's experience.
"Have you thought about getting [remarried, pregnant again, another pet, another job]?"	"Your loved one was irreplaceably special."	Grievers are not seeking a replacement. They want their loved ones back. Suggesting moving on too soon may feel dismissive of their pain.
"She is with [God, in heaven] now."	"I can only imagine how much you are missing her."	Implying that the loss was an act of a higher power may make the griever feel betrayed or punished by God. This statement also assumes Christian beliefs, which may not align with the griever's faith or worldview.
"You can be grateful for the time you had together."	"You were married for 36 years."	Suggesting gratitude may imply that the griever is ungracious or should feel satisfied with the time they had. In reality, they still long for their loved one and the future they lost.
"Let me know if there is anything I can do for you."	"I would like to take the flowers from the funeral home to your house."	The grieving person is often overwhelmed. Suggesting that they find something for you to do is an additional burden. Make a concrete offer of assistance.

b. Making telephone calls

c. Driving to the funeral home

d. Taking care of children or other family members

Grieving individuals often struggle to identify or articulate their needs. Family and friends can help by managing routine tasks, reducing stress, and providing practical support during an overwhelming time.

7. Refer the individual who is grieving to a grief, loss, and bereavement support group. Support groups provide a structured space to share loss, offering connection and understanding—even for those with strong family or social support.

8. Offer spiritual support and referrals when needed. *Dealing with an illness or catastrophic loss can cause profound spiritual pain.*

9. When the patient is experiencing intense emotions, provide understanding and support. *Empathetic words that reflect acceptance of an individual's feelings promote healing.*

Dysfunctional Grief

Related to

- Lack of support systems
- Preexisting psychiatric disorders
- Death of a significant other
- Other risk factors (e.g., substance use, multiple losses, poor physical health, other mental health risks)
- Violent death of a loved one
- Death of child
- Death of a nonsocially sanctioned significant other

Desired Outcome The patient will verbalize a realistic appraisal of the deceased and return to a baseline level of functioning.

Assessment/Interventions and *Rationales*

1. Assess for suicidal thoughts or ideation. *Individuals who have severe depression or suicidal thoughts following a loss may require hospitalization and protection from self-neglect and self-harm.*

2. Talk with the grieving individual in realistic terms. Discuss concrete changes that have occurred and how they may affect the person's future. *Discussing the death and how it has and will continue to affect the*

person's life can help the death become more concrete and real.

3. If the individual who is grieving has difficulty talking about the death, encourage other means of expression (e.g., keeping a journal, drawing, reading literature about grief). *Talking is usually the most important tool for resolving initial pain. However, any expression of feelings can help the individual to identify, accept, and process the loss.*

4. Explore negative feelings toward the deceased, feelings of guilt, or feelings of resentment. *Understanding that negative feelings are normal and experienced by most people can make the patient aware of such feelings and then process them.*

5. Encourage the patient to recall memories (happy ones, sad ones, difficult ones), listen actively, and stay silent when appropriate. *Reviewing memories is an important stage in mourning. Being with the grieving individual and sharing painful feelings supports healing.*

6. Encourage the patient to talk to others individually, in small groups, or through community-based bereavement groups. *Talking and listening are the most important activities to activate the mourning process and help resolve grief.*

7. Avoid false reassurances that the grieving individual will recover from the loss. *For some, separation through death is never okay. Even when the grieving process is complete, the person might be deeply missed.*

8. Provide referrals for comprehensive grief and bereavement services. *Complicated grief treatment includes both interpersonal and cognitive behavior approaches to mitigate the effects of trauma and reduce stress.*

9. Identify the person's religious or spiritual background and determine whether religious or spiritual counseling might be helpful. *For many people, religious and spiritual support, and sharing feelings with a trusted and empathetic religious or spiritual figure are extremely comforting at this time.*

10. Offer written guidelines for coping with overwhelming grief. *When one is grieving, even simple tasks can become monumental, life becomes confusing, and normal routines are often interrupted. These guidelines offer simple reminders and help validate the grieving individual's experience.*

Box 20.1 provides guidelines that can be provided to people who are grieving.

Box 20.1 Caring for Yourself While Grieving

Take the time you need to grieve. The hard work of grief uses psychological energy. Resolution of the "numb state" that occurs after loss requires a few weeks at least. A minimum of 1 year—to cover all the birthdays, anniversaries, and other important dates without your loved one—is expected before you can "learn to live" with your loss. Many local hospitals or hospice agencies offer a version of "How to Handle the Holidays" seminar that can be helpful.

Express your feelings. Remember that anger, anxiety, loneliness, and even guilt are normal reactions and that everyone needs a safe place to express them. Tell your personal story of loss as many times as you need to—this repetition is a helpful and necessary part of the grieving process.

Make a daily structure and stick to it. Although it is hard to do, keeping some semblance of structure makes the first few weeks after a loss easier. Getting through each day helps restore the confidence you need to accept the reality of loss.

At some point, you might want to read books about how others have dealt with loss. They often have helpful suggestions for a person in your situation.

As hard as it is, try to take good care of yourself. Eat well, talk with friends, and get plenty of rest. Make use of exercise. It can help you vent pent-up frustrations.

Expect the unexpected. You may begin to feel a bit better, only to have a brief "emotional collapse." These are expected reactions. You also might dream, visualize, think about, or search for your loved one. This, too, is a part of the grief process.

If you are losing weight, sleeping excessively or intermittently, or still experiencing deep depression after 3 months, seek professional help. If you have or have experienced a psychiatric disorder in the past (e.g., major depressive disorder, substance use), be sure to get the additional support you need.

👪 NURSE, PATIENT, AND FAMILY RESOURCES

American Academy of Hospice and Palliative Medicine (AAHPM)
AAHPM is the professional organization for physicians, nurses, and other healthcare providers specializing in hospice and palliative medicine.
www.aahpm.org

American Association of Retired People (AARP)
AARP is a nonprofit, nonpartisan organization that empowers people to choose how they live as they age.
www.aarp.org

GriefShare (Support Groups)
A support group to help individuals move through the grief process.
www.griefshare.org

Hospice Foundation of America
A trusted source of information on end-of-life, hospice care, and grief. Includes information about living with advanced life-limiting illness, options for care, and helpful resources for caregivers.
www.hospicefoundation.org

National Institute on Aging (NIA)
NIA, one of the 27 Institutes and Centers of NIH, leads a broad scientific effort to understand the nature of aging and to extend the healthy, active years of life.
www.nia.nih.gov

CHAPTER 21

Attention-Deficit/ Hyperactivity Disorder Medications

Attention-deficit/hyperactivity disorder (ADHD) affects both children and adults, manifesting as persistent patterns of inattention, impulsivity, and hyperactivity that can interfere with daily functioning. Treatment often includes a combination of behavioral interventions and pharmacotherapy. Medications prescribed for ADHD fall into two primary categories: stimulants and nonstimulants. Additionally, certain medications are used adjunctively to manage co-occurring symptoms such as anger, aggression, and emotional dysregulation.

STIMULANTS

Paradoxically, ADHD symptoms are effectively managed with stimulant drugs. These drugs often produce dramatic improvements, quickly enhancing attention and task-directed behavior while reducing impulsivity, restlessness, and distractibility.

Methylphenidate (Ritalin and other brand names) and mixed amphetamine salts (Adderall) are the most widely used stimulants due to their relative safety and ease of use. Not surprisingly, insomnia is a common side effect of stimulant medications. Using the minimum effective dose is essential, and administering the medication no later than 4 p.m. or reducing the last dose of the day can help mitigate sleep disturbances. The long-acting versions allow for a single morning dose, providing sustained medication release throughout the day and reducing the incidence of insomnia. Other common side effects include appetite suppression, headache, abdominal pain, and lethargy.

Concerns with stimulant medications include side effects such as agitation, exacerbation (worsening) of psychotic symptoms, hypertension, and growth suppression. As with any controlled substance, there is a risk of misuse, including illicit sales or the use by individuals for whom the medication was not prescribed.

NONSTIMULANTS

Unlike stimulants, nonstimulants are not controlled substances and have a lower risk of misuse. The FDA has approved four nonstimulants for the treatment of ADHD: atomoxetine, viloxazine, clonidine, and guanfacine. Unlike stimulants, nonstimulants are not controlled substances and have a lower risk of misuse. The FDA has approved four nonstimulants for the treatment of ADHD: atomoxetine, viloxazine, guanfacine, and clonidine.

Atomoxetine (Strattera) is a norepinephrine reuptake inhibitor approved for use in children 6 years and older. Common side effects include gastrointestinal disturbances, urinary retention, fatigue, dizziness, and insomnia. It may also cause liver injury in some patients and a slight increase in blood pressure and heart rate. Therapeutic responses develop slowly, and it may take up to 6 weeks for full improvement. This medication is preferable for individuals whose anxiety is exacerbated by stimulants. It is also useful for those with comorbid anxiety, active substance use disorders, or tics.

Ongoing monitoring of vital signs and regular screening of liver function are important when using atomoxetine. Rarely, serious allergic reactions occur. Patients and their families should be educated on the risks and benefits of treatment before starting this medication. Atomoxetine is used with extreme caution in patients with comorbid major depressive disorder, as it has been associated with increased suicidal ideation.

Viloxazine (Qelbree) is another nonstimulant norepinephrine reuptake inhibitor with FDA approval for ADHD.

Common side effects include somnolence, decreased appetite, fatigue, nausea, vomiting, dry mouth, and irritability. In adults, additional side effects may include headache, constipation, and insomnia. Viloxazine is dosed once daily, and therapeutic effects typically emerge within a few weeks of treatment initiation.

As with atomoxetine, viloxazine requires careful monitoring, particularly in patients with comorbid conditions. It carries a boxed warning for an increased risk of suicidal thoughts and behaviors, especially in pediatric patients. Regular assessment of mood and behavioral changes is essential. While viloxazine may be a beneficial option for individuals who do not tolerate stimulants, its sedative effects should be considered when determining the optimal dosing schedule. Educate patients and their families on the potential risks and benefits before starting treatment.

Two centrally acting alpha-2 adrenergic agonists, clonidine (Kapvay, Catapres) and guanfacine (Intuniv, Tenex) have FDA approval for the treatment of ADHD. Both medications should be increased gradually and not discontinued abruptly. They may be used alone or in conjunction with other ADHD medications.

Of the two, clonidine is associated with more side effects: somnolence, fatigue, insomnia, nightmares, irritability, constipation, respiratory symptoms, and dry mouth. Guanfacine tends to cause somnolence, lethargy, fatigue, insomnia, nausea, dizziness, hypotension, and abdominal pain.

See Table 21.1 for a summary of the FDA-approved medications used to treat ADHD.

MANAGING AGGRESSIVE BEHAVIORS IN ATTENTION-DEFICIT/HYPERACTIVITY DISORDER

To manage aggressive behaviors individuals with ADHD, pharmacological agents-including stimulants, mood stabilizers, alpha-adrenergic agonists, and antipsychotics-may be used. Stimulants have a dose-dependent effect: at low doses, they can paradoxically increase aggression, whereas moderate to high doses suppress aggressive behaviors. Mood stabilizers such as lithium and anticonvulsants reduce aggressive behavior and are recommended for impulsivity, explosive temper, and mood lability.

Table 21.1 FDA-Approved Drugs for Attention-Deficit/Hyperactivity Disorder

Generic and Trade Names	Ages	Duration in Hours	Doses Per Day
STIMULANTS			
Amphetamine			
Adzenys XR-ODT	6+	12	1
Dyanavel XR	6+	12	1
Evekeo	3+	4-6	2-3
Dexmethylphenidate			
Focalin	6+	4-5	2
Focalin XR	6+	8-12	1
Dextroamphetamine			
Dexedrine	3-16	4-6	2-3
Procentra	3-16	4-6	2-3
Zenzedi	3-16	4-6	2-3
Lisdexamfetamine			
Vyvanse	6+	10-12	1
Methamphetamine			
Desoxyn	6+	6-8	1-2
Methylphenidate			
Adhansia XR	6+	10-12	1
Aptensio XR	6+	10-12	1
Concerta, Relexxii	6-65	10-12	1
Cotempla XR-ODT	6-17	12	1
Daytrana (transdermal patch)	6-17	10-12	1
Jornay PM	6+	10-12	1 (evening)
Metadate ER	6-15	6-8	1-2
Metadate CD	6-15	6-8	1
Methylin ER	6+	6-8	1
Mydayis	13+	Up to 16h	1
QuilliChew ER	6+	12	1
Quillivant XR	6-17	12	1
Ritalin	6-12	6-8	1-2
Ritalin LA	6-12	7-9	1
Ritalin SR	6-12	6-8	1-2
Mixed salts of a single-entity amphetamine product			
Adderall	6+	4-6	2
Adderall-XR	6+	10-12	1-2
NONSTIMULANTS			
Atomoxetine			
Straterra	6-65	24	1-2
Viloxazine			
Qelbree	6-17	24	1

Table 21.1 FDA-Approved Drugs for Attention-Deficit/Hyperactivity Disorder—cont'd

Generic and Trade Names	Ages	Duration in Hours	Doses Per Day
Clonidine			
Kapvay, Catapres	6-17	24	2
Guanfacine			
Intuniv, Tenex	6-17	24	1

Data from Food and Drug Administration (2019). FDA online label repository. https://labels.fda.gov.

Mood stabilizers such as lithium and anticonvulsants help reduce aggression and are recommended for individuals with impulsivity, explosive temper, and mood lability. Due to their sedative effects, clonidine and guanfacine are beneficial in reducing agitation and rage while improving frustration tolerance.

Antipsychotic medications have been shown to decrease violent behavior, hyperactivity, and social unresponsiveness. However, their use is generally reserved for severe aggression due to the risk of tardive dyskinesia and other adverse effects associated with long-term treatment.

CHAPTER 22

Antipsychotic Medications

Antipsychotic medications are used to treat psychotic symptoms in disorders such as schizophrenia and bipolar mania. Before their development, medications like antihistamines provided sedation but did not alleviate psychosis. Individuals with schizophrenia often spent months or years in state or private hospitals, leading to significant emotional and financial burdens to patients, families, and society.

In 1951 the first antipsychotic, chlorpromazine, was developed in France for use as a general anesthetic. The following year, its antipsychotic properties were discovered. Marketed under the trade name **Thorazine**, chlorpromazine and subsequent antipsychotic drugs provided symptom control, allowing many patients to live and receive treatment in the community.

Antipsychotic medications typically require 2 to 6 weeks to achieve their full therapeutic effects. While they are not addictive, they should be discontinued gradually to minimize discontinuation syndrome, which may include dizziness, nausea, tremors, insomnia, electric shock-like sensations, and anxiety. Unlike some other psychotropic medications, antipsychotics are unlikely to be lethal in overdose.

Some antipsychotics are available in short-acting intramuscular injection form, primarily used for agitation, emergencies such as aggression, or when a patient refuses court-mandated medication. However, when administered directly into the system, side effects can be intensified and less easily managed. Additionally, the **inhaled antipsychotic loxapine (Adasuve)** can help reduce agitation but requires some level of patient cooperation for effective use.

Antipsychotics are classified into two major categories:

1. First-generation antipsychotics (FGAs), also known as *typical* antipsychotics, were the original antipsychotic medications. They are also known as *typical* antipsychotics. These drugs act as dopamine (D_2 receptor) antagonists and include such medications as chlorpromazine (Thorazine) and haloperidol (Haldol).

2. Second-generation antipsychotics (SGAs), also known as *atypical* antipsychotics, were developed after FGAs. They are also known as *atypical* antipsychotics. These drugs function as serotonin (5-HT_{2A} receptor) and dopamine (D_2 receptor) antagonists, with clozapine (Clozaril) being a notable example. Some SGAs, such as aripiprazole (Abilify), act as dopamine antagonists in areas of high dopamine activity but as dopamine agonists in areas of low dopamine activity.

FIRST-GENERATION ANTIPSYCHOTICS

FGAs primarily reduce positive symptoms of psychosis but have little effect on negative symptoms.

- Positive symptoms refer to the presence of abnormal experiences that should not be there, such as hallucinations, delusions, and disorganized thoughts.
- Negative symptoms refer to the absence of normal functions—qualities that should be present but are not. These include the ability to experience joy, motivation, and interest in social interactions. Instead, individuals may exhibit anhedonia (inability to feel pleasure), avolition (lack of motivation), and a sociality (disinterest in engaging with others)

FGAs are used less frequently today due to their limited effect on negative symptoms and high incidence of side effects. However, they remain effective in treating positive symptoms and are relatively inexpensive. For patients who tolerate their side effects, FGAs remain a viable treatment option.

Drug-Induced Movement Disorders

FGAs act as dopamine (D_2) antagonists in both limbic and motor centers. Blockage of D_2 receptors in motor areas can cause extrapyramidal symptoms (EPSs), which include the following symptoms:

- Acute dystonia: Sudden, sustained contractions of one or more muscle groups, typically in the head and neck. While acute dystonia can be frightening and painful, it is not dangerous unless it affects the airway. It often causes significant anxiety and should be treated promptly.
- Akathisia: An inner restlessness or an inability to stay still or remain in one place. Akathisia can be severe and distressing to patients and may be mistaken for anxiety or agitation. These symptoms may lead to administering more of the drug that originally caused the akathisia, making it worse.
- Parkinsonism: Temporary symptoms that look like Parkinson's disease. These symptoms include tremor, reduced accessory movements (e.g., less arm swinging when walking), gait impairment, reduced facial expressiveness (i.e., facial masking), and slowing of motor behavior (bradykinesia).

EPSs can be extremely distressing. They impact medication adherence, reduce quality of life, impair social relationships, and interfere with daily activities such as driving a car. EPSs can be minimized by lowering doses and can be prevented by using antipsychotics less likely to cause EPSs. Fortunately, these side effects may diminish over time.

EPSs can also be treated with the addition of other drugs. Anticholinergic medications are useful but come with their own side effects, including dry mouth, constipation, urinary hesitancy, tachycardia, thickening of secretions, and dry skin. Misuse of anticholinergic drugs is also a potential problem because they can produce an enjoyable altered sensorium. Drugs used for dystonia, akathisia, and parkinsonism are listed in Table 22.1.

Tardive dyskinesia is a delayed and persistent drug-induced movement disorder characterized byf involuntary, rhythmic movements. It develops in about 25% of patients after chronic exposure to dopamine receptor blockers, resulting in hyperactive dopamine signaling. Unlike acute movement disorders, tardive dyskinesia often persists even after the medication is discontinued.

Early symptoms typically begin in the mouth and facial muscles and may progressively involve the fingers, toes, neck, trunk, or pelvis. More common in women, the severity of tardive dyskinesia varies from mild to severe and can be disfiguring or incapacitating.

Table 22.1 Medications Used for Drug-Induced Movement Disorders

Generic (Brand) Name	Indications
Anticholinergic Benztropine (Cogentin) Trihexyphenidyl (Artane)	Dystonias, parkinsonism
Dopaminergic Amantadine (Symmetrel)	Parkinsonism
Antihistamine Diphenhydramine (Benadryl)	Dystonias, parkinsonism
Beta-Adrenergic Antagonist Propranolol (Inderal)	Akathisia
Alpha-Adrenergic Agonist Clonidine (Catapres)	Akathisia
Antianxiety Agents Clonazepam (Klonopin) Lorazepam (Ativan)	Akathisia, dystonia

The National Institute of Mental Health (NIMH) developed the Abnormal Involuntary Movement Scale (AIMS; Fig. 22.1) to identify and track involuntary movements. Administering the AIMS is a key nursing responsibility when caring for individuals taking FGAs. This scale is typically used every 3 to 6 months or as clinically indicated. A positive AIMS examination is defined as a score of 2 in two or more movement categories or a score of 3 or 4 in a single movement category.

Primary prevention of tardive dyskinesia involves using the lowest effective dose of antipsychotic medication for the shortest duration possible. If tardive dyskinesia is detected, reducing or discontinuing the medication is recommended when feasible. Some clinicians suggest switching to clozapine (Clozaril), as it has a lower risk of causing tardive dyskinesia. When making treatment decisions, the risk of a permanent movement disorder must be carefully weighed against the potential for worsening psychosis.

Tardive dyskinesia in adults is treated with valbenazine (Ingrezza) and deutetrabenazine (Austedo), both of which are selective vesicular monoamine transporter inhibitors. The drugs reduce the severity of abnormal involuntary movements. Individuals can continue to take antipsychotics while on these medications.

ABNORMAL INVOLUNTARY MOVEMENT SCALE (AIMS)

Public Health Service
Alcohol, Drug Abuse, and Mental Health Administration
National Institute of Mental Health

Name: ____________________
Date: ____________________
Prescribing Practitioner: ____________________

Code: 0 = None
1 = Minimal, may be extreme normal
2 = Mild
3 = Moderate
4 = Severe

Instructions: Complete Examination Procedure before making ratings.

	Movement ratings: Rate highest severity observed. Rate movements that occur upon activation one *less* than those observed spontaneously. Circle movement as well as code number that applies.	Rater Date	Rater Date	Rater Date	Rater Date
Facial and Oral Movements	1. **Muscles of facial expression** (e.g., movements of forehead, eyebrows, periorbital area, cheeks, including frowning, blinking, smiling, grimacing)	0 1 2 3 4	0 1 2 3 4	0 1 2 3 4	0 1 2 3 4
	2. **Lips and perioral area** (e.g., puckering, pouting, smacking)	0 1 2 3 4	0 1 2 3 4	0 1 2 3 4	0 1 2 3 4
	3. **Jaw** (e.g., biting, clenching, chewing, mouth opening, lateral movement)	0 1 2 3 4	0 1 2 3 4	0 1 2 3 4	0 1 2 3 4
	4. **Tongue:** Rate only increases in movement both in and out of mouth — *not* inability to sustain movement. Darting in and out of mouth.	0 1 2 3 4	0 1 2 3 4	0 1 2 3 4	0 1 2 3 4
Extremity Movements	5. **Upper (arms, wrists, hands, fingers):** Include choreic movements (i.e., rapid, objectively purposeless, irregular, spontaneous) and athetoid movements (i.e., slow, irregular, complex, serpentine). *Do not include tremor* (i.e., repetitive, regular, rhythmic).	0 1 2 3 4	0 1 2 3 4	0 1 2 3 4	0 1 2 3 4
	6. **Lower (legs, knees, ankles, toes)** (e.g., lateral knee movement, foot tapping, heel dropping, foot squirming, inversion and eversion of foot)	0 1 2 3 4	0 1 2 3 4	0 1 2 3 4	0 1 2 3 4
Trunk Movements	7. **Neck, shoulder, hips** (e.g., rocking, twisting, squirming, pelvic gyrations)	0 1 2 3 4	0 1 2 3 4	0 1 2 3 4	0 1 2 3 4
Global Judgments	8. **Severity of abnormal movements overall**	0 1 2 3 4	0 1 2 3 4	0 1 2 3 4	0 1 2 3 4
	9. **Incapacitation due to abnormal movements**	0 1 2 3 4	0 1 2 3 4	0 1 2 3 4	0 1 2 3 4
	10. **Patient's awareness of abnormal movements:** Rate only patient's report. No awareness 0 Aware, no distress 1 Aware, mild distress 2 Aware, moderate distress 3 Aware, severe distress 4	0 1 2 3 4	0 1 2 3 4	0 1 2 3 4	0 1 2 3 4
Dental Status	11. **Current problems with teeth and/or dentures**	No Yes	No Yes	No Yes	No Yes
	12. **Are dentures usually worn?**	No Yes	No Yes	No Yes	No Yes
	13. **Edentia**	No Yes	No Yes	No Yes	No Yes
	14. **Do movements disappear in sleep?**	No Yes	No Yes	No Yes	No Yes

A

Fig. 22.1 Abnormal Involuntary Movement Scale (*AIMS*). Instructions: Rate highest severity observed. Rate movements that occur upon activation as one point *less* than those observed spontaneously. Circle movement as well as code number that applies. Scoring: 0 = Absent, 1 = Minimal, 2 = Mild, 3 = Moderate, 4 = Severe.

Common adverse effects include sleepiness and QT prolongation, which can increase the risk of fainting, seizures, or sudden death. These drugs are contraindicated in individuals with congenital or acquired long-QT syndrome or other related dysrhythmias. Caution is advised for individuals who drive, operate heavy machinery, or engage in other hazardous activities until they understand how the

---

AIMS Examination Procedure

Either before or after completing the Examination Procedure, observe the patient unobtrusively, at rest (e.g., in waiting room).

The chair to be used in this examination should be a hard, firm one without arms.

1. Ask patient to remove shoes and socks.
2. Ask patient whether there is anything in his or her mouth (e.g., gum, candy) and, if there is, to remove it.
3. Ask patient about the *current* condition of his or her teeth. Ask patient if he or she wears dentures. Do teeth or dentures bother the patient *now*?
4. Ask patient whether he or she notices any movements in mouth, face, hands, or feet. If yes, ask to describe and to what extent they *currently* bother patient or interfere with his or her activities.
5. Have patient sit in chair with hands on knees, legs slightly apart, and feet flat on floor. Look at entire body movements while in this position.
6. Ask patient to sit with hands hanging unsupported: if male, between legs; if female and wearing a dress, hanging over knees. Observe hands and other body areas.
7. Ask patient to open mouth. Observe tongue at rest within mouth. Do this twice.
8. Ask patient to protrude tongue. Observe abnormalities of tongue movement. Do this twice.
9. Ask patient to tap thumb, with each finger, as rapidly as possible for 10 to 15 seconds, separately with right hand, then with left hand. Observe each facial and leg movement.
10. Flex and extend patient's left and right arms (one at a time). Note any rigidity.
11. Ask patient to stand up. Observe in profile. Observe all body areas again, hips included.
12. Ask patient to extend both arms outstretched in front with palms down. Observe trunk, legs, and mouth.
13. Have patient walk a few paces, turn, and walk back to chair. Observe hands and gait. Do this twice.

B

Fig. 22.1, cont'd

medication affects them. Caution is advised for individuals who drive, operate heavy machinery, or engage in other hazardous activities until they understand how the medication affects them.

Ideally, patients should be screened for undiagnosed movement disorders, such as Parkinson's disease, before starting antipsychotic therapy. Underlying conditions may be mistaken for drug side effects, leading to missed diagnoses and untreated symptoms.

Anticholinergic Side Effects

The FGAs cause anticholinergic side effects by blocking muscarinic acetylcholine receptors. These effects include urinary retention, dilated pupils, reduced visual accommodation (blurred near vision), tachycardia, and dry mucous membranes. Reduced peristalsis may resulting in constipation and, in rare cases, paralytic ileus and bowel obstruction. Cognitive impairment is also a potential concern.

Taking multiple medications with anticholinergic effects increases the risk of anticholinergic toxicity, which is covered later in this chapter. In general, FGAs tend to have either strong EPS potential or strong anticholinergic potential. That is, when one side effect is prominent, the other is not.

Other First-Generation Antipsychotic Side Effects

FGAs commonly cause sedation, though this effect typically diminishes over time. Orthostatic (postural) hypotension increases the risk of falls when standing suddenly. A lowered seizure threshold increases the risk of seizures.

Visual changes such as photosensitivity and cataracts are associated with chlorpromazine (Thorazine) and thioridazine (Mellaril). Hyperprolactinemia (elevated prolactin levels) can lead to sexual dysfunction (e.g., impotence, anorgasmia, impaired ejaculation), galactorrhea (breast milk production), gynecomastia (enlargement of male breast tissue), and amenorrhea (cessation of menstruation).

Significant weight gain-often exceeding 50 pounds in a year-can cause psychological distress. It also increases the risk of cardiovascular disorders and diabetes mellitus.

Serious side effects are uncommon. However, anticholinergic toxicity, neuroleptic malignant syndrome prolongation of the QT interval, and liver impairment may occur during FGA therapy. FGAs increase mortality in older adults with major neurocognitive disorders. Food and Drug Administration (FDA)-approved FGAs and specific side effects are listed in Table 22.2.

SECOND-GENERATION ANTIPSYCHOTICS

Like FGAs, SGAs can cause sedation, sexual dysfunction, seizures, and increased mortality in older adults with major neurocognitive disorders. However, most SGAs are less likely to cause significant EPS, particularly tardive dyskinesia. While SGAs share many of the same potential side effects as FGAs, they are generally fewer, milder, and better tolerated. Serious risks associated with SGAs include anticholinergic toxicity, neuroleptic malignant syndrome (NMS), and QT interval prolongation.

Some SGAs also have antidepressant properties and are FDA-approved for adjunctive use in the treatment of major depressive disorder as well as bipolar disorder. As with all antidepressants, they carry a theoretical risk of increased suicidality, particularly in adolescents.

Table 22.2 FDA-Approved First-Generation Antipsychotics

Generic (Trade) Name	Specific Side Effects
Chlorpromazine (Thorazine)	Sedation, weight gain, hypotension, constipation, hyperprolactinemia, photosensitivity, NMS, akathisia, EPS, tardive dyskinesia
Fluphenazine (Prolixin)	Sedation, weight gain, hyperprolactinemia, NMS, EPS, akathisia, tardive dyskinesia, dystonia
Haloperidol (Haldol)	Sedation, hypotension, constipation, hyperprolactinemia, NMS, akathisia, EPS, tardive dyskinesia, dystonia
Loxapine	Sedation, hypotension, constipation, hyperprolactinemia, dystonia, NMS, akathisia, EPS, tardive dyskinesia
Loxapine (Adasuve)	Altered taste, sedation, bronchospasm. Contraindicated with asthma and chronic obstructive pulmonary disease
Molindone (Moban)	Sedation, constipation, hyperprolactinemia, dystonia, NMS, akathisia, EPS, tardive dyskinesia,
Perphenazine (Trilafon)	Sedation, weight gain, hypotension, constipation, hyperprolactinemia, dystonia, NMS, akathisia, EPS, tardive dyskinesia
Thioridazine (Mellaril)	Sedation, weight gain, hypotension, constipation, hyperprolactinemia, dystonia, pigmentary retinopathy, NMS, akathisia, EPS, tardive dyskinesia,
Thiothixene (Navane)	Sedation, hypotension, constipation, hyperprolactinemia, dystonia, NMS, akathisia, EPS, tardive dyskinesia
Trifluoperazine (Stelazine)	Sedation, hypotension, constipation, hyperprolactinemia, dystonia, NMS, akathisia, EPS, tardive dyskinesia

EPS, Extrapyramidal symptom; *NMS*, neuroleptic malignant syndrome

The first SGA, clozapine (Clozaril), was approved in 1989 and produced dramatic improvements in patients whose treatment had been resistant to FGAs. It also helped alleviate negative symptoms. However, clozapine carries a 1% risk of agranulocytosis, or severe neutropenia. Other serious side effects are myocarditis, life-threatening bowel emergencies, new-onset type 2 diabetes, and, rarely, ketoacidosis. Due to these risks, clozapine use has declined in the United States, and many clinicians reserve it as a last resort. Despite its risks, it remains one of the few drugs with FDA approval for reducing suicidality in schizophrenia.

Metabolic Syndrome

All SGAs carry a risk of metabolic syndrome, which includes weight gain (particularly in the abdominal area), dyslipidemia, elevated blood glucose, and insulin resistance. This condition significantly increases the risk of diabetes, certain cancers, hypertension, and cardiovascular disease, making its prevention and monitoring critical nursing responsibilities.

A subset of the SGAs is sometimes referred to as third-generation antipsychotics. This group includes aripiprazole (Abilify), brexpiprazole (Rexulti), cariprazine (Vraylar), and lumateperone (Caplyta). These medications are dopamine system stabilizers, meaning they reduce dopamine activity in some brain regions while increasing it in others.

Aripiprazole and brexpiprazole act as D_2 partial agonists, meaning they bind to D_2 receptors without fully activating them, effectively modulating dopamine levels rather than completely blocking dopamine activity. Cariprazine is a partial agonist with a stronger affinity for D_3 receptors than D_2 receptors, which may contribute to improving cognitive symptoms in some patients.

FDA-approved SGAs and specific side effects are listed in Table 22.3

Table 22.4 summarizes the side effects of antipsychotic medication and the nursing care that is associated with these side effects.

Serious Antipsychotic Side Effects

Although rare, serious and potentially fatal side effects of antipsychotics include anticholinergic toxicity, neuroleptic malignant syndrome, agranulocytosis, QT prolongation, and liver impairment. Nurses in psychiatric, primary care, and emergency settings must recognize early signs and educate patients and families on when to seek urgent care.

Anticholinergic toxicity is a potentially life-threatening condition caused by antipsychotics or other medications with anticholinergic effects, including many antiparkinsonian drugs. Older adults and those taking multiple

Table 22.3 **FDA-Approved Second- and Third-Generation Antipsychotics**

Generic (Trade) Name	Specific Side Effects
Aripiprazole (Abilify, Abilify Discmelt, Abilify Maintena)	Dizziness, insomnia, akathisia, activation, nausea, vomiting, sedation
Aripiprazole lauroxil (Aristada, Aristada Initio)	Akathisia, injection site pain, sedation
Aripiprazole lauroxil (Aristada, Aristada Initio)	
Asenapine (Saphris, Secuado)	Risk of diabetes and dyslipidemia, EPS, hyperprolactinemia, sedation weight gain, akathisia, NMS, tardive dyskinesia, oral hypoesthesia/tongue numbing (sublingual tablet), application site reaction (patch)
Brexpiprazole (Rexulti)	Headache, EPS, dyspepsia
Cariprazine (Vraylar)	EPS, insomnia, nausea, sedation
Clozapine (Clozaril, Versacloz, FazaClo)	Risk of diabetes and dyslipidemia, increased salivation, sweating, agranulocytosis, sedation, weight gain, constipation, hypotension, seizures
Iloperidone (Fanapt)	Risk of diabetes and dyslipidemia, EPS, hyperprolactinemia, sedation, weight gain, akathisia, NMS, tardive dyskinesia
Lumateperone (Caplyta)	Risk of diabetes and dyslipidemia, weight gain, complete blood counts in patients with preexisting low white blood cell count or history of leukopenia or neutropenia, tardive dyskinesia, sedation
Lurasidone (Latuda)	Risk of diabetes and dyslipidemia, EPS, hyperprolactinemia, sedation, weight gain, akathisia, NMS, tardive dyskinesia
Olanzapine (Zyprexa, Zyprexa Zydis, Zyprexa Relprevv)	Risk of diabetes and dyslipidemia, sedation, weight gain, hyperprolactinemia, constipation, hypotension, seizures. Zyprexa Relprevv risk of a postinjection delirium/sedation syndrome

(Continued)

Table 22.3 FDA-Approved Second- and Third-Generation Antipsychotics—cont'd

Generic (Trade) Name	Specific Side Effects
Paliperidone (Invega, Invega Sustenna, Invega Trinza)	Risk of diabetes and dyslipidemia, EPS, hyperprolactinemia, sedation, weight gain, tachycardia, headache
Quetiapine (Seroquel, Seroquel XR)	Risk of diabetes and dyslipidemia, dizziness, sedation, weight gain, constipation, hypotension
Risperidone (Risperdal, Risperdal Consta, Perseris, Risperdal M-Tab)	Risk of diabetes and dyslipidemia, EPS, hyperprolactinemia, sedation, weight gain, akathisia, NMS, tardive dyskinesia
Ziprasidone (Geodon)	Activating, sedation, hypotension, akathisia

EPS, Extrapyramidal symptom

Table 22.4 Antipsychotic Medication Side Effects and Nursing Care

Side Effect	Nursing Care
Extrapyramidal Symptoms (EPSs)	
Acute dystonic reactions	
Acute painful contractions of tongue, face, neck, and back (usually tongue and jaw first)	Monitor and ensure an open airway.
Spasm of muscles causing backward arching of the head, neck (torticollis), and spine	Administer intramuscular antiparkinsonian agent. Consider intramuscular or intravenous diphenhydramine (Benadryl).
Eyes rolling back (oculogyric crisis)	Provide prophylactic oral antiparkinsonian agent as ordered.
Laryngeal dystonia could threaten airway (rare)	Offer reassurance and maintain a supportive presence for the patient.

Table 22.4 **Antipsychotic Medication Side Effects and Nursing Care—cont'd**

Side Effect	Nursing Care
Akathisia Motor restlessness, characterized by: • Pacing • Inability to stand still or stay in one place • Rocking while seated • Shifting from one foot to the other while standing	Differentiate akathisia (i.e., inability to sit still, generalized muscle restlessness) from anxious repetitive movement (usually involves only the extremities). Ask specific questions such as "Do you feel anxious about something?" Consult the prescriber regarding possible medication adjustments. Administer propranolol (Inderal), lorazepam (Ativan), or diazepam (Valium) as ordered. Encourage relaxation exercises to help reducerestlessness. Monitor for suicidality, particularly in severe cases.
Parkinsonism Masklike face Stiff, stooped posture Shuffling gait Drooling Tremor "Pill-rolling" finger movements Dysphagia or reduced spontaneous swallowing	Administer antiparkinsonian agents such as trihexyphenidyl (Artane) or benztropine (Cogentin), as ordered. If symptoms are intolerable, consult the prescriber about dose reduction or medication change. Provide a towel to manage excess saliva. Education the patient on fall prevention strategies.
Tardive Dyskinesia **Face:** Protruding or writhing tongue Blowing, smacking, or licking movements Facial distortion **Limbs:** **Chorea:** Rapid, purposeless, irregular movements **Athetoid movements**: Slow, complex, serpentine motions **Trunk**: Neck and shoulder movements Hip jerks and rocking Twisting pelvic thrusts	Screen with the AIMs scale at least every 3 months. Consult the provider about adjusting medication choice or lowering the dose. Teach the patient that purposeful muscle movement can override and masks involuntary movements. Encourage strategies to conceal involuntary movements, such as holding one hand with the other. Administer valbenazine (Ingrezza) or deutetrabenazine (Austedo) as ordered.

(Continued)

Table 22.4 Antipsychotic Medication Side Effects and Nursing Care—cont'd

Side Effect	Nursing Care

Hypotension and Orthostatic (Postural)

Hypotension

When standing, systolic blood pressure rises, diastolic blood pressure decreases, and pulse increases	Monitor blood pressure and pulse in both lying (or sitting) and standing positions.
	Hold the dose and consult the prescriber if systolic pressure is <80 mm Hg when standing.
	Advise the patient to rise slowly to reduce dizziness and to hold on to railings or furniture while rising.
	If lying down, instruct the patient to move slowly to a sitting position, pause until dizziness subsides, then standi.
	Explain that symptoms typically resolve within 1–2 weeks.
	Encourage adequate hydration.

Anticholinergic

Dry mouth	Encourage ice chips or frequent sips of water.
	Suggest sugarless candy or gum to stimulate salivation.
	Recommend xylitol-containing moisture supplements or other saliva substitutes.
	Educate the patient on substances that worsen dry mouth including caffeine, alcohol, tobacco, antihistamines, and decongestants.
	Discuss with the provider the potential use of pilocarpine (Salagen) or cevimeline (Evoxac) to stimulate saliva production with the provider.
	Promote dental hygiene and regular dental care.

Table 22.4 **Antipsychotic Medication Side Effects and Nursing Care—cont'd**

Side Effect	Nursing Care
Urinary retention and hesitancy	Assess for distended bladder. Suggest running water and a warm moist towel on abdomen. Catheterization may be necessary.
Constipation	Encourage adequate fluid and fiber intake. Promote physical activity. Consider stool softeners, laxatives, or natural dietary options such as prune juice.
Blurred vision	Inform the patient that blurred vision may improve in 1–2 weeks. Encourage the use of reading or magnifying glasses. If intolerable, consult prescriber regarding medication change.
Dry eyes	Encourage the use of artificial tears.
Sexual dysfunction	Discuss the use of an alternative medication with the provider. Suggest artificial lubricants to alleviate vaginal dryness.
Metabolic Syndrome	
Antipsychotic-Induced weight gain Dyslipidemia (abnormal lipid levels) Increased insulin resistance leading to a higher risk of cardiovascular disease, diabetes, and other medical conditions	Monitor weight, blood pressure, fasting lipids, and blood glucose. Encourage proper nutrition and regular physical activity to minimize weight gain. Assist the patient in identifying low-calorie snack options and engaging in activities such as walking or cycling. Educate the patient on the importance of regular medical evaluations to detect early signs of metabolic syndrome. Discuss with the provider the potential off-label use of metformin or topiramate to reduce weight gain.

anticholinergic drugs are at greatest risk. Symptoms include autonomic nervous system instability, dilated pupils, urinary retention, and delirium with altered mental status. Mental status changes can include hallucinations and may be mistaken for a worsening of the patient's psychosis. Individuals whose psychosis is inexplicably worsening should be evaluated for anticholinergic toxicity.

ANTICHOLINERGIC TOXICITY

This life-threatening condition results from antipsychotics or other anticholinergic medications, especially in older adults and those on multiple anticholinergic drugs. Symptoms include autonomic instability, dilated pupils, urinary retention, and delirium with altered mental status. Hallucinations may occur, mimicking worsening psychosis. If a patient's psychosis suddenly worsens, evaluate for anticholinergic toxicity.

Neuroleptic Malignant Syndrome

Neuroleptic malignant syndrome (NMS) occurs in 0.2% to 1% of patients, primarily with FGAs but also with SGAs. Caused by excessive dopamine receptor blockade, it presents with reduced consciousness, generalized muscle rigidity, autonomic instability, and high fever (>103°F/39°C). Fatal in ~6% of cases, NMS requires immediate discontinuation of the antipsychotic, aggressive fluid management, temperature reduction, and monitoring for complications such as deep vein thrombosis and rhabdomyolysis (muscle breakdown that can cause organ failure).

Agranulocytosis

Severe neutropenia (ANC <100/μL) occurs most often with clozapine (Clozaril) but is possible with other antipsychotics. This condition greatly increases infection risk, with symptoms such as fever, chills, and sore throat. Untreated, it leads to septicemia and death. Monitoring absolute neutrophil count (ANC) testing is essential for early detection.

QT Prolongation

QT prolongation delays ventricular repolarization, increasing the risk of tachycardia, fainting, seizures, and sudden death. High-risk FGAs include chlorpromazine (Thorazine), haloperidol (Haldol), and thioridazine (Mellaril). SGAs associated with QT prolongation include iloperidone (Fanapt), quetiapine (Seroquel), risperidone (Risperdal), and ziprasidone (Geodon). An ECG should be

Table 22.5 **Serious Side Effects of Antipsychotics and Associated Nursing Care**

Side Effect	Nursing Care
Anticholinergic Toxicity	
Potentially life-threatening medical emergency	Hold all medications.
Reduced or absent peristalsis (risk of bowel obstruction); urinary retention; mydriasis (pupillary dilation); hyperpyrexia without diaphoresis (hot dry skin); delirium with tachycardia, unstable vital signs, agitation, disorientation, hallucinations, reduced responsiveness; worsening of psychotic symptoms; seizure; repetitive motor movements.	Contact the prescriber immediately. Implement emergency cooling measures as ordered (cooling blanket, alcohol, or ice bath). Use urinary catheterization if needed. Administer a benzodiazepine or other sedative as ordered. Physostigmine may reverse anticholinergic toxicity. Evaluate for toxicity any time psychosis unexpectedly worsens.
Neuroleptic Malignant Syndrome (NMS)	
Rare but life-threatening medical emergency (early detection improves survival)	Hold all medications. Contact prescriber immediately.
A sudden drop in dopamine activity due to **D2 receptor blockade or abrupt withdrawal of D2 receptor stimulation.**	Transfer to a critical care unit; if in the community, call 911 for emergency transport.
Hyperpyrexia (fever > 103 °F) is the most diagnostic symptom.	Dantrolene (Dantrium), a muscle relaxant, may be ordered to relieve muscle rigidity and reduce fever caused by muscle contractions.
Severe muscle rigidity, dysphasia, flexor–extensor posturing, reduced or absent speech and movement, decreased responsiveness.	Bromocriptine (Parlodel), a dopamine agonist, helps restore dopamine balance. Implement emergency cooling measures (cooling blanket, alcohol, or ice bath).
Autonomic dysfunction: hypertension, tachycardia, diaphoresis, incontinence.	Maintain hydration with oral or IV fluids. Monitor and correct electrolyte imbalance.
Delirium, stupor, or coma.	Monitor and report cardiac dysrhythmias. Heparin may be ordered to decrease the possibility of pulmonary emboli.

(Continued)

Table 22.5 Serious Side Effects of Antipsychotics and Associated Nursing Care—cont'd

Side Effect	Nursing Care
Agranulocytosis *Potentially fatal blood disorder characterized by dangerously low neutrophil counts* Increases susceptibility to infections, which may be severe. Early symptoms may include sorethroat, fever, malaise, and body aches.	Monitor neutrophil counts weekly for 6 months, then twice monthly for 6 more months, and monthly thereafter. If neutropenia develops, hold the drug and consult the prescriber. Moderate neutropenia (ANC <500/μL) and severe neutropenia (ANC <100/μL) require treatment interruption. In some cases, clozapine may be reinstituted once ANC returns to normal. Implement temporary reverse isolation may be initiated. Provide education regarding signs of infection reporting these symptoms promptly to the prescriber.
QT Prolongation *Medical emergency, potentially fatal* Increases the risk of ventricular tachyarrhythmias, which can lead to syncope, cardiac arrest, or sudden death. Tachycardia, irregular pulse, fainting. Seizures may occur due to erratic heartbeats resulting in brain oxygen deprivation.	Evaluate all patients for existing QT prolongation with electrocardiogram, as ordered, before beginning antipsychotic therapy. Monitor pulse for tachycardia and irregularities. Recognize that fainting or seizures in a person taking antipsychotics may indicate impending cardiac arrest. Be prepared to initiate life-saving emergency interventions.

Table 22.6 **Long-Acting Injectable Antipsychotics**

Generic (Trade) Name	Nursing Considerations
Aripiprazole monohydrate[b] (Abilify Maintena)	Oral supplementation for 14 days after first injection Once monthly\ Administer by IM or SC (deltoid or gluteal)
Aripiprazole lauroxil[b] (Aristada)	Oral supplementation for 21 days after first injection Every 4, 6, or 8 weeks Administer by IM (deltoid or gluteal) injection
Aripiprazole lauroxil[b] (Aristada Initio)	One-time injection Deltoid or gluteal site. One-time initiation dose combined with a 30 mg dose of aripiprazole and a selected dose of Aristada.
Fluphenazine decanoate[a] (generic only)	Decrease oral dose by half after 1st injection, then discontinue after 2nd injection Every 2-4 weeks Oil-base viscous solution Administer by IM or SC Z-track (deltoid or gluteal) injection
Haloperidol decanoate[a] (Haldol Decanoate)	Taper oral dose and discontinue after 2-3 injections Once monthly Oil-based, viscous solution Administer by IM Z-track (gluteal) injection
Olanzapine pamoate[b] (Zyprexa Relprevv)	Every 2 or 4 weeks Monitor the patient for excess sedation for 3 hours postinjection Administer by IM (gluteal) injection Shake vigorously just before administering.
Paliperidone palmitate[b] (Invega Sustenna)	Once monthly When initiating, the first two injections are given deltoid on days 1 and 8 Administer by IM (deltoid or gluteal) injection
Paliperidone palmitate[b] (Invega Trinza)	Every 3 months Must be established on monthly paliperidone for at least 4 months Administer by IM (deltoid or gluteal) injection

(Continued)

Table 22.6 **Long-Acting Injectable Antipsychotics—cont'd**

Generic (Trade) Name	Nursing Considerations
Risperidone microspheres[b] (Risperdal Consta)	Oral supplementation for 21 days Every 2 weeks Administer by IM (deltoid or gluteal) injection
Risperidone polymer[b] (Perseris)	Once monthly Administer by SC (abdomen or back of upper arm) injection Lump at injection site will decrease in size over time - o not rub or massage

[a]First generation.
[b]Second generation.

performed before starting antipsychotic therapy in high-risk patients.

Liver Impairment

More common with FGAs, liver impairment can occur in early therapy and may cause elevated liver enzymes, jaundice, abdominal pain, ascites, edema, dark urine, pale stools, and easy bruising. Patients may also report itching, fatigue, nausea, and appetite loss. Routine liver function monitoring is crucial for early detection.

Table 22.5 summarizes serious side effects of antipsychotics and the nursing care to respond to these side effects.

Long-Acting Injectable Antipsychotics

Some antipsychotics are available in long-acting injectable (LAI) formulations, requiring administration every 2 to 4 weeks or even months (Table 22.6). Certain formulations have specific administration protocols that must be followed. LAIs offer several advantages, including improved adherence by reducing the need for frequent dosing and minimized conflict over medication compliance. However, drawbacks include limited dosing flexibility once administered and the possibility that patients may feel a loss of control or perceive coercion in their treatment.

CHAPTER 23

Mood-Stabilizers

Mood stabilizers are a class of medications used to manage symptoms of bipolar disorder. Originally, the term "mood stabilizer" referred to drugs effective in treating both mania and depression. However, while most of the medications in this category are effective in treating mania, not all of them effectively treat depression.

Table 23.1 summarizes medications used for the treatment of bipolar disorder.

LITHIUM

In 1970, lithium was given FDA approval for the treatment of acute mania, and in 1974 for maintenance therapy in bipolar disorder. Until the mid-1990s, lithium was the only drug approved for both acute and maintenance treatment. Lithium is sold as Eskalith, Eskalith CR, and Lithobid.

Lithium is a soft natural silvery metal, and most of the lithium in the United States is derived from dry lake beds in South America. Lithium is found in trace amounts in vegetables, grains, spices, and drinking water. Trace amounts are present in most rocks, and weathering processes release lithium into the soil, ground, and standing water, and even into the public water supply. Notably, regions with high levels of lithium in public drinking water are associated with lower suicide rates (Memon et al., 2020).

Lithium is particularly effective in reducing the following:
- Elation, grandiosity, and expansiveness
- Flight of ideas
- Irritability and manipulative behaviors
- Anxiety
- Self-injurious behavior
  To a lesser extent, lithium helps control:
- Insomnia
- Psychomotor agitation

Table 23.1 **FDA-Approved Drugs for Bipolar Disorder**

Generic (Trade) Name	Bipolar Depression	Acute Mania	Bipolar Maintenance
Mood Stabilizers			
Lithium (Eskalith, Eskalith CR, Lithobid)	—	FDA-approved	FDA-approved
Antiseizure Medications			
Carbamazepine (Equetro)	—	FDA-approved	—
Divalproex sodium delayed-release (Depakote), divalproex sodium extended-release (Depakote ER)	—	FDA-approved	—
Lamotrigine (Lamictal)	—	—	FDA-approved
First-Generation Antipsychotics			
Chlorpromazine (Thorazine)	—	FDA-approved	—
Loxapine (Adasuve) orally inhaled	—	FDA-approved[a]	—
Second-Generation Antipsychotics			
Aripiprazole (Abilify)	—	FDA-approved[b]	FDA-approved
Aripiprazole (Abilify Maintena)	—	—	FDA-approved
Asenapine (Saphris)	—	FDA-approved[b]	FDA-approved
Cariprazine (Vraylar)	FDA-approved	FDA-approved[b]	—
Lumateperone (Caplyta)	FDA-approved	FDA-approved[b]	—
Lurasidone (Latuda)	FDA-approved	—	—
Olanzapine (Zyprexa)	—	FDA-approved[b]	FDA-approved
Quetiapine (Seroquel, Seroquel XR)	FDA-approved	FDA-approved[b]	FDA-approved
Risperidone (Risperdal)	—	FDA-approved[b]	—
Risperidone (Risperdal Consta)	—	—	FDA-approved

Table 23.1 **FDA-Approved Drugs for Bipolar Disorder—cont'd**

Generic (Trade) Name	Bipolar Depression	Acute Mania	Bipolar Maintenance
Ziprasidone (Geodon)	—	FDA-approved	FDA-approved
Combination Second-Generation Antipsychotic and Antidepressant			
Olanzapine (Zyprexa) + fluoxetine (Prozac) = Symbyax	FDA-approved	—	—

[a]Bipolar I acute agitation
[b]Bipolar I mixed episode
From U.S. Food and Drug Administration (2016). FDA online label repository. Retrieved from http://labels.fda.gov/.

- Threatening or assaultive behavior
- Distractibility
- Paranoia
- Hypersexuality

Lithium's antimanic effects typically take 7 to 14 days to achieve. Therefore, during the initial stages of treatment, other medications such as a second-generation antipsychotic may be given to help decrease psychomotor activity, manage aggression, and prevent exhaustion.

A narrow range exists between the therapeutic dose and toxic dose of lithium. The lithium level is drawn every 2 to 3 days after beginning lithium therapy and after any dosage change until the therapeutic level has been reached. Blood levels are then checked every 3 to 6 months. Initially, levels should be from 0.8 to 1.2 mEq/L during acute manic states.

Maintenance blood levels are lower ranging from 0.6 to 0.8 mEq/L. Even lower levels of lithium—0.4 to 0.6 mEq/L—may be considered in some cases, such as adjunctive treatment for bipolar I patients or monotherapy for bipolar II patients. To prevent serious toxicity, lithium levels should not exceed 1.5 mEq/L. Lithium side effects, signs of toxicity, and interventions are listed in Table 23.2.

Lithium treatment is associated with a decline in renal and thyroid function, and with hypercalcemia. Women

Table 23.2 Lithium Side Effects, Signs of Toxicity, and Interventions

Side Effects and Signs of Lithium Toxicity		Interventions
Expected Side Effects	<1.5 mEq/L	Symptoms often subside during treatment. Doses should be kept low. Kidney function and thyroid levels should be assessed before treatment and then on an annual basis.
	Nausea, vomiting, diarrhea, thirst, polyuria (increased urination), polydipsia (excessive thirst), lethargy, sedation, and fine hand tremor.	
	Long-term use may result in renal toxicity, goiter, and hypothyroidism may occur with long-term use.	
Early Signs of Toxicity	1.5–2.0 mEq/L	Medication should be withheld, blood lithium levels measured, and dosage reevaluated.
	Gastrointestinal upset, coarse hand tremor, confusion, hyperirritability of muscles, electroencephalographic changes, sedation, and incoordination.	
Advanced Signs of Toxicity	2.0–2.5 mEq/L	Hospitalization is indicated. The drug is stopped, and excretion is hastened. Whole bowel irrigation may be done to prevent further absorption of lithium.
	Ataxia, giddiness, serious electroencephalographic changes, blurred vision, clonic movements, large output of dilute urine, seizures, stupor, severe hypotension, and coma. Death is usually secondary to pulmonary complications.	
Severe Toxicity	2.0–2.5 mEq/L	In addition to the previously listed interventions, hemodialysis may be necessary.
	Convulsions, oliguria (producing no or small amounts of urine), and death can occur.	

younger than 60 years and people with lithium concentrations higher than median are at greatest risk. Individuals need baseline measures of renal, thyroid, and parathyroid function and regular long-term monitoring.

Lithium therapy is generally contraindicated in patients with cardiovascular disease, brain damage, renal disease, thyroid disease, or myasthenia gravis. Whenever possible, lithium is not given to women who are pregnant because it may harm the fetus. There is controversy regarding the use of lithium in breastfeeding mothers. Some sources list lithium as a contraindication in breastfeeding, while other sources do not, particularly if the infant is older than 2 months. The amount of lithium excreted into breast milk and absorbed by the infant varies widely, but it is generally considered low. If lithium therapy is continued during breastfeeding, maternal, and sometimes infant, serum levels are monitored closely. Lithium use is also contraindicated in children younger than 12 years. Box 23.1

A fine hand tremor, polyuria, and mild thirst may occur early in therapy for the acute manic phase and may persist throughout treatment. Transient and mild nausea and general discomfort may also appear during the first few days of lithium administration. Because lithium is a salt, patients are advised to maintain balanced hydration by drinking an adequate amount of water and consuming a normal level of dietary salt. Dehydration from exercise, heat, vomiting, or diarrhea may result in toxic levels of lithium in the bloodstream. Patient and family teaching is provided in Box 23.1.

ANTISEIZURE MEDICATIONS

Antiseizure medications, also known as anticonvulsants, were initially developed to treat convulsions associated with epilepsy. However, early epilepsy trials revealed that patients treated with these medications experienced improvements in mood, prompting investigations into their potential psychiatric benefits. Antiseizure medications are now commonly used to treat acute bipolar depression, acute mania, and/or bipolar maintenance. They generally share several key characteristics including:

- Superior in treating patients with rapid cycling bipolar disorders.
- Effective in diminishing impulsive and aggressive behavior in patients without psychosis.

Box 23.1 Patient and Family Teaching: Lithium Therapy

Give the patient and the patient's family the following information, both verbally and in written form, and encourage them to ask questions

- Lithium is a mood stabilizer that helps prevent relapse. It is important to continue taking the drug even after the current episode subsides.
- Lithium is not addictive.
- Blood lithium levels are monitored until a therapeutic level is reached. Initially, more frequent testing is required, followed by checks every 3 to 6 months thereafter.
- Fluid and sodium balance are important since lithium is a salt.
- Maintain a consistent fluid intake of six 12-oz glasses of fluid a day (1500–3000 mL). High fluid intake leads to lower levels of lithium and less therapeutic effect. Lower fluid intake leads to higher lithium levels, which could produce toxicity.
- Aim for consistency in sodium intake. High sodium intake leads to lower levels of lithium and less therapeutic effect. Low sodium intake leads to higher lithium levels, which could produce toxicity.
- Stop taking lithium if you experience excessive diarrhea, vomiting, or sweating. All of these symptoms can lead to dehydration and increase blood lithium to toxic levels. Inform your care provider if you have any of these problems.
- Lithium levels may be increased while taking angiotensin-converting enzyme (ACE) inhibitors, angiotensin receptor blockers, thiazide diuretics, and nonsteroidal anti-inflammatory drugs. Inform your prescriber if you are taking any of these medications.
- Talk to your prescriber about having renal (kidney), thyroid, and parathyroid function checked periodically due to potential side effects.
- Do not take over-the-counter medicines without checking with your prescriber. Even nonsteroidal anti-inflammatory drugs (e.g., ibuprofen, naproxen) may increase serum lithium levels, diminish renal lithium clearance, and possibly induce lithium toxicity.
- Take lithium with meals to reduce stomach irritation.
- You may gain up to 5 pounds of water weight in the first week. Additional weight gain may occur,

---

Box 23.1 Patient and Family Teaching: Lithium Therapy—cont'd

> particularly in women. Discuss how much weight gain is acceptable with your prescriber.
> - Support groups are available for individuals with bipolar disorder and their friends, family, and caregivers. A local self-help group is [provide name and phone number].
> - Online support groups specific to the population being served (e.g., veterans, young adults, older adults, and minorities) are also available.

- Beneficial in controlling mania within 2 weeks and depressive symptoms within 3 weeks or earlier.
- More effective when there is no family history of bipolar disorder.
- Helpful in cases of alcohol and benzodiazepine withdrawal.

Valproate

Valproate, available as divalproex (Depakote), and valproic acid have FDA approval for treating acute mania. This group of drugs is one of the most widely prescribed mood stabilizers in psychiatry. Valproate and valproic acid are first-line mood stabilizers. They work quickly, and most people tolerate them well. It takes about a week for an adequate serum level of the drug to be reached. Patients typically experience symptom reduction within 1 to 4 days after reaching the adequate serum level.

Common side effects of valproate include gastrointestinal irritation, nausea, diarrhea, vomiting, weakness, sedation, tremor, weight gain, and hair loss. The FDA features a black box warning for several adverse responses. Box 23.2 contains the warning on the valproic acid label.

The warning is essentially identical on the divalproex label. Hepatotoxicity is the first warning. Although rare, it is important to monitor liver function. Low platelets (thrombocytopenia) may also occur, so platelet counts and coagulation studies are also monitored.

Another warning on the FDA label is the risk of valproate use in pregnancy due to teratogenicity (i.e., a drug that interferes with the development of the fetus). Pregnancy screening is recommended before starting this medication

Box 23.2 FDA Black Box Warning for Valproic Acid

Warning: Life-Threatening Adverse Reactions
  See full prescribing information for complete boxed warning.

- Hepatotoxicity, including fatalities, usually during first 6 months of treatment. Children under the age of 2 years are at considerably higher risk of fatal hepatotoxicity. Monitor patients closely, and perform liver function tests prior to therapy and at frequent intervals thereafter.
- Teratogenicity, including neural tube defects.
- Pancreatitis, including fatal hemorrhagic cases.

From U.S. Food and Drug Administration. (2008). Approved label – FDA. Retrieved from https://www.accessdata.fda.gov/drugsatfda_docs/label/2009/022152s002lbl.pdf.

and birth control should be used to prevent pregnancy while taking it. Fetal valproate syndrome is the result of exposure to valproate during the first three months of pregnancy. It includes neural tube defects such as spina bifida, distinctive facial features, congenital heart defects, and musculoskeletal abnormalities. There have been rare, spontaneous reports of polycystic ovary disease associated with these drugs.

Pancreatitis, including fatal hemorrhagic cases, has been reported while using valproate. Symptoms of pancreatitis include abdominal pain or tenderness, vomiting, abdominal distention, fever, and chills. Notably, there is no correlation between the serum level of the drug or the duration of therapy and the onset of symptoms. After successful management of pancreatitis, the reintroduction of valproate is avoided.

Carbamazepine

Carbamazepine (Equetro) is indicated as a second-line treatment for acute mania and mixed states. It seems to work better for mania with rapid cycling, paranoia, and anger than in mania with euphoria and hyperactivity., paranoia, and anger.

Liver enzymes are monitored at least weekly for the first 8 weeks of treatment. Carbamazepine can increase drug metabolizing enzymes which can speed up its metabolism.

Liver function studies are also important because this drug can cause hepatitis. The FDA provides a black box warning for aplastic anemia and agranulocytosis. Pretreatment hematological testing is recommended along with periodic complete blood counts. Carbamazepine is discontinued if significant bone marrow suppression is detected.

Carbamazepine also carries a black box warning for serious dermatologic reactions. These include toxic epidermal necrolysis and Stevens-Johnson syndrome. Both conditions result in erythema and death of the epidermis and mucous membranes, resulting in serious exfoliation and possible sepsis. Involvement of the mucous membranes can result in gastrointestinal hemorrhage, respiratory failure, ocular abnormalities, and genitourinary complications. These reactions occur in up to 6 per 10,000 new users who are of Western European descent. The risk in some people of Asian descent is 10 times higher because of an inherited variation of the HLA-B gene. At-risk individuals are screened for this gene before beginning treatment with carbamazepine.

Lamotrigine

Lamotrigine (Lamictal) is an FDA-approved maintenance therapy medication. Patients usually tolerate lamotrigine well. It is more effective in lengthening the time between depressive episodes. The most common side effects are dizziness, ataxia, somnolence, headache, diplopia, blurred vision, and nausea.

Like carbamazepine, the FDA provides a black box warning for life-threatening rashes such as Stevens-Johnson syndrome and toxic epidermal necrolysis. About 1 in 10 patients develop a rash within 8 weeks of starting treatment with lamotrigine. Even though usually benign, the medication is discontinued if a rash occurs. About 1% of this group progresses to toxic epidermal necrolysis or Stevens-Johnson syndrome. Instruct patients to seek immediate medical attention if a rash appears.

FIRST-GENERATION ANTIPSYCHOTICS

First-generation antipsychotics used to be the treatment of choice for acute mania with or without psychosis.

However, because these first-generation agents may cause severe side effects and may worsen depressive symptoms in patients with bipolar disorder, they have limited use.

Two of these first-generation antipsychotics have FDA approval for the treatment of acute mania. They are chlorpromazine (Thorazine) and inhaled loxapine (Adasuve). Loxapine is available only in supervised settings with clinician administration.

SECOND-GENERATION ANTIPSYCHOTICS

Many of the second-generation antipsychotics are FDA-approved for acute mania. In addition to showing sedative properties during the early phase of treatment thereby decreasing insomnia, anxiety, and agitation, the second-generation antipsychotics seem to have mood-stabilizing properties.

Second-generation antipsychotics may also cause serious side effects. These side effects stem from a tendency toward weight gain that may lead to insulin resistance, diabetes, dyslipidemia, and cardiovascular impairment. See Chapter 22 for a more complete discussion of antipsychotic medications and their side effects.

Benzodiazepines

Though not considered a core treatment in bipolar disorder, some benzodiazepines (e.g., clonazepam [Klonopin] and lorazepam [Ativan]) can rapidly help control manic symptoms such as restlessness, agitation, or insomnia until mood-stabilizing drugs take effect. These drugs are used for a limited time in treatment-resistant mania.

BIPOLAR DEPRESSION

Treatment of bipolar depression with a common antidepressant alone may increase the risk of triggering a manic episode. However, this risk is significantly reduced when the antidepressant is combined with a mood stabilizer.

Specific medications are indicated for bipolar depression. The second-generation antipsychotics lurasidone (Latuda), quetiapine (Seroquel), lumateperone (Caplyta), and cariprazine (Vraylar) have FDA approval for the treatment of bipolar depression. Symbyax is another drug with approval for this type of depression. It is a combination of medication consisting of the second-generation antipsychotic olanzapine (Zyprexa) and the selective serotonin reuptake inhibitor fluoxetine (Prozac).

CHAPTER 24

Antidepressants

Major depressive disorder is the most common psychiatric disorder, affecting nearly 14.5% of people at least once in their lifetime. Symptoms include a long-lasting depressed mood along with feelings of guilt, anxiety, and recurrent thoughts of death and suicide. The monoamine hypothesis, developed in the 1950s, posits that depression results from a deficiency or imbalance in the monoamine neurotransmitters, such as serotonin, dopamine, and norepinephrine. Most currently used antidepressants are thought to act based on this hypothesis, which continues to provide a basis for pharmacotherapy.

One concern with the monoamine hypothesis is that it does not explain why antidepressants have a delayed or latent response. While antidepressants act relatively quickly to improve the levels or balance of monoamines, they generally require 2 to 4 weeks, or longer, to show therapeutic effects on depressive symptoms. Another challenge is that up to 30% of individuals do not respond to medications. These delayed responses and lack of effectiveness in some individuals suggest that alternative hypotheses may be needed to better understand the pathophysiology of depression. Ongoing research into these alternate hypotheses could pave the way for the development of new treatments for major depressive disorder.

ANTIDEPRESSANT MEDICATIONS

Antidepressant medications can have a positive impact on poor self-concept, social withdrawal, vegetative signs of depression, and activity levels. Target symptoms include:
- Sleep disturbance (decreased or increased)
- Appetite disturbance (decreased or increased)
- Fatigue
- Decreased or absent libido
- Psychomotor retardation or agitation

- Diurnal mood variations (often worse in the morning)
- Impaired concentration or memory
- Anhedonia (inability to experience pleasure)
- Feelings of guilt and self-loathing

A drawback of antidepressant drugs is that improvement in mood may take 2 to 4 weeks or longer. If a patient has acute suicidal ideation, electroconvulsive therapy (discussed in Chapter 30) may be a reliable and effective alternative.

The goal of antidepressant therapy is the complete remission of symptoms. Often, the first antidepressant prescribed may not be the one that ultimately leads to remission. An aggressive approach to treatment can help identify the most effective medication. While opinions vary on what constitutes adequate drug trial for treating depression, 6 weeks is commonly used in clinical trials.

For individuals experiencing their first depressive episode, antidepressant therapy is typically continued for 6 to 12 months after remission. Afterward, the decision to maintain pharmacotherapy is made collaboratively between the individual and the clinician. The risk of relapse following antidepressant discontinuation is high, though not universal. Some individuals may experience multiple depressive episodes or have chronic depression and may benefit from long-term or indefinite antidepressant therapy.

Antidepressants may precipitate a manic episode with bipolar disorder. If an antidepressant is indicated, patients with bipolar disorder often receive a mood-stabilizing drug along with the antidepressant to reduce the possibility of this event.

CHOOSING AN ANTIDEPRESSANT

Antidepressants generally work by increasing the availability of one or more neurotransmitters—serotonin, norepinephrine, and dopamine. While clinical trials show that antidepressants demonstrate similar efficacy (i.e., the ability to produce the desired result), differ in adverse effects, cost, safety profiles, and maintenance considerations. Selecting the appropriate antidepressant depends based on several factors, including:

- The patient's symptom profile
- Side effect profile (e.g., sexual dysfunction, weight gain)
- Ease of administration

- History of past response
- Safety and medical considerations

Advanced practice providers, such as advanced practice psychiatric-mental health nurses and psychiatrists, may use pharmacogenetic testing to guide medication decisions. One type of genetic test assesses drug metabolism. The human body relies on cytochrome P450 (CYP) enzymes to process medications including the CYP2D6 enzyme, which plays a key role in metabolizing many antidepressants. One type of genetic test assesses drug metabolism. The human body relies on cytochrome P450 (CYP) enzymes to process medications, including the CYP2D6 enzyme, which plays a key role in metabolizing many antidepressants. Polymorphisms in CYP2D6 influence how an individual responds to a medication.

Genetic testing can help determine an individual's drug metabolism profile, classifying them into one of four categories:

1. Poor metabolizers lack a functional enzyme, leading to slow drug processing. This can cause the medication accumulation, increasing the risk of side effects. Lower doses may be required.
2. Intermediate metabolizers have reduced enzyme function, resulting in slower drug metabolism. This can lead to heightened side effects and an increased risk of drug interactions.
3. Normal metabolizers (also called extensive metabolizers) process medications as expected, making them more likely to experience therapeutic benefits with minimal side effects.
4. Ultra-rapid metabolizers break down medications too quickly, often before they can exert their full effect. These individuals may require higher doses or alternative treatments.

DISCONTINUING AN ANTIDEPRESSANT

An underrecognized problem may occur with abrupt discontinuation of antidepressant medications. This withdrawal reaction, known as discontinuation syndrome, occurs at a high rate—about 20%—in patients after taking medication for at least 6 weeks. Symptoms include flu-like aching, insomnia, nausea, imbalance, sensory disturbances, and hyperarousal. These symptoms tend to last 1 or 2 weeks or are eliminated quickly if the drug is restarted.

The syndrome is more common with longer duration of treatment and with drugs with a shorter half-life. All approved antidepressant drugs carry the potential for this problem. Nurses need to be aware of this syndrome and provide education on how to prevent it, such as slow tapering off of the antidepressant.

ANTIDEPRESSANT CLASSIFICATION

This chapter reviews several classifications of antidepressants, beginning with the most commonly prescribed groups. Table 24.1 provides an overview of antidepressants used in the United States and discussed in this chapter.

Selective Serotonin Reuptake Inhibitors

The selective serotonin reuptake inhibitors (SSRIs) work by blocking the reabsorption (reuptake) of serotonin into neurons, increasing its availability in the synaptic cleft. Some SSRIs tend to be more activating, while others tend to be more sedating. The choice of drug depends, in part, on the patient's symptoms.

Fluoxetine (Prozac), the first SSRI, was to be introduced in 1987 and quickly became popular due to its effectiveness and tolerability. Within 2 years, US, pharmacies were filling 65,000 fluoxetine prescriptions per month. By 2022, that number had risen to approximately 24 million prescriptions annually.

Indications

SSRIs are commonly the first-line treatment for treating major depressive disorder. In addition to their use in treating depressive disorders, the SSRIs are prescribed for anxiety disorders. Generalized anxiety disorder, panic disorder, social anxiety disorder, and obsessive–compulsive disorder are all treated with US Food and Drug Administration (FDA)–approved SSRIs. Fluoxetine (Prozac) has FDA approval for bulimia nervosa. Fluoxetine, sertraline (Zoloft), and controlled-release paroxetine (Paxil CR) have FDA approval for the treatment of premenstrual dysphoric disorder. Another paroxetine, Brisdelle, is used to treat

Table 24.1 FDA-Approved Drugs for Major Depressive Disorder

Generic (Trade) Name	Side Effects	Warnings
Selective Serotonin Reuptake Inhibitors (SSRIs)		
Citalopram (Celexa) Escitalopram (Lexapro) Fluoxetine (Prozac, Prozac Weekly) Paroxetine (Paxil, Paxil CR, Pexeva) Sertraline (Zoloft)	Agitation, insomnia, headache, nausea and vomiting, sexual dysfunction, hyponatremia	Discontinuation syndrome—dizziness, insomnia, nervousness, irritability, nausea, and agitation—may occur with abrupt withdrawal (depending on half-life); taper slowly.
Serotonin Norepinephrine Reuptake Inhibitors (SNRIs)		
Desvenlafaxine (Pristiq)	Nausea, headache, dizziness, insomnia, diarrhea, dry mouth, sweating, constipation	Neonates with *in utero* exposure may require respiratory support and tube feeding.
Duloxetine (Cymbalta, Drizalma)	Nausea, dry mouth, insomnia, somnolence, constipation, reduced appetite, fatigue, sweating, blurred vision	May reduce pain associated with depression, approved for fibromyalgia, pain of diabetic peripheral neuropathy, and chronic musculoskeletal pain.
Levomilnacipran (Fetzima)	Nausea, orthostatic hypotension, constipation, sweating, increased heart rate, palpitations, difficulty urinating, decreased appetite, sexual dysfunction	May cause urinary hesitancy.
Venlafaxine (Effexor, Effexor XR)	Hypertension, nausea, insomnia, dry mouth, sedation, sweating, agitation, headache, sexual dysfunction	Monitor blood pressure, especially at higher doses and with a history of hypertension. Discontinuation syndrome.

Serotonin Antagonists and Reuptake Inhibitors (SARIs)

Nefazodone	Sedation, hepatotoxicity, dizziness, hypotension, paresthesia	Life-threatening liver failure is possible but rare. Priapism of the penis or clitoris is a rare but serious side effect.
Trazodone	Severe sedation, hypotension, nausea	Risk of prolonged erections and priapism. Palpitations, ventricular premature beats, serotonin syndrome.
Vilazodone (Viibryd)	Diarrhea, nausea, vomiting, dry mouth, dizziness, insomnia	

Serotonin Modulator and Stimulator

Vortioxetine (Trintellix)	Constipation, nausea, vomiting	Hyponatremia, rare induction of manic states, serotonin syndrome.

Serotonin Receptor Agonist

Gepirone (Exxua XR)	Dizziness, nausea, insomnia, abdominal pain, dyspepsia.	Contraindicated with prolonged QT interval, severe hepatic impairment, or current use of strong CCYP 3A4 inhibitors.

Norepinephrine Dopamine Reuptake Inhibitor (NDRI)

Bupropion (Wellbutrin, Aplenzin XL, Forfivo XL)	Agitation, insomnia, headache, nausea, and vomiting; sexual dysfunction is rare.	High doses increase seizure risk, especially in individuals who are predisposed to them.

(Continued)

Table 24.1 FDA-Approved Drugs for Major Depressive Disorder—cont'd

Generic (Trade) Name	Side Effects	Warnings
Noradrenergic and Specific Serotonergic Antidepressant (NaSSA)		
Mirtazapine (Remeron)	Weight gain/appetite stimulation, sedation, dizziness, and headache. Sexual dysfunction is rare.	Somnolence is exaggerated by alcohol, benzodiazepines, and other central nervous system depressants.
Tricyclic Antidepressants (TCAs)		
Amitriptyline	Dry mouth, constipation, urinary retention, blurred vision, hypotension, cardiac toxicity, sedation	Lethal in overdose. Use cautiously in older adults and patients with cardiac disorders, elevated intraocular pressure, urinary retention, hyperthyroidism, seizure disorders, and liver or kidney dysfunction.
Amoxapine		
Desipramine (Norpramin)		
Doxepin (Sinequan)		
Imipramine (Tofranil)		
Nortriptyline (Aventyl, Pamelor)		
Protriptyline (Vivactil)		
Trimipramine (Surmontil)		
Monoamine Oxidase Inhibitors (MAOIs)		
Isocarboxazid (Marplan)	Insomnia, nausea, agitation, and confusion; hypertensive crisis	Contraindicated with most antidepressants. Tyramine-rich food may result in a hypertensive crisis. There are many drug and dietary interactions.
Phenelzine (Nardil)		
Tranylcypromine (Parnate)		
Selegiline (Emsam transdermal patch)		
N-Methyl-d-Aspartate (NMDA) Receptor Antagonists		
Esketamine (Spravato)	Dissociation, dizziness, nausea, sedation, vertigo, hypoesthesia (loss of sensation), anxiety, lethargy, increased blood pressure, vomiting, and feeling drunk	Monitor for sedation, dissociation, and hypertension for 2 hours when using the nasal spray. Controlled substance schedule III. Extremely expensive. Available only through an FDA Risk Evaluation and Mitigation Strategy (REMS) program.

Dextromethorphan/Bupropion (Auvelity)	Dizziness, headache, diarrhea, somnolence, dry mouth, sexual dysfunction, and hyperhidrosis.	Dose-related seizure risk Increased blood pressure and hypertension Activation of mania and hypomania Psychosis Angle-closure glaucoma with untreated anatomically narrow angles.

Gamma-Aminobutyric Acid (GABA) A Receptor Positive Modulator

Brexanolone (Zulresso)	Sedation/somnolence, dry mouth, loss of consciousness, and flushing/hot flush	FDA-approved for postpartum depression. Schedule IV controlled substance. There is a risk of excessive sedation or sudden loss of consciousness during administration. Patients must be accompanied during interaction with children. It is available only through an FDA REMS program.
Zuranolone (Zurzuvae)	Drowsiness, dizziness, diarrhea, fatigue, nasopharyngitis, and urinary tract infection.	FDA-approved for postparpartum depression. Schedule IV controlled substance. Monitor for confusion or trouble walking. Patients should not drive or operate machinery, until at least 12 hours after taking each dose. Avoid alcohol. Potential for fetal harm; the use of contraceptives is recommended.

From US Food and Drug Administration. FDA online label repository. www.labels.fda.gov.

moderate to severe vasomotor symptoms (e.g., hot flashes, night sweats) associated with menopause.

Common Adverse Reactions

Medications that enhance synaptic serotonin within the central nervous system (CNS) may result in agitation, anxiety, sleep disturbance, tremor, sexual dysfunction (primarily anorgasmia), or tension headache. Autonomic nervous system reactions such as dry mouth, sweating, weight change, mild nausea, and loose stools may also be experienced with the SSRIs.

Potential Toxic Effect

A rare and life-threatening event associated with SSRIs, and with any medications that increase serotonin, is serotonin syndrome. This syndrome is related to overactivation of the central serotonin receptors caused by either too high a dose or interaction with other drugs. These other drugs include the following:

- Antimigraine medications, such as lasmiditan and triptans, (almotriptan, naratriptan, and sumatriptan)
- Pain medications, such as opioid pain medications including codeine, fentanyl, hydrocodone, meperidine, oxycodone, and tramadol
- Lithium, a mood stabilizer
- Amphetamines in overdose
- Illicit drugs, including lysergic acid diethylamide (LSD), ecstasy, and cocaine.
- Herbal supplements, including St. John's wort, ginseng, and nutmeg
- Cough and cold medications containing dextromethorphan
- Antinausea medications such as granisetron, metoclopramide, droperidol, and ondansetron
- Linezolid, an antibiotic
- Skeletal muscle relaxants such as cyclobenzaprine and metaxalone

Symptoms of serotonin syndrome are abdominal pain, diarrhea, sweating, fever, tachycardia, elevated blood pressure, altered mental state (delirium), myoclonus (muscle spasms), increased motor activity, irritability, hostility, and mood change. Severe manifestations are hyperpyrexia (excessively high fever), cardiovascular shock, and death.

Box 24.1 **Signs of Serotonin Syndrome and Treatments**

Signs
- Hyperactivity or restlessness
- Tachycardia → cardiovascular shock
- Fever → hyperpyrexia
- Elevated blood pressure
- Altered mental states (delirium)
- Irrationality, mood swings, hostility
- Seizures → status epilepticus
- Myoclonus, incoordination, tonic rigidity
- Abdominal pain, diarrhea, bloating
- Apnea → death

Treatments
- Discontinue serotonergic medications
- Initiate symptom management:
- Serotonin receptor blockade with cyproheptadine, methysergide, propranolol
- Cooling blankets, chlorpromazine for hypothermia
- Dantrolene, diazepam (Valium) for muscle rigidity or rigors
- Anticonvulsants
- Artificial ventilation
- Induction of paralysis

The risk of this syndrome seems to be greatest when an SSRI is administered in combination with a second serotonin-enhancing agent, especially monoamine oxidase inhibitors (MAOIs). SSRIs are discontinued for 2 to 5 weeks before starting an MAOI. Box 24.1 lists the signs of serotonin syndrome and provides a summary of emergency treatments.

Serotonin Norepinephrine Reuptake Inhibitors

Serotonin norepinephrine reuptake inhibitors (SNRIs) inhibit the reuptake of both serotonin and norepinephrine. The SNRIs include venlafaxine (Effexor), desvenlafaxine (Pristiq), duloxetine (Cymbalta), and levomilnacipran (Fetzima). All are FDA-approved and are first-line treatments of major depressive disorder, and several have indications for anxiety disorders. Another SNRI, milnacipran (Savella), is indicated only for fibromyalgia.

The SNRIs have a similar side effect profile to the SSRIs, but SNRIs are more likely to cause excessive sweating. In addition, SNRIs cause dose-dependent increases in blood pressure and heart rate due to their norepinephrine reuptake blockade. Monitor blood pressure and heart rate at baseline and periodically thereafter, particularly at dose changes.

Venlafaxine is a serotonergic agent at lower therapeutic doses, and norepinephrine reuptake blockage only occurs at higher doses (i.e., over 150 mg/day). Of the SNRIs, venlafaxine is the most likely to produce discontinuation syndrome (i.e., flu-like symptoms, insomnia, nausea, dizziness, paresthesia, anxiety).

Desvenlafaxine (Pristiq) is the primary active metabolite of venlafaxine. When an individual takes venlafaxine, it will eventually be metabolized into desvenlafaxine. Therefore, the mechanism of action and side effects of the two antidepressants are similar. Nausea is a prominent side effect of this drug.

Duloxetine (Cymbalta) is an SNRI that has FDA approval for both major depressive disorder and generalized anxiety disorder. It is also approved for treating diabetic peripheral neuropathy, fibromyalgia, and chronic musculoskeletal pain.

Levomilnacipran (Fetzima) is the most noradrenergic SNRI. It causes urinary hesitancy in up to 6% of patients secondary to the actions of norepinephrine on the genitourinary tract. Levomilnacipran is the most selective for norepinephrine reuptake of all the SNRIs.

Serotonin Antagonist and Reuptake Inhibitors

Nefazodone (Serzone) and trazodone (Desyrel) belong to the serotonin antagonist and reuptake inhibitor, or SARI, class of antidepressants. Both medications inhibit neuronal uptake of serotonin and antagonize 5-HT2A receptors. Nefazodone also inhibits norepinephrine reuptake. Common side effects include sedation, headache, nausea, dizziness, and blurred vision.

Nefazodone is not commonly prescribed. Sexual dysfunction is minimal with its use, but it is associated with rare, life-threatening liver failure. Avoid nefazodone in patients with preexisting liver impairment. Nefazodone is also contraindicated with several medications due to its inhibition of CYP3A4, a common drug-metabolizing enzyme.

Trazodone is FDA-approved for major depressive disorder, but it is most commonly prescribed off-label as a hypnotic. Due to its sedating effects, it is prescribed at bedtime for insomnia.

Trazodone is a potent α1 receptor antagonist, which contributes to dizziness and orthostatic hypotension. Educate patients to rise slowly when awakening to avoid falls. Potent α1 antagonists with little anticholinergic activity, such as trazodone, can cause priapism, a painful prolonged erection caused by the inability for detumescence (subsidence of erection).

Vilazodone (Viibryd) enhances serotonin neurotransmission via 5-HT_{1A} receptor partial agonism (similar to buspirone) and neuronal inhibition of serotonin reuptake (similar to SSRIs). Weight gain is not associated with this drug, and sexual side effects are limited.

Patients are instructed to take this antidepressant with food for better bioavailability and avoid nighttime doses to prevent sleep disruption. Common side effects include diarrhea, nausea, insomnia, and vomiting. Vilazodone should be used with caution in people taking medications that affect coagulation because it can increase the risk of bleeding. The decision to use vilazodone in pregnant or nursing women should consider the potential risks to the fetus or baby versus the benefit to the mother.

Serotonin Modulator and Stimulator

Vortioxetine (Trintellix) has a similar side effect and contraindication profile to vilazodone. Nausea is the most common reason identified for discontinuing vortioxetine treatment. Constipation and vomiting have also been reported. Some studies suggest that vortioxetine may have cognitive benefits, improving processing speed and executive function in individuals with depression.

Unlike traditional SSRIs, vortioxetine acts as a serotonin modulator and stimulator, targeting multiple serotonin receptors in addition to inhibiting serotonin reuptake. It is typically taken once daily, with or without food. Due to its long half-life, withdrawal symptoms may be less severe compared to other serotonergic antidepressants, but gradual discontinuation is still recommended.

Serotonin Receptor Agonist

The only medication in this novel classification is gepirone (Exxua XR). Gepirone acts as a partial agonist at the serotonin 1A receptor and an antagonist at the serotonin 2A receptor. Because it functions differently than commonly used serotonin reuptake inhibitors, it may have a distinct side effect profile. Specifically, it may have less impact on sexual functioning and weight gain. Common side effects occurring in more than 5% of those treated with Gepirone include dizziness, nausea, insomnia, abdominal pain, and dyspepsia.

Gepirone is contraindicated in patients with congenital long QT syndrome and those with severe hepatic impairment. It should also not be used in individuals taking strong CYP3A4 inhibitors, as these can significantly increase plasma concentrations of the antidepressant.

Norepinephrine and Dopamine Reuptake Inhibitor

Bupropion (Wellbutrin) is a norepinephrine and dopamine reuptake inhibitor (NDRI). It is also FDA-approved for smoking cessation as Zyban. With no serotonergic activities, it carries a lower risk of sexual dysfunction than most other antidepressants. Side effects include insomnia, tremor, anorexia, and weight loss. Contraindications include seizure disorders or eating disorders, or the abrupt discontinuation of alcohol or sedatives (including benzodiazepines) secondary to the increased risk of seizures.

Noradrenergic and Specific Serotonergic Antidepressant

Mirtazapine (Remeron) is a noradrenergic and specific serotonergic antidepressant (NaSSA). Mirtazapine enhances norepinephrine and serotonin neurotransmission by antagonizing both presynaptic $\alpha2$ receptors and postsynaptic 5-HT2 and 5-HT3 receptors. This drug provides both antianxiety and antidepressant effects with minimal sexual dysfunction, limited gastrointestinal symptoms, and improved sleep. Common side effects are sedation, appetite stimulation, and weight gain. This drug is used with caution in patients with renal and hepatic insufficiency.

Tricyclic Antidepressants

Tricyclic antidepressants (TCAs) inhibit the reuptake of norepinephrine and serotonin by the presynaptic neurons in the CNS. They also block the actions of acetylcholine, and some TCAs also affect histamine.

The first TCAs were imipramine (Tofranil) and amitriptyline (formerly sold as Elavil). These TCAs were introduced in the early 1960s.

Positive effects on some symptoms of depression, such as insomnia and anorexia, may be experienced within 10 to 14 days. Full effects may not be seen for 4 to 8 weeks.

Indications

Most TCAs are indicated for the treatment of major depressive disorder. Side effect profiles are considered when choosing a particular TCA. A stimulating TCA, such as desipramine (Norpramin) or protriptyline (Vivactil), may be best for a patient who is lethargic and fatigued. If a more sedating effect is needed for agitation or restlessness, drugs such as amitriptyline and doxepin (Sinequan) may be more appropriate choices. Regardless of which TCA is given, the initial dose should always be low and be increased gradually.

Common Adverse Reactions

Many of the side effects of TCAs are due to their secondary pharmacological actions. The TCAs antagonize several receptors, including H1, α1, and M1, and these receptor effects are responsible for several side effects. By blocking H1 receptors in the brain, sedation and weight gain occur. Blockade of α1 receptors on blood vessels results in vasodilation and the side effects of dizziness and orthostatic hypotension. The effects of acetylcholine are blunted by M1 receptor blockade, and this leads to anticholinergic effects such as blurred vision, dry mouth, tachycardia, urinary retention, and constipation. In older adults, anticholinergic activity causes memory difficulties or confusion.

Administering the total daily dose of TCA at night is beneficial for two reasons. First, most TCAs have sedative effects and thereby aid sleep. Second, the minor side effects occur while the individual is sleeping, which increases adherence to drug therapy.

Toxicity/Overdose

TCA overdose carries a risk of death from cardiac conduction abnormalities: dysrhythmias, tachycardia, myocardial infarction, and heart block. Initial symptoms are CNS stimulation, including hyperpyrexia, delirium, hypertension, hallucinations, seizures, hyperreflexia, and Parkinsonian symptoms. This phase is followed by CNS depression. Immediate medical care is essential for TCA overdose. The TCAs are used cautiously in patients with suicidal history or ideation because they are lethal in overdoses.

Contraindications

People who have recently had a myocardial infarction or other cardiovascular problems, those with narrow-angle glaucoma or a history of seizures, and women who are pregnant are not typically treated with TCAs except with extreme caution and careful monitoring. TCAs are contraindicated for use with MAOIs.

Monoamine Oxidase Inhibitors

The enzyme monoamine oxidase is responsible for inactivating, or breaking down, monoamine neurotransmitters in the brain such as norepinephrine, serotonin, dopamine, and tyramine in the brain. When a person takes an monoamine oxidase inhibitor (MAOI), the activity of this enzyme is reduced, leading to a decreased breakdown of these neurotransmitters. As a result, there is an increase in the levels of mood-elevating neurotransmitters, which can help alleviate depressive symptoms.

Indications

MAOIs are considered third-line antidepressants due to their significant drug interactions and dietary restrictions. MAOIs with FDA approval are phenelzine (Nardil), tranylcypromine (Parnate), and isocarboxazid (Marplan). A transdermal patch, selegiline (EMSAM), does not require strict dietary restrictions at its lowest dose.

Common Adverse Reactions

Some common and troublesome long-term side effects of the MAOIs are orthostatic hypotension, weight gain, edema, change in cardiac rate and rhythm, constipation, urinary hesitancy, sexual dysfunction, vertigo, overactivity, muscle twitching, insomnia, weakness, and fatigue. Hypomania and mania may be activated with MAOIs.

Potential Toxic Effects

Inhibiting MAO results in the inability to break down tyramine sufficiently. Individuals who take MAOIs and eat tyramine-rich foods are at risk for a hypertensive crisis. This crisis results in severe hypertension that can lead to such events as a cerebrovascular accident, intracranial hemorrhage, and death. Blood pressure is monitored during treatment with these drugs. Also, a reduction or elimination of foods and drugs that contain high amounts of tyramine is essential (Table 24.2).

The hypertensive crisis usually occurs within 15 to 90 minutes of ingestion of the offending substance. Early symptoms include irritability, anxiety, flushing, sweating, and a severe headache. The patient then becomes anxious and restless, and he or she develops a fever. Eventually, the fever becomes severe, seizures ensue, and coma or death is possible.

When a hypertensive crisis is suspected, immediate medical attention is crucial. If ingestion is recent, gastric lavage and charcoal may be helpful. Pyrexia is treated with hypothermic blankets or ice packs. Fluid therapy is essential, particularly with hyperthermia. A short-acting antihypertensive agent such as nitroprusside, nitroglycerine, or phentolamine may be used. Intravenous benzodiazepines are useful for agitation and seizure control.

Table 24.3 identifies common side effects and toxic effects of the MAOIs.

Contraindications

The use of MAOIs may be contraindicated with the following:

- Cerebrovascular disease
- Hypertension and congestive heart failure
- Liver disease
- Consumption of foods containing tyramine, L-tryptophan, and dopamine
- Use of certain medications
- Recurrent or severe headaches
- Surgery in the previous 10 to 14 days
- Younger than 16 years old

Table 24.2 Safe and Unsafe Foods With Monoamine Oxidase Inhibitors

Unsafe Foods (High Tyramine Content)	Safe Foods (Little or No Tyramine)
Vegetables and beans	
Avocados, especially if overripe; fermented bean curd; fermented soybean; soybean paste; snow peas, broad beans (fava beans) and their pods	Most fresh, frozen, canned, or dried vegetables, leafy salad greens, lentils, and beans; most veggie burgers that contain no soy product
Fruits	
Dried fruits (e.g., figs); overripe fruit	Most fresh, frozen, or canned fruits and fruit juices
Meats	
Meats that are fermented, smoked, or otherwise aged; spoiled meats; liver, unless very fresh; fermented meats (e.g., pepperoni, salami)	Fresh meats that are known to be fresh (exercise caution in restaurants where meat may not be fresh)
Fish	
Dried or cured fish; fish that is fermented, smoked, or otherwise aged; spoiled fish	Fish that is known to be fresh; vacuum-packed fish, if eaten promptly or refrigerated only briefly after opening
Milk, milk products	Milk, yogurt, cottage cheese, cream cheese
Practically all cheeses	
Breads, cereals, and crackers	
Yeast extract (e.g., Marmite, Bovril); sourdough bread; crackers and breads that contain aged cheese	Commercial yeast breads, hot and cold cereals, most crackers
Beer, wine	
Beer that contains yeast (e.g., draft or homemade beer), red wine, sherry, liqueurs, vermouth	Majority of canned and bottled
Other foods	
Protein dietary supplements; soups (may contain protein extract); shrimp paste; soy sauce	

Table 24.2 Safe and Unsafe Foods With Monoamine Oxidase Inhibitors—cont'd

Unsafe Foods (High Tyramine Content)	Safe Foods (Little or No Tyramine)
Foods That Contain Other Nontyramine Vasopressors	
Chocolate	
It contains phenylethylamine, a pressor agent; large amounts can cause a reaction.	
Fava beans	
They contain dopamine, a pressor agent; reactions are most likely with overripe beans.	
Ginseng	
Headache, tremulousness, and mania-like reactions have occurred.	
Caffeine	
Caffeine is a weak pressor agent; large amounts may cause an increase in blood pressure.	

Table 24.3 Adverse Reactions to and Toxic Effects of Monoamine Oxidase Inhibitors

Adverse Reactions	Comments
Hypotension Sedation, weakness, fatigue Insomnia Changes in cardiac rhythm Muscle cramps Anorgasmia or sexual impotence Urinary hesitancy or constipation Weight gain	Hypotension is an expected side effect. Orthostatic blood pressures should be taken— first lying down, then sitting or standing after 1–2 minutes. This may be a dangerous side effect, especially in older adults who may fall and sustain injuries as a result of dizziness from the blood pressure drop.
Toxic Effects	**Comments**
Hypertensive crisis: Severe headache Tachycardia, palpitations Hypertension Nausea and vomiting	Transport the individual to the emergency department— monitor blood pressure. Agents that may be given are 5-mg intravenous phentolamine or sublingual nifedipine to promote vasodilation. Individuals may be prescribed a 10-mg nifedipine capsule to carry in case of emergency.

N-METHYL-D-ASPARTATE (NMDA) RECEPTOR ANTAGONISTS

Two N-methyl-D-aspartate (NMDA) receptor antagonists are esketamine (Spravato) and dextromethorphan/bupropion (Auvelity). These are **fast-acting antidepressants**. Spravato is a nasal spray that typically works 2 to 4 hours after being administered. Auvelity is an oral tablet that begins working in about 1 week.

Esketamine (Spravato)

Esketamine, a derivative of ketamine, is an NMDA receptor antagonist used for treatment-resistant depression and major depressive disorder with acute suicidal ideation. It works by blocking glutamate's effects on the NMDA receptor, though its precise mechanism in depression is unclear.

Esketamine is FDA-approved for use with an oral antidepressant, administered under healthcare provider supervision in certified facilities. Patients are monitored for dissociation, sedation, and increased blood pressure, with treatment occurring twice weekly for four weeks, then less frequently.

It is available only as an intranasal spray, and patients must be educated on its use. Common side effects include dissociation, dizziness, nausea, increased blood pressure, and cognitive impairments, requiring caution with driving or operating machinery. Pregnancy prevention is advised, as esketamine may cause embryo–fetal toxicity. Treatment costs $600–$900 per session, with potential insurance coverage and payment assistance.

Dextromethorphan/bupropion (Auvelity)

Auvelity combines the cough suppressant dextromethorphan with the antidepressant bupropion to offer a novel treatment for major depressive disorder (MDD). Dextromethorphan modulates NMDA receptors, which play a role in depression, while bupropion targets norepinephrine and dopamine receptors. This dual-action approach may enhance therapeutic outcomes while potentially reducing side effects.

Although bupropion has long been used as an antidepressant, its combination with dextromethorphan represents an innovative expansion of treatment options. Clinical trials have shown encouraging results, confirming Auvelity's effectiveness in alleviating depression symptoms.

Common side effects of Auvelity include dizziness, headache, diarrhea, and drowsiness, along with dry mouth, sexual dysfunction, and excessive sweating. Serious side effects include a dose-related risk of seizures, which requires discontinuation if one occurs, increased blood pressure, and hypertension. Blood pressure should be monitored before and during treatment. The drug may trigger mania or hypomania, so patients should be screened for bipolar disorder. Psychotic reactions should prompt contact with a healthcare provider, and angle-closure glaucoma may occur in those with untreated narrow angles.

GAMMA-AMINOBUTYRIC ACID (GABA) A RECEPTOR POSITIVE MODULATORS

Brexanolone (Zulresso)

Brexanolone (Zulresso) was the first medication to receive FDA approval for postpartum depression. The pharmacology of brexanolone is not fully known, but it appears to interact with GABA type A receptors. It is a neuroactive steroid and identical to a metabolite of progesterone, called allopregnanolone. Brexanolone is a DEA schedule IV substance with limited potential for misuse.

Like esketamine, this drug is available only through a REMS program to mitigate the risk of harm resulting from excessive sedation and loss of consciousness. Pharmacies and healthcare settings that dispense brexanolone are required to be certified. All patients who use this therapy are included in a national registry to identify risks and to support its safe use.

Brexanolone is administered over a total of 60 hours (2.5 days) through continuous intravenous infusion. Patients are at risk of excessive sedation and sudden loss of consciousness during the administration. The infusion is stopped if excessive sedation occurs. The infusion may then be resumed at the same or a lower dose. Patients are monitored for hypoxia using continuous pulse oximetry equipped with an alarm. Mothers are accompanied during interactions with their children, for support if excessive sedation and sudden loss of consciousness occur.

The most common side effects are sedation/somnolence, dry mouth, loss of consciousness, and flushing/hot flashes. Brexanolone is discontinued if postpartum depression becomes worse or if new suicidal thoughts and behaviors occur. Improved symptoms are noticeable within a few hours and last at least a month.

Like esketamine, the cost of brexanolone may be a barrier to its use. This financial limitation is unfortunate given that low-income women are at the greatest risk for postpartum depression. The pharmaceutical company that produces this drug does advertise financial support and guidance.

Zuranolone (Zurzuvae)

Zuranolone (Zurzuvae) is the first oral medication approved to treat postpartum depression. Like brexanolone, it is also a neuroactive steroid that interacts with GABA type A receptors.

Zuranolone is also a Schedule IV drug. It is taken orally for 14 days in the evening with a fatty meal. The most common side effects include drowsiness, dizziness, diarrhea, fatigue, nasopharyngitis, and urinary tract infections. Women should use effective contraception during treatment with zuranolone, while taking the medication, and for one week after discontinuation due to the potential for fetal harm.

FDA labeling includes a boxed warning that Zurzuvae can impact a person's ability to drive and perform other potentially hazardous activities. At the same time, individuals may not be able to assess their degree of impairment. To reduce the risk of harm, patients should not drive or operate heavy machinery for at least 12 hours after taking Zurzuvae.

ANTIDEPRESSANT USE IN SPECIAL POPULATIONS

Use of Antidepressants by Pregnant Women

Antidepressants cross the placenta. The decision to treat severe depression, particularly with suicidal ideation, must weigh the risks versus the benefits. If antidepressant therapy is used during pregnancy, it is typically a single medication (monotherapy) at the lowest effective dose, especially during the first trimester. SSRIs are considered an option, except for paroxetine (Paxil), which has a small association with fetal heart defects.

Antidepressant Use by Children and Adolescents

Although antidepressants can be effective in treating depression in children and adolescents, concerns have been raised about their potential to induce suicidal behavior in some young patients. In response, the FDA issued a black-box warning in 2005—the most serious type of prescription drug warning—stating that antidepressants may increase the risk of suicidal thoughts and behaviors in this population.

By 2024, evidence suggested that this warning had unintended consequences, leading to decreased use of essential medications and reduced mental health treatment for pediatric depression. This decline in care was linked to an increase in suicide attempts and deaths among young patients.

Regardless of these findings, young people prescribed antidepressants should be closely monitored for worsening depression, suicidal thoughts or behaviors, or unusual changes in mood, such as agitation. Close supervision is especially important during the first four weeks of treatment and following any dose adjustments.

Use of Antidepressants by Older Adults

Polypharmacy and the metabolic changes associated with aging raises concerns when prescribing antidepressants for older adults. SSRIs are typically first-line treatment, though they can have for side effects. Alternative options include tricyclic antidepressants, mirtazapine (Remeron), bupropion (Wellbutrin), and venlafaxine (Effexor). To minimize risks, starting doses should be half the usual adult dose, with adjustments made no more frequently than every 7 days ("start low and go slow").

CHAPTER 25

Antianxiety Medications

Anxiety disorders result in chronic fears and distressing thoughts that interfere with everyday living. However, most cases are treatable. Pharmacotherapy is an important adjunct to other therapies, especially cognitive behavioral therapy (CBT). Several classes of medications are effective in the treatment of anxiety disorders.

- Selective serotonin reuptake inhibitors (SSRIs) are the first-line treatment for all anxiety disorders, especially panic disorders.
- Serotonin-norepinephrine reuptake inhibitors (SNRIs) are also used as first-line treatment for anxiety disorders.
- Antianxiety agents such as benzodiazepines are effective but are only recommended to be used short term. These medications are not recommended for patients with substance use disorders.
- Buspirone (BuSpar) is a suitable option for the long-term management of generalized anxiety disorder (GAD). With minimal abuse potential, it is particularly useful for individuals with a history of substance use disorders.

Table 25.1 summarizes medications approved by the FDA for the treatment of anxiety disorders.

ANTIDEPRESSANTS

SSRIs are considered a first line of treatment for most anxiety. These include paroxetine (Paxil), fluoxetine (Prozac), escitalopram (Lexapro), and sertraline (Zoloft). Some of these antidepressants have more of an activating effect than others and may initially increase anxiety. Fluoxetine and sertraline tend to be the most activating, while paroxetine has a more calming effect, SSRIs also provide the secondary benefit of treating comorbid depressive disorders.

Table 25.1 FDA-Approved Drugs for the Treatment of Anxiety Disorders

	Generalized Anxiety Disorder	Panic Disorder	Social Anxiety Disorder
Selective serotonin reuptake inhibitors	Escitalopram (Lexapro) Paroxetine (Paxil)	Fluoxetine (Prozac) Paroxetine (Paxil) Sertraline (Zoloft)	Paroxetine (Paxil) Sertraline (Zoloft)
Serotonin-norepinephrine reuptake inhibitors	Venlafaxine (Effexor) Duloxetine (Cymbalta)[a]	Venlafaxine (Effexor)	Venlafaxine (Effexor)
Benzodiazepines	Alprazolam (Xanax) Chlordiazepoxide (Librium) Clorazepate (Tranxene) Diazepam (Valium) Lorazepam (Ativan) Oxazepam (Serax)	Alprazolam (Xanax) Clonazepam (Klonopin)	
Other	Buspirone (BuSpar)		

From US Food and Drug Administration. (various dates). *FDA label online repository.* www.labels.fda.gov.
[a]Approved for children and adolescents aged 7 to 17 years.

Venlafaxine (Effexor), an SNRI, is another first-line treatment for several anxiety disorders. Another SNRI, duloxetine (Cymbalta), is effective in the treatment of GAD.

Monoamine oxidase inhibitors (MAOIs) are reserved for treatment-resistant conditions. A life-threatening hypertensive crisis can occur if patients do not follow dietary restrictions to avoid tyramine-containing foods. Patients are given specific dietary instructions. The risk of hypertensive crisis also makes the use of MAOIs contraindicated in patients with comorbid substance use disorders. See Chapter 24 for more information about MAOIs and other antidepressant medications.

ANTIANXIETY DRUGS

Antianxiety drugs are often used to treat the somatic and psychological symptoms of anxiety disorders. Benzodiazepines are the most commonly used medication because of their rapid onset of action. By reducing moderate or severe anxiety, these medications help patients better engage in treatment for underlying problems. However, due to their potential for misuse, benzodiazepines are prescribed only for short-term use or until other medications or therapies become effective.

An important nursing intervention is to monitor for benzodiazepine side effects, including sedation, ataxia, and decreased cognitive function. Paradoxical reactions—reactions that are the exact opposite of intended responses—sometimes occur. Symptoms such as anxiety, agitation, talkativeness, and loss of impulse control may occur when using this classification of medications.

Benzodiazepines are not recommended for older adults due to an increased risk of delirium, falls, and fractures. In pregnancy, maternal benzodiazepines use is associated with a 2.5 times higher likelihood of cesarean delivery (Yonkers et al., 2017). They are almost 3 times more likely to result in a need for ventilatory support for the newborn. Maternal benzodiazepine use during pregnancy has also been shown to be associated with other adverse outcomes such as:

- Cleft lip and palate
- Preterm birth
- Low birth weight
- Neonatal respiratory distress

Benzodiazepines may be used during breastfeeding when anxiety is severe. Among them, lorazepam (Ativan) is preferred, as it has not been shown to cause adverse effects in infants, likely due to its shorter half-life. If benzodiazepines are used during breastfeeding, it is crucial to monitor the infant for adverse effects and to limit the duration of maternal benzodiazepine use. Healthcare providers should engage in shared decision-making with breastfeeding mothers, considering both the therapeutic benefits and potential risks.

If used long-term, benzodiazepines require gradual tapering to prevent withdrawal effects. Tapering can last weeks to months depending on factors such as dosage, half-life, and duration of therapy. Because these drugs are central nervous system depressants, sudden discontinuation can lead to rebound hyperactivity, tremors, insomnia, psychomotor agitation, anxiety, and, in severe cases, grand mal seizures. Unlike other withdrawal syndromes, benzodiazepine withdrawal symptoms tend to fluctuate, varying from day to day and week to week.

Buspirone (BuSpar) is a nonbenzodiazepine alternative with little potential for misuse. Buspirone takes 2 to 4 weeks to reach its full effects. This medication may be used for long-term treatment and is taken on a regular schedule.

OTHER CLASSES OF MEDICATIONS

Other medications used to treat anxiety disorders include beta-blockers, anticonvulsants, antihistamines, and antipsychotics. These agents are often added if the first course of treatment is ineffective.

Beta-blockers block the receptors that, when stimulated, cause the heart to beat faster and have been used to treat social anxiety disorder (SAD). Medications such as propranolol (Inderal) reduce physical manifestations of anxiety by slowing the heart rate and reducing blushing.

Anticonvulsants such as gabapentin (Neurontin) and pregabalin (Lyrica) are commonly prescribed off-label for SAD and GAD. Pregabalin is particularly beneficial due to its relatively tolerable side effect profile compared to SSRIs and SNRIs and its ability to treat comorbid conditions like neuropathic pain and substance use disorders, potentially reducing the need for multiple medications. Its different mechanism of action may also help patients who have not found relief with other anxiety treatments. However, neither medication is FDA-approved for these uses.

Antihistamines can be a safe, nonaddictive alternative to benzodiazepines for managing anxiety. They may help treat patients with concurrent substance use disorders. Hydroxyzine (Vistaril) is an effective short-term (up to 4 months) antianxiety agent. A commonly used antihistamine, diphenhydramine (Benadryl), commonly used to treat sleep disturbances associated with anxiety due to its sedative properties, is not recommended by healthcare professionals as a primary treatment for anxiety.

The antihistamines are also anticholinergics, meaning they block the binding of acetylcholine to neural receptors. As a result, anticholinergic side effects, including dry mouth, constipation, and cognitive effects, should to be monitored. These drugs are avoided or used with caution in older adults because the body's production of acetylcholine diminishes with age.

Antipsychotic medications are primarily prescribed for managing severe symptoms of schizophrenia or schizoaffective disorder. Their use in treating **anxiety disorders** is generally considered when first-line treatments are ineffective. The risks of metabolic side effects, as well as the consequences of the dopamine blockade, significantly reduce the use of antipsychotics for anxiety disorders. The FDA has not approved any antipsychotics specifically for the treatment of anxiety disorders.

HERBAL THERAPY AND INTEGRATIVE APPROACHES

Herbal therapy and dietary supplements are commonly used, however they are not subject to the same rigorous testing as prescription medications. Also, herbs and dietary supplements may not be uniformly prepared or dosed, and there is no guarantee of bioequivalence of the active compound among preparations. Problems that can occur with the use of psychotropic herbs include toxic side effects and herb–drug interactions.

Since the use of herbal products has become more mainstream, the importance of better oversight of safety has been heightened. Despite these concerns, the American Association of Poison Control indicates that most major classes of prescribed medications are associated with significantly more adverse effects and fatalities than vitamins, dietary supplements, herbs, and homeopathic remedies

Table 25.2 **Essential Oils Used in Mental Health–Related Concerns**

Essential Oil	Use
Clary sage	Relaxing, relieves anxiety
Ginger	Emotionally and physically warming
Lavender	Calming, decreases anxiety
Lemon	Reduces anxiety
Mandarin	Calming
Neroli	Relieves and decreases anxiety
Roman chamomile	Relieving anxiety
Rose	Relieves and decreases anxiety
Vetiver	Calming, grounding

From National Association of Holistic Aromatherapy. (2024). *Most commonly used essential oils.* www.naha.org/explore-aromatherapy/about-aromatherapy/most-commonly-used-essential-oils.

(Gummin et al., 2022). In 2022, the top 25 categories of poisoning fatalities did not include vitamins/supplements.

Herbal supplements are widely used and generally considered safe, but some herbs may have negative effects on certain individuals and interactions with other medications. Kava (*Piper methysticum*), native to the Pacific Islands, is traditionally consumed as a beverage made from the root of the plant and is known for its sedative and anxiolytic properties.

Kava is known to dramatically inhibit a liver enzyme (P450), which is critical for the metabolism of many medications. This inhibition could result in liver failure, especially when taken along with alcohol or other medications such as central nervous system depressants (antianxiety agents fall into this category). Long-term use of high doses of kava has also been associated with dry, scaly skin or even jaundice (yellowing of the skin).

Valerian is a perennial flowering plant commonly used for conditions related to anxiety, psychological stress, and insomnia. Although it has proven effective for insomnia, there is insufficient scientific evidence to fully assess its long-term safety. Unlike kava, valerian is considered safe for most people when used in medicinal amounts on a short-term basis. However, some individuals may experience side effects such as headaches, excitability, restlessness, or, in some cases, worsening insomnia. As with any supplement, it is important to use valerian with caution, especially when combined with other sedatives or medications.

German chamomile is an herb whose flowers are used to make supplements commonly used for GAD. While chamomile is generally considered safe, there have been reports of allergic reactions, including rare cases of anaphylaxis, following its use. Individuals with allergies to ragweed or related plants are particularly prone to such reactions.

Essential oils, when inhaled or massaged into the skin, may help reduce anxiety. Table 25.2 provides an overview of essential oils commonly used for anxiety- and stress-relief.

ANXIETY TREATMENT IN SPECIAL POPULATIONS

Anxiety Treatment in Children

A few medications are FDA-approved specifically for anxiety disorders in children and adolescents. The SNRI duloxetine (Cymbalta) is approved for children aged 7 to 17 years for GAD. Medications approved for other age groups, such as SSRIs, are commonly prescribed off-label for anxiety disorders in children, including GAD, panic disorder, and SAD, with good results.

Anxiety Treatment in Older Adults

Anxiety disorders are prevalent in older adults, with GAD being the most common. Although the prevalence is similar to that in younger populations, the treatment approach for older adults requires careful consideration due to physiological changes associated with aging. The adage "start low and go slow" is critical, as the absorption, distribution, metabolism, and elimination of medications may differ in older individuals. As a result, medications like antidepressants are typically started at a lower dose—often half or a quarter of the usual starting dose—and are gradually increased to minimize potential side effects and ensure efficacy.

CHAPTER 26

Sleep Promoting Medications

Sleep is a fundamental aspect of life, and essential for recharging the mind and enabling proper cognitive function. Sleep is impacted and implicated in virtually every psychiatric disorder and condition. This chapter begins by exploring medications used to promote sleep in individuals with insomnia. On the other end of the sleep spectrum is narcolepsy, a chronic disorder characterized by excessive daytime sleepiness and sudden sleep attacks. Pharmacotherapy for this disorder is also discussed.

INSOMNIA

Insomnia is characterized by dissatisfaction with the quantity or quality of sleep. It is the most prevalent sleep disorder, affecting nearly half of all adults. Women and older adults are more frequently impacted by insomnia.

Table 26.1 provides an overview of FDA-approved medications for insomnia. With the exception of ramelteon (Rozerem) and doxepin (Silenor), all drugs in this table are US Drug Enforcement Administration (DEA) schedule IV drugs.

Over-the-counter, herbal, and dietary sleep aids are briefly discussed in this section. Additionally, certain drug classes are used off-label to promote sleep, even though they are not specifically FDA-approved for this purpose. These include antidepressants, anticonvulsants, and antihistamines. Second-generation antipsychotics, typically prescribed for conditions like schizophrenia, may also improve sleep in people using them for other psychiatric problems.

Table 26.1 **FDA-Approved Drugs for Insomnia**

Generic (Trade) Name	Onset of Action (min)	Duration of Action	Use in Insomnia	
			DFA	DMS
Benzodiazepines				
Estazolam	15–60	Intermediate	✓	✓
Flurazepam[a]	30–60	Long	✓	✓
Quazepam (Doral)[a]	20–45	Long	✓	✓
Temazepam (Restoril)	45–60	Intermediate	—	✓
Triazolam (Halcion)	15–30	Short	✓	—
Nonbenzodiazepine Receptor Agonists				
Eszopiclone (Lunesta)	60	Intermediate	✓	✓
Zaleplon (Sonata)	15–30	Ultra short	✓	—
Zolpidem immediate release (Ambien)	30	Short	✓	—
Immediate release (Intermezzo)[b]	30	Short	—	✓
Extended release (Ambien CR)	30	Intermediate	✓	✓
Oral spray (Zolpimist)	10	Short	✓	—
Melatonin Receptor Agonist				
Ramelteon (Rozerem)	30	Short	✓	—
Orexin Receptor Antagonists				
Daridorexant (Quviviq)	30	Intermediate	✓	✓
Lemborexant (Dayvigo)	15–20	Intermediate	✓	✓
Suvorexant (Belsomra)	30	Intermediate	✓	✓
Tricyclic Antidepressant				
Doxepin (Silenor)	>60	Intermediate	—	✓

DFA, Difficulty falling asleep; *DMS*, difficulty maintaining sleep.
[a]Generally not recommended due to its long duration of action.
[b]A sublingual tablet taken in the middle of the night when there are at least 4 hours left to sleep.
From US Food and Drug Administration. (various dates). Drugs@ FDA: FDA-approved drugs. https://www.accessdata.fda.gov/ scripts/cder/daf/.

BENZODIAZEPINES

Benzodiazepines have antianxiety, hypnotic (sleep-inducing), anticonvulsant, amnestic (loss of memory), and muscle relaxant properties. Benzodiazepines potentiate, or promote, the activity of gamma-aminobutyric acid (GABA) by binding to a specific site on the GABA receptor complex. This binding results in an increased frequency of chloride channel opening causing membrane hyperpolarization, and reducing cellular excitation. If cellular excitation is decreased, the result is a calming effect.

All benzodiazepines cause sedation at higher therapeutic doses. Several benzodiazepines are FDA-approved for the treatment of insomnia with a predominantly hypnotic effect: estazolam, flurazepam, temazepam (Restoril), quazepam (Doral), and triazolam (Halcion).

Nurses caution patients about taking benzodiazepines when engaging in activities that require mental alertness, such as driving or operating machinery, due to the risk of sedation, ataxia, and slowed reflexes. Central nervous system (CNS) depressants such as alcohol intensify these effects. In older adults, benzodiazepine use is associated with falls, bone fractures, and delirium, and these medications are avoided.

This class of drugs is categorized as Schedule IV by the DEA. Craving, tolerance, and withdrawal can develop even when taken for their intended indication. Chapter 12 provides a discussion of sedative-, hypnotic-, and anxiolytic-related substance use disorders.

When used alone, benzodiazepines rarely inhibit the brain to the degree of respiratory depression and death. However, when combined with other CNS depressants such as alcohol and opioids, they may lead to a coma or fatal overdose.

SHORT-ACTING SEDATIVE-HYPNOTIC SLEEP AGENTS

Nonbenzodiazepine receptor agonists, or Z-hypnotics, include eszopiclone (Lunesta), zaleplon (Sonata), and zolpidem (Ambien). Zolpidem comes in additional formulations. Intermezzo is an immediate-release drug and is used to help people fall back to sleep if they wake in the middle of the night. Ambien CR has two separate layers, one that dissolves quickly and promotes falling asleep, and the other dissolves more slowly to help in continuing sleep. Zolpimist is an oral spray that takes effect within 10 minutes, so it should be used right before bedtime for optimal results and safety.

The Z-hypnotics possesses hypnotic and amnestic effects without the antianxiety, anticonvulsant, or muscle relaxant properties of benzodiazepines. This is due to their selectivity for $GABA_A$ receptors containing an alpha-1 subunit. Similar to benzodiazepines, nonbenzodiazepine receptor agonists can cause sedation, ataxia, and harmful effects in older people, including falls, bone fractures, and delirium. They are controlled substances but seem to cause less tolerance and dependence than benzodiazepines. Nevertheless, exercise caution or consider alternatives for patients with substance use disorders. Eszopiclone can cause an unpleasant, bitter taste upon awakening in about one-third of patients.

Compared to benzodiazepines, the nonbenzodiazepines generally have shorter half-lives and no active metabolites. Zaleplon has the short half-life, approximately 1 hour, and helps patients to fall asleep, whereas eszopiclone has a half-life of approximately 6 hours and will also assist patients with staying asleep. Zolpidem is metabolized more slowly in women than in men, leading to higher blood levels in female patients. In response to this finding, the FDA reduced the starting dose for all zolpidem products for female patients to minimize the risk of side effects, including excessive sedation and impaired alertness.

The FDA has issued warnings for all approved hypnotic medications regarding complex sleep-related behaviors such as sleepwalking, driving, cooking, or eating. These activities occur while the patient is not fully awake, and they may have no memory of engaging in them. Although these events are rare, the use of other CNS depressants, including alcohol, may increase this risk.

MELATONIN RECEPTOR AGONIST

Melatonin (MT) is a hormone that is excreted by the pineal gland at night as part of the normal circadian rhythm. Ramelteon (Rozerem) is an MT receptor agonist and acts similarly to endogenous MT. It has a high selectivity and potency at the MT_1 receptor site—which regulates sleepiness—and at the MT_2 receptor site—which regulates circadian rhythms.

Ramelteon is not classified as a scheduled substance and lacks misuse potential. Side effects include headache and dizziness. This medication may decrease testosterone and increase prolactin levels, possibly causing a decreased interest in sex or problems with fertility. Ramelteon and fluvoxamine, a selective serotonin reuptake inhibitor (SSRI), interact and use together is contraindicated.

OREXIN RECEPTOR ANTAGONISTS

Orexins (OXs), neuropeptides produced in the hypo-thalamus, play a key role in promoting wakefulness. These peptides naturally bind to OX1 and OX_2 receptors. Orexin receptor antagonists, such as Suvorexant (Belsomra), daridorexant (Quviviq), and lemborexant (Dayvigo), are FDA-approved for insomnia characterized by difficulty falling asleep or staying asleep. In patients with narco-lepsy, OX-containing neurons appear to be diminished, so suvorexant and lemborexant are contraindicated. Rare side effects associated with these medications include sleep paralysis, hallucinations during sleep onset or awaken-ing or falling asleep, and cataplexy-like symptoms (loss of muscle tone prompted by strong emotions, such as laughter or surprise) have occurred with use. OX recep-tor antagonists are controlled substances, so they are used with caution in patients with substance use disorders.

TRICYCLIC ANTIDEPRESSANT

A low-dose formulation of the tricyclic antidepressant doxepin, under the brand name Silenor, is FDA-approved for the treatment of insomnia characterized by difficulty staying asleep. It does not decrease the time to sleep onset. Doxepin has a high affinity for the H1 receptor, making it a selective H1 antagonist in low doses. This affinity results in sedating properties.

Silenor is not recommended for use in patients with severe urinary retention or glaucoma, or those taking monoamine oxidase inhibitors (MAOIs). Because this medication does not carry misuse potential, it is not a controlled substance.

OVER-THE-COUNTER SLEEP AIDS

Individuals use a variety of over-the-counter sleep aids to get a good night's sleep. Many of these drugs contain diphenhydramine (Benadryl), an antihistamine commonly used for allergy symptoms. One of its side effects is drowsiness, making this a popular option as a sleep aid. These sleep aids can cause unwanted sleepiness in the morning, difficulty urinating, confusion, and delirium. Some of the over-the-counter products that contain diphenhydramine include the following:

- Excedrin PM
- Nytol
- Tylenol PM
- ZzzQuil
- Sominex

Doxylamine is another antihistamine commonly used as a sleep aid and is found in Unisom. Common side effects include dry mouth, ataxia, urinary retention, drowsiness, and memory problems. In higher doses, more severe side effects can occur, such as hallucinations, psychosis, and an increased sensitivity to external stimuli.

Antihistamines are also anticholinergics, that is, they block the binding of acetylcholine to neural cholinergic receptors. Anticholinergic side effects, including dry mouth, constipation, and cognitive effects, should be monitored. These drugs are avoided or used with caution in older adults because the body's production of acetylcholine diminishes with age. Older adults taking anticholinergic drugs are at risk for brain atrophy, delirium, and clinical decline. Therefore their use is strongly discouraged in this population.

Over-the-counter drugs work best when used for mild and infrequent insomnia. Despite "nonhabit-forming" labels, there is still reason for concern. Most over-the-counter sleep aids result in habituation and, therefore, are not recommended to be used longer than 2 weeks.

HERBAL AND DIETARY SUPPLEMENTS FOR INSOMNIA

Valerian is a tall, flowering plant native to Asia and Europe. Its roots are used as a dietary supplement for conditions such as insomnia, anxiety, depression, and menopause symptoms. However, the evidence supporting its efficacy in treating insomnia is insufficient. There is no information available regarding the long-term safety of valerian, or its safety in children younger than 3 years, pregnant women, or nursing mothers. Mild side effects could include morning fatigue, headaches, dizziness, and upset stomach.

Melatonin is a hormone produced by the pineal gland in the brain, playing a crucial role in regulating the sleep-wake cycle. The production and release of melatonin are closely linked to light exposure. In response to darkness, the pineal gland increases melatonin production, while light exposure slows or halts its production. Melatonin supplements are commonly used for sleep disorders, such as jet lag, circadian rhythm disruptions, and sleep issues related to night shift work sleep problems. In the US, melatonin is considered a dietary supplement and not a drug, therefore it is less strictly regulated by the FDA.

German chamomile, often called "sleep tea," has been used for centuries to treat conditions like insomnia, gastrointestinal issues, and skin ailments. It is generally well-tolerated, though allergic reactions may occur, especially in those allergic to ragweed or similar plants. Other side effects can include drowsiness, nausea, or vomiting if consumed in large amounts. Chamomile may also interact with blood thinners, so caution is advised for those with allergies or on certain medications, such as warfarin or cyclosporine.

NARCOLEPSY

Individuals with narcolepsy experience uncontrollable daytime sleepiness and sudden sleep attacks, which can significantly impair functioning. A hallmark of narcolepsy is cataplexy, a sudden, bilateral loss of muscle tone often triggered by strong emotions. These can lead to symptoms such as slurred speech, weak knees, or in more severe cases, complete paralysis, resembling the sleep paralysis seen during rapid-eye-movement (REM) sleep.

Treatment for narcolepsy includes naps, exercise, and a balanced diet. Medications with FDA approval for excessive daytime sleepiness include CNS stimulants such as modafinil (Provigil), armodafinil (Nuvigil), methylphenidate, and amphetamine. The CNS depressants sodium oxybate (Xyrem), and calcium, magnesium, potassium, and sodium oxybate (Xywav) are indicated for the treatment of both excessive daytime sleepiness and cataplexy in patients with narcolepsy. Another nonstimulant medication, pitolisant (Wakixis), is also indicated for both excessive daytime sleepiness and cataplexy in patients with narcolepsy. A nonstimulant, noncontrolled substance solriamfetol (Sunosi) may improve wakefulness in patients with narcolepsy.

Modafinil (Provigil) is indicated to improve wakefulness and reduce sleepiness in adults with narcolepsy, sleep apnea, and shift work disorder. It is a nonamphetamine, DEA Schedule IV controlled substance with moderate misuse potential. Modafinil is taken first thing in the morning with or without food. Common side effects include headache, nausea, nervousness, rhinitis, diarrhea, back pain, anxiety, insomnia, dizziness, and dyspepsia. A serious rash, including Stevens-Johnson syndrome and toxic epidermal necrolysis, has been reported. Individuals are instructed to discontinue modafinil at the first sign of rash, unless the rash is clearly not drug related.

Armodafinil (Nuvigil) is a longer-lasting isomer of modafinil, resulting in higher plasma concentration later in the day. This may lead to improved wakefulness throughout the day compared with modafinil. However, there is no difference in safety or efficacy between the two. Armodafinil is a DEA Schedule IV controlled substance. It should be taken early in the day with or without food. Common side effects include headache, nausea, dizziness, and insomnia. Rare cases of serious or life-threatening rash have been reported and patients are instructed to discontinue armodafinil if a rash appears.

Methylphenidate (Ritalin) is a CNS stimulant used to treat narcolepsy and also commonly prescribed for attention-deficit/hyperactivity disorder (ADHD). It has a high potential for misuse and is a DEA schedule II substance. Immediate-release formulations are generally taken two or three times a day, preferably 30 to 45 minutes before meals.

Common side effects include tachycardia, palpitations, headache, insomnia, anxiety, hyperhidrosis (excessive sweating), weight loss, decreased appetite, dry mouth, nausea, and abdominal pain. Serious side effects include hypertension, tachycardia, myocardial infarction, and stroke. It can also worsen psychiatric disorders such as bipolar mania or psychosis, and may induce new manic symptoms.

Amphetamine (Adderall) is a CNS stimulant indicated for narcolepsy and ADHD. Like methylphenidate, it is a DEA Schedule II controlled substance with a high misuse potential. Immediate-release versions are taken two or three times daily with or without food. Common side effects include stomachache, decreased appetite, and nervousness.

Sodium oxybate (Xyrem) is a CNS depressant FDA-approved for both excessive daytime sleepiness and cataplexy in individuals 7 years of age and older with narcolepsy. It helps to restore normal sleep architecture, especially slow-wave sleep, which improves daytime alertness. Sodium oxybate is a sodium salt of gamma-hydroxybutyrate (GHB), a Schedule I controlled substance, also known as a date rape drug. Sodium oxybate is a schedule III medication with low-moderate misuse potential. It can only be prescribed under an FDA program called a Risk Evaluation and Mitigation Strategy (REMS), with prescription only by certified prescribers, and dispensed only to a patient enrolled by a certified pharmacy.

Xyrem should be taken 2 hours after eating while in bed and lying down after dosing. Patients need to set an alarm to wake them 3 hours after the first dose. The second dose is then taken, and a deep sleep should follow. The most common side effects of sodium oxybate in adults are nausea, dizziness, vomiting, somnolence, enuresis (bedwetting), and tremor. In children, the most common adverse reactions were enuresis, nausea, headache, vomiting, weight loss, decreased appetite, and dizziness.

CNS depression for the first 6 hours after dosing contraindicates hazardous activities requiring mental alertness. This medication may also increase depression and suicidality, and it is important to monitor patients carefully. Due to its high sodium content, patients are monitored for heart failure, hypertension, or impaired renal function. Sodium oxybate is contraindicated with concurrent use of sleep medications and alcohol.**Xywavcalcium, magnesium, potassium, and sodium oxybate**

Xywav is a **calcium, magnesium, potassium, and sodium oxybate** oral medication used for the treatment of cataplexy and excessive daytime sleepiness in individuals with narcolepsy. It is also the first and only medication approved for idiopathic hypersomnia. Xywav is closely related to Xyrem, although it contains 92% less sodium. Like sodium oxybate, Xywav is approved for children as young as 7, is a Schedule III controlled substance, requires two doses of an oral solution, and requires an REMS protocol for prescribing and dispensing. In patients transitioning from sodium oxybate to Xywav, the dose should be identical.

Common side effects in adults include headache, nausea, dizziness, decreased appetite, parasomnia, diarrhea, hyperhidrosis (excessive sweating), anxiety, and vomiting. Common side effects in children include enuresis, nausea, headache, vomiting, weight loss, decreased appetite, and dizziness.

Pitolisant (Wakix) is a nonstimulant histamine-3 (H3) receptor antagonist/inverse agonist medication with FDA approval for excessive daytime sleepiness in narcolepsy and cataplexy. Pitolisant is an H3 receptor antagonist/inverse agonist and is not scheduled as a controlled substance by the DEA. Pitolisant is taken once a day in the morning. It is contraindicated in patients with hepatic impairment and has the potential to prolong the QT interval. Its use is not recommended in patients with end-stage renal disease. Common side effects include insomnia, nausea, and anxiety.

Solriamfetol (Sunosi) is a nonstimulant dopamine and norepinephrine reuptake inhibitor. Since both dopamine and norepinephrine are wakefulness neurotransmitters, individuals taking this medication experience less sleepiness. Solriamfetol is indicated to improve wakefulness in adults with excessive daytime sleepiness associated with narcolepsy and obstructive sleep apnea. Like pitolisant, Solriamfetol is not classified as a controlled substance. It is contraindicated with the use of MAOIs. Sunosi is administered once daily upon waking. Common side effects include headache, nausea, decreased appetite, insomnia, and anxiety. Monitor blood pressure and heart rate in patients receiving solriamfetol.

CHAPTER 27

Medications for Substance Use Disorders

Pharmacotherapy for substance use disorders is primarily focused on managing acute intoxication and overdose, alleviating withdrawal symptoms, and supporting long-term abstinence. Medication-assisted treatment (MAT) refers to the combination of pharmacological interventions with counseling and behavioral therapies. The goal of MAT is to restore balance to brain chemistry, diminish the euphoric effects of alcohol and substances, curb physiological cravings, and support the body's recovery to its normal functioning.

ALCOHOL

Alcohol Overdose

An alcohol overdose occurs after drinking more than the body can safely process. Blood alcohol levels can continue to rise even when a person is no longer drinking due to continued absorption from the stomach and intestines. Signs of alcohol poisoning are listed in Box 27.1.

The patient is at risk for death from an alcohol overdose, so it is dangerous to assume that the patient will be able to "sleep it off." Medical care should focus on managing breathing problems, which may require an artificial airway, monitoring cardiac status, administering fluids to increase hydration and blood glucose levels, and using gastric lavage to clear alcohol from the body. Heated blankets may also be used to manage hypothermia.

Alcohol Withdrawal

Alcohol is a central nervous system depressant that affects two key neurotransmitters:

> ### Box 27.1 **Signs of Alcohol Poisoning**
>
> - Vomiting
> - Reduced responses, such as an absence of the gag reflex (which can lead to choking and asphyxiation)
> - Slow respirations (fewer than 8 breaths per minute)
> - Irregular breathing (more than 10 seconds between breaths)
> - Hypothermia (low body temperature)
> - Bluish, pale, or clammy skin
> - Mental confusion, stupor, coma, or inability to awaken
> - Seizures

1. Gamma-aminobutyric acid (GABA): A major inhibitory (calming) neurotransmitter. Chronic alcohol exposure reduces GABA receptor sensitivity, leading to decreased inhibitory tone when alcohol use stops.
2. Glutamate: A major excitatory (stimulating) neurotransmitter. Chronic alcohol use increases glutamate receptors to compensate for alcohol's depressant effects. When alcohol is withdrawn, this results in excessive, unregulated excitation.

Mild alcohol withdrawal begins 6 to 8 hours after alcohol cessation and is characterized by tremors (the "shakes"), increased blood pressure and pulse, insomnia, anxiety, panic, muscle twitching, sweating, and nausea. In mild withdrawal, supportive care (hydration, nutrition, monitoring) may be sufficient, and benzodiazepines are not always necessary.

Moderate alcohol withdrawal typically occurs 24 to 36 hours after cessation, presenting with intense anxiety, pronounced tremors, insomnia, seizures, hallucinations, hypertension, and tachycardia. Benzodiazepines, such as chlordiazepoxide (Librium), diazepam (Valium), and lorazepam (Ativan), are the primary treatment for moderate alcohol withdrawal and can help alleviate symptoms, including anxiety, tremors, and seizures."

Psychotic and perceptual symptoms may begin in 8 to 10 hours. If a patient is undergoing withdrawal to the point of psychosis, it is considered a medical emergency due to the risks of unconsciousness, seizures, and delirium. Benzodiazepines such as lorazepam (Ativan) can be given either orally or intramuscularly and tapered over the next 5 to 7 days.

Alcohol withdrawal delirium, also known as delirium tremens (DTs), is a medical emergency that can occur within the first 72 hours of alcohol cessation and may last up to 5 days (Rahman & Paul, 2023). If left untreated, it has a 37% mortality rate. Symptoms include autonomic hyperactivity, leading to tachycardia, diaphoresis, fever, anxiety, insomnia, and hypertension, as well as delusions and visual or tactile hallucinations.

Withdrawal seizures typically occur within 6 to 48 hours after alcohol cessation and are generally generalized tonic-clonic. Additional seizures may occur within hours of the first episode. Intravenous diazepam (Valium) is a common and effective treatment for managing these seizures.

Delusions and hallucinations can lead to unpredictable behaviors as patients try to protect themselves from what they believe are genuine dangers. After three days of heavy alcohol cessation, all patients are at risk for this condition and may pose a danger to themselves and others. However, it is rare in individuals in good physical health. The risk increases significantly in those with serious medical conditions such as hepatitis or pancreatitis.

Prevention of alcohol withdrawal delirium is the primary goal. Oral diazepam (Valium) may help alleviate acute agitation, tremors, impending or active DTs, and hallucinosis. Chlordiazepoxide (Librium) is also commonly used to manage symptoms. However, if delirium develops, intravenous lorazepam (Ativan) is the preferred treatment. In some cases, seclusion may be necessary to ensure safety. Dehydration, often worsened by diaphoresis and fever, should be corrected with oral or intravenous fluids.

Wernicke-Korsakoff Syndrome

People with long-term heavy alcohol use may experience short-term memory disturbances, often due to thiamine deficiency caused by poor nutrition or nutrient malabsorption. One such condition is Wernicke's encephalopathy, an acute and reversible condition. If left untreated, it can progress to Korsakoff's syndrome, a chronic condition with a low recovery rate (about 20%).

Along with memory disturbances, symptoms of Wernicke's encephalopathy are an altered gait, vestibular (balance) dysfunction, confusion, and ocular motility abnormalities (horizontal nystagmus, lateral orbital palsy, and gaze palsy). Sluggish reaction to light and unequal pupil size are also symptoms. Wernicke's encephalopathy responds rapidly to large doses of intravenous thiamine two to three times daily for 1 or 2 weeks. Treatment of Korsakoff's syndrome is thiamine for 3 to 12 months. Although patients with Korsakoff's syndrome may never fully recover, cognitive improvement may occur with thiamine and nutritional support.

Alcohol Relapse Prevention

For many years, disulfiram was the only medication available for long-term treatment of alcohol use disorder. However, its use was limited due to adverse side effects. Now there are two additional medications to prevent cravings in people recovering from alcohol use disorder: naltrexone and acamprosate.

Disulfiram

Disulfiram, formerly sold under the brand name Antabuse, is a medication used to support the treatment of chronic alcoholism by producing an acute sensitivity to ethanol (drinking alcohol). It works by inhibiting the enzyme aldehyde dehydrogenase (ALDH), specifically the ALDH2 enzyme, leading to an accumulation of acetaldehyde in the blood when alcohol is consumed. The elimination half-life of disulfiram varies among individuals, with estimates ranging from approximately 7 hours to 60–120 hours. This variability means that disulfiram can remain active in the body for several days, influencing its effectiveness and the duration of its interaction with alcohol.

Disulfiram is designed to deter alcohol consumption by inducing severe discomfort upon alcohol intake, mimicking a severe hangover. Symptoms of this reaction include nausea, vomiting, sweating, flushing, headache, chest pain, shortness of breath, rapid heart rate, dizziness, and blurred vision. These effects typically occur quickly after alcohol consumption and can last from 30 minutes to several hours. This aversion therapy aims to motivate individuals to abstain from drinking due to the fear of experiencing these unpleasant symptoms.

Consuming alcohol while taking **disulfiram** can lead to severe reactions. These reactions can range from mild to life-threatening, including:

- **Mild to Moderate Symptoms**: Nausea, vomiting, sweating, flushing, headache, chest pain, shortness of breath, rapid heart rate, dizziness, and blurred vision.
- **Severe and Life-Threatening Reactions**: Respiratory depression, cardiovascular collapse, arrhythmias, myocardial infarction, acute congestive heart failure, unconsciousness, convulsions, and death.

These adverse effects typically begin within 10 to 30 minutes of alcohol consumption and can last for several hours. The severity depends on factors such as the amount of alcohol ingested, the dose of disulfiram, and individual health conditions.

In the absence of alcohol, disulfiram is generally well tolerated. Common side effects include fatigue, dermatitis, impotence, optic neuritis, and cognitive changes and it may exacerbate psychosis in some individuals. While disulfiram is associated with a low risk of serum aminotransferase elevations, it can, in rare cases, cause severe and even fatal liver injury. Because of this risk, it is typically prescribed at low doses and is now used less frequently than alternative medications.

Disulfiram is contraindicated in individuals with myocardial disease, coronary occlusion, psychosis, or pregnancy and in those with high levels of impulsivity and suicidality. Disulfiram is not recommended for patients who are taking metronidazole, paraldehyde, and alcohol-containing products such as cough syrups or using aftershave.

Naltrexone

Naltrexone is used once abstinence has been achieved. It is an opiate antagonist with FDA approval for managing both alcohol and opioid use disorders. It works by competitively binding to opioid receptors, reducing the pleasure associated with drinking and the cravings to use.

Naltrexone is available in two forms: the oral tablet and the long-acting, monthly intramuscular (IM) injection. Oral dosing begins with a single dose, and most individuals can remain on this dose for maintenance. Taking naltrexone with or after meals can help reduce gastrointestinal side effects.

The IM depot injection, administered in the gluteal muscle, is often preferred for patients with substance use disorders, as it improves adherence compared to the oral formulation. However, IM injection may not be suitable if excess body mass prevents the use of a 2-inch needle, and subcutaneous administration should be avoided, as it may cause severe injection site reactions.

This medication is well tolerated by most people recovering from alcohol use disorder, and most people will not experience serious side effects after the first few days. Common side effects include nausea, headache, dizziness, nervousness, fatigue, insomnia, vomiting, anxiety, and somnolence. Hepatitis and liver dysfunction have been associated with the use of naltrexone.

For patients using naltrexone to support alcohol abstinence, treatment typically begins in the early months of sobriety, when cravings are strongest. However, for individuals who also have a history of opioid use, they must be opioid-free for 7 to 10 days before starting naltrexone. Even small amounts of opioids, including codeine-containing cough syrups, must be avoided while taking naltrexone, as it may precipitate withdrawal. A naloxone challenge test may be used to confirm the absence of opioids i a patient's system before starting therapy, particularly in those with dual substance use disorders. If opioid withdrawal symptoms occur, it indicates the presence of opioids in the system.

Acamprosate

Acamprosate works to reduce the intensity of cravings in individuals who have quit drinking. Its mechanism of action is thought to counteract the imbalance between the excitatory glutamatergic and the inhibitory GABA activity, helping the brain to recover slowly while reducing some of the discomfort of withdrawal symptoms.

Acamprosate is available in an oral tablet form and is typically taken three times a day, which may require commitment and consistency from the patient. However, for those dedicated to their recovery, the medication can be a helpful tool.

Along with reducing alcohol cravings, acamprosate also seems to help people sleep better during recovery. Improved sleep is significant in alcohol use disorder since insomnia is a major contributor to relapse.

Common side effects are usually mild and transient. They include headache, diarrhea, flatulence, abdominal pain, paresthesia, and skin reactions. Acamprosate may be discontinued abruptly without causing withdrawal symptoms, and is not addictive. Acamprosate is contraindicated in individuals with renal impairment and should not be used in patients with significant kidney dysfunction.

Table 27.1 identifies medications used in the treatment of alcohol withdrawal and relapse prevention.

Table 27.1 Common Medications Used for Treatment of Alcohol Use Disorder

Generic (Brand Name)	Uses	Implications for the Therapeutic Process
Disulfiram	Maintenance, relapse prevention, aversion therapy	Physical effects when alcohol is used: Intense nausea and vomiting, headache, diaphoresis (sweating), flushing, dyspnea (respiratory difficulties), and confusion. Avoid all alcohol and substances such as cough syrup and mouthwash containing alcohol.
Naltrexone	Relapse prevention, reduces pleasurable effects of alcohol and cravings	Available in oral or long-acting (once monthly) injectable form. Common side effects include nausea (often improving after the first month), headache, and sedation. Injection site pain may occur with the IM form. Patients who use opioids needs to abstain 7-10 days before starting naltrexone to avoid precipitated withdrawal.

(Continued)

Table 27.1 Common Medications Used for Treatment of Alcohol Use Disorder—cont'd

Generic (Brand Name)	Uses	Implications for the Therapeutic Process
Acamprosate	Relapse prevention	Begin taking on the fifth day of abstinence from alcohol. Tablets are taken three times a day. Side effects include diarrhea, gastrointestinal upset, appetite loss, dizziness, anxiety, and difficulty sleeping. Contraindicated in patients with renal impairment.
Topiramate (Topamax)	Off-label use for alcohol reduction	Adverse effects associated with topiramate include cognitive impairment (e.g., word-finding difficulties), paresthesias, weight loss, headache, fatigue, dizziness, and depression

US Food and Drug Administration. (2024). Drugs. Retrieved from https://www.fda.gov/drugs.

CANNABIS

Cannabis is a plant from the *Cannabaceae* family, containing the potent compounds delta-9-tetrahydrocannabinol (THC) and cannabidiol (CBD). THC is primarily responsible for the psychoactive effects of cannabis, while CBD is non-intoxicating and is being explored for its therapeutic potential.

Cannabis intoxication can lead to clinically significant behavioral and psychological changes, including impaired motor coordination, euphoria, anxiety, distorted sense of time, impaired judgment, and social withdrawal. In some cases, delirium and psychosis may occur. Most instances of cannabis intoxication do not require medical intervention and resolve on their own. Supportive care in a calm, non-stimulating environment is typically sufficient.

If symptoms are severe or distressing, symptomatic treatment may be considered, such as α-2-adrenergic agonists or β-blockers for tachycardia. Benzodiazepines may be used short-term for panic attacks, and antihistamines may be used off-label for anxiety or restlessness. Antipsychotics may be needed for psychosis.

Cannabis withdrawal occurs with the cessation of heavy, prolonged use (typically daily or nearly daily use over several months). Symptoms begin within one week of cessation and may include:

- Irritability, anger, or aggression
- Nervousness or anxiety
- Sleep disturbances (insomnia, vivid or disturbing dreams)
- Decreased appetite or weight loss
- Restlessness
- Depressed mood
- Abdominal pain
- Tremors or shakiness
- Sweating, fever, chills, headache
- Clinically significant distress or impairment in social, occupational, or other important areas of functioning.

While cannabis withdrawal is generally self-limited, treatment strategies may focus on symptom relief and support. No specific medications have been proven effective for cannabis withdrawal, but short-term symptomatic treatments, such as diazepam (Valium) for up to 7-10 days, may be useful.

OPIOIDS

Opioid Overdose

Overdose is a common risk among individuals who misuse illicit substances such as heroin or prescription pain medications like oxycodone, hydrocodone, and morphine. An opioid overdose is a medical emergency and requires immediate intervention. Signs of opioid overdose are listed in Box 27.2.

Naloxone should be administered to any patient with signs of opioid overdose, or those suspected of overdose. It is a safe and effective drug that has no clinical effects in individuals who are intoxicated with opioids.

Box 27.2 Signs of Opioid Overdose

- Extreme sleepiness
- Unresponsive to verbal stimuli or sternal rub
- Blue or purple discoloration of the fingernails or lips
- Slow pulse and/or low blood pressure
- Slow, shallow breathing in a patient who cannot be awakened
- Respiratory death rattle—distinct, labored exhalation from the throat
- Hallmark symptoms: coma, pinpoint pupils, respiratory depression

---

Treatment for an opioid overdose focuses on ensuring the patient's breathing. This includes aspirating secretions, inserting an airway, using mechanical ventilation, and providing oxygen. In the absence of medical equipment, rescue breathing is recommended.

Naloxone, an opioid antagonist, can be delivered by intranasal spray, intramuscular, subcutaneous, or intravenous routes. The intravenous route provides the most rapid onset of action, making it the preferred method in emergencies. Naloxone should be administered in the smallest effective dose to maintain normal respiratory drive, as too much naloxone may induce withdrawal symptoms. The duration of action for naloxone is short compared with many opioids (20–90 minutes), so repeated administration may be required.

Naloxone usually results in a rapid response of increased respirations and pupillary dilation within 3 to 5 minutes. Methods of naloxone delivery are listed in Table 27.2.

Patients should be monitored for at least 4 hours after naloxone administration to assess for recurrence of opioid toxicity. Those who have overdosed on long-acting opioids are monitored for a longer duration, as naloxone's effects may wear off before the opioid's effects have dissipated.

Opioid Withdrawal and Relapse Prevention

The principles of opioid detoxification and withdrawal are as follows:

1. Substitute a longer-acting, pharmacologically equivalent drug.
2. Stabilize the patient on the substituted drug.
3. Gradually taper and withdraw the substituted drug.

Table 27.2 **Methods of Naloxone Delivery**

Brand Name	Delivery Method	Notes
Narcan	Subcutaneous, intramuscular, intravenous	Most rapid onset of action is intravenous administration
Narcan Nasal Spray	Intranasal	Prefilled device that requires no assembly Delivers a single dose into one nostril Two doses per package
Naloxone Auto-Injector	Intramuscular or subcutaneous	Hand-held automatic injection into outer thigh, through clothing if necessary Device provides verbal instruction on how to deliver the medication.

The following drugs include opioid agonists, partial agonists, and antagonists. Agonists and partial agonists are typically used for medically supervised withdrawal and maintenance. Antagonists are used to accelerate detoxification and then to prevent relapse.

Methadone

Methadone (Dolophine, Methadose) is a synthetic narcotic opioid used to alleviate the painful symptoms of opioid withdrawal and for the maintenance of abstinence. Methadone is a full opioid agonist that tricks the brain by activating opioid receptors and reducing craving. It also blocks the euphoric effects of other opiate drugs such as heroin, morphine, and codeine, as well as semisynthetic opioids like oxycodone and hydrocodone.

Methadone is classified as a DEA Schedule II drug with high misuse potential. It can only be dispensed through an opioid treatment program certified by a government substance use agency. The duration of methadone therapy can be fairly long. In pregnancy, a low dose of methadone may be the safest course. Neonatal withdrawal is usually mild and can be managed with morphine.

Serious side effects may occur with methadone use. Patients are instructed to seek medical care if they experience difficulty breathing. Symptoms such as lightheadedness, fainting, chest pain, and a pounding heartbeat may indicate QT prolongation, a potentially dangerous cardiac arrhythmia. Hives, rash, or swelling of the face, lips, tongue, or throat could signal an allergic reaction. Hallucinations or confusion should be reported to a care provider.

Alpha Agonists

Two alpha-agonist antihypertensives are often used to reduce the symptoms of opioid withdrawal. Clonidine (Catapres) works by blocking neurotransmitters that trigger sympathetic nervous system activity. It eases sweating, hot flashes, watery eyes, and restlessness. This drug also decreases anxiety and may even shorten the detox process.

Lofexidine (Lucemyra) has FDA approval for mitigating opioid withdrawal symptoms during abrupt discontinuation. It allows individuals to withdraw at home over a few days rather than a week. However, lofexidine is relatively expensive. A 96-tablet bottle costs approximately $1,185 to $1,872 depending on the pharmacy.

Buprenorphine

Buprenorphine reduces or eliminates withdrawal symptoms and drug cravings without the dangerous side effects of heroin and other opioids. It is used to help people reduce or stop their use of heroin or other opiates such as pain relievers like morphine. Buprenorphine both blocks and activates opiate receptors and is known as a partial opioid agonist.

A DEA schedule III drug, buprenorphine, can be prescribed by providers who have completed special education. Some buprenorphine products also contain naloxone. The naloxone in the combined formulation causes a withdrawal reaction if it is intravenously injected, thereby deterring misuse. The FDA has approved the following schedule III buprenorphine products, some of which contain naloxone:

- Suboxone (buprenorphine and naloxone) sublingual tablets or sublingual film
- Zubsolv (buprenorphine and naloxone) sublingual tablets
- Sublocade (buprenorphine) is supplied as a prefilled syringe for subcutaneous administration once a month;

available only through an FDA supervised program (REMS)

- Brixadi: Extended-release subcutaneous injection of buprenorphine, available in weekly and monthly formulations.

Side effects of buprenorphine include nausea, vomiting, constipation, muscle aches and cramps, insomnia, irritability, and fever. This drug is used only after abstaining from opioids for 12 to 24 hours and in the early stages of opioid withdrawal. If administered too soon or to patients who still have opioids in their system, buprenorphine may precipitate acute withdrawal symptoms. This is due to its partial agonist properties, which can displace other opioids from receptors in the brain and induce withdrawal in patients who are not in the early stages of opioid detoxification.

Naltrexone

Naltrexone is an opioid antagonist that prevents intoxication. Naltrexone is available as a tablet form of the drug, and as a long-acting injectable given once a month. If a person using naltrexone relapses and uses the misused drug, naltrexone blocks the euphoric and sedative effects.

Side effects of naltrexone include gastrointestinal (GI) distress, muscle cramps, dizziness, sedation, and appetite disturbances. Injection site reactions are common. About 70% of users experience reactions that range from pain, swelling, and bruising to more serious complications like cellulitis, induration, and, more rarely, abscess and necrosis.

Table 27.3 identifies medications used in the treatment of opioid use disorder.

HALLUCINOGENS

Treatment for hallucinogen intoxication includes reassurance that the symptoms are caused by the drug and that the symptoms will subside. Patient and provider safety are essential goals. Physical restraint may be necessary. In severe cases, an antipsychotic such as haloperidol (Haldol) or a benzodiazepine such as diazepam (Valium) can be used in the short term.

Patients who have ingested phencyclidine (PCP) cannot be talked down and may require restraint. A calming medication such as a benzodiazepine may be administered

Table 27.3 FDA-Approved Medications for Opioid Use Disorder

Medication and Action	Form	Use
Methadone (opioid agonist)		Withdrawal and maintenance treatment
• Dolophine	Tablet	
• Methadose	Tablet, oral concentrate	
Buprenorphine (partial opioid agonist)		Withdrawal and maintenance treatment
• Suboxone (buprenorphine and naloxone)	Sublingual tablets or sublingual film	
• Zubsolv (buprenorphine and naloxone)	Sublingual tablet	
• Sublocade (buprenorphine XR)	Long-acting injectable	Maintenance treatment
• Brixadi	Subcutaneous injection	
Naltrexone (opioid antagonist)		Relapse prevention
	Tablet	
	Long-acting injectable	

FDA, Food and Drug Administration.

intramuscularly or intravenously. Mechanical cooling may be necessary for severe hyperthermia.

INHALANTS

Inhalant intoxication usually does not require any treatment. However, serious and potentially fatal responses such as coma, cardiac arrhythmias, or bronchospasm do happen. A psychotic response can be induced by inhalant intoxication.

SEDATIVES, HYPNOTICS, AND BENZODIAZEPINES

Like alcohol, repeated sedative, hypnotic, and benzodiazepine use results in repeated dampening of the central nervous system, causing rebound hyperactivity. Symptoms such as autonomic hyperactivity, tremor, insomnia, psychomotor agitation, anxiety, and grand mal seizures occur. The degree and timing of the withdrawal syndrome depend on the specific substance. Half-life is an important predictor of withdrawal time.

Gradual reduction of these substances will prevent seizures and other withdrawal symptoms. Benzodiazepine withdrawal can be supported by using a long-acting barbiturate such as phenobarbital.

AMPHETAMINES

Depending on the amphetamine used, specific drugs are used short-term to treat withdrawal symptoms. Antipsychotics may be prescribed for a few days. If there is no psychosis, diazepam (Valium) is useful in treating agitation and hyperactivity. Once the patient has been withdrawn from the amphetamine, depression can be treated with antidepressants.

TOBACCO

Withdrawal from and treatment for tobacco use disorder are facilitated by nicotine replacement therapies. This highly effective approach is available in various forms, including gum, lozenges, nasal sprays, inhalers, and patches. For patients using the gum, it's important to instruct them not to chew continuously, as this may cause gastrointestinal upset. Instead, they should chew a few times until they feel a tingling sensation in their mouth. Then, the gum should be placed between the cheek and gums until the tingling almost stops, after which they can resume chewing. This process is repeated until the tingling sensation stops, usually within about 30 minutes.

Non-nicotine therapy options include the antidepressant bupropion sustained-release (Zyban), which helps reduce cravings for nicotine. Another option is varenicline (previously marketed as the now-discontinued Chantix), a nicotinic receptor partial agonist that mimics nicotine's effects, helping to reduce cravings and withdrawal symptoms. Additionally, varenicline partially blocks nicotine receptors, which reduces the effects of nicotine if smoking is resumed.

CHAPTER 28

Neurocognitive Medications

There are three main types of FDA-approved medications used in the treatment of Alzheimer's disease and other dementias. These include drugs that aim to slow disease progression, those that help manage cognitive symptoms such as memory loss and impaired thinking, and those that treat noncognitive symptoms such as insomnia and agitation. A detailed overview of these medications is provided in Table 28.1.

SLOWING DISEASE PROGRESSION

These medications are the first to target the underlying pathology of dementia by reducing amyloid plaques, which are implicated in disease progression. The FDA granted accelerated approval for aducanumab (Aduhelm) in 2021, but it was discontinued by the manufacturer in 2024. Two other amyloid-targeting drugs, lecanemab (Leqembi) and donanemab (Kisunla), were approved in 2023 and 2024 respectively.

These drugs are indicated for early Alzheimer's disease, including mild cognitive impairment and mild dementia stage of disease. While lecanemab and donanemab are not cures and do not restore lost memories or cognitive function, clinical trials have shown they can slow disease progression, with the most significant benefits observed after 18 months of treatment.

Before starting anti-amyloid treatment, clinicians must confirm the presence of beta-amyloid plaques. While the FDA does not mandate a specific diagnostic tool, common options include amyloid PET scans or lumbar puncture (CSF tests).

Lecanemab (Leqembi) is administered as an intravenous infusion every two weeks, while donanemab (Kisunla) is

Table 28.1 **FDA-Approved Drugs for Alzheimer's Disease**

Generic (Trade)	Indications	Side Effects
Slows Disease Progression		
Amyloid Targeting Approaches		
Donanemab (Kisunla) IV infusion every 4 weeks	Mild cognitive impairment or mild dementia with confirmed elevated beta-amyloid in the brain	Infusion-related and allergic reactions Amyloid-related imaging abnormalities (ARIA)—brain swelling that usually resolves over time. Symptoms include headache, dizziness, nausea, confusion, and vision changes Serious hemorrhages have occurred
Lecanemab (Leqembi) IV infusion every 2 weeks	Mild cognitive impairment or mild dementia with confirmed elevated beta-amyloid in the brain	
Manages Cognitive Symptoms		
Cholinesterase Inhibitors		
Donepezil (Aricept, Aricept ODT[a])	Mild, moderate, and severe Alzheimer's disease (AD)	Nausea, vomiting, muscle cramps, increased frequency of bowel movements, loss of appetite.
Rivastigmine (Exelon) Rivastigmine transdermal system (Exelon Patch)	Mild to moderate AD	Nausea, vomiting, increased frequency of bowel movements, loss of appetite.
Galantamine (Razadyne, Razadyne ER)	Mild to moderate AD	Nausea, vomiting, increased frequency of bowel movements, loss of appetite.
Glutamate Regulator		
Memantine (Namenda, Namenda XR)	Moderate to severe AD	Dizziness, headache, confusion, constipation
Cholinesterase Inhibitor + Glutamate Regulator		
Memantine/ donepezil (Namzaric)	Moderate to severe AD after a trial of donepezil	Side effects of Memantine, plus nausea, vomiting, frequency of bowel movements, loss of appetite.

(Continued)

Table 28.1 FDA-Approved Drugs for Alzheimer's Disease—cont'd

Generic (Trade)	Indications	Side Effects
Treats Noncognitive Symptoms		
Suvorexant (Belsomra)	Insomnia in mild to moderate AD	Impaired alertness and motor coordination, increased depression/suicidal thoughts, complex sleep behaviors/paralysis, comprised respiratory function.
Brexpriprazole (Rexulti)	Agitation associated with dementia	Headache, dizziness, urinary tract infection, nasopharyngitis, and sleep disturbances (both somnolence and insomnia)

[a]Orally disintegrating tablet.
US Food and Drug Administration. (Various dates). FDA online label repository. Retrieved from https://labels.fda.gov/.

given as an intravenous infusion every four weeks. Both medications require confirmation of elevated beta-amyloid in the brain before initiation.

Common side effects include headache, dizziness, nausea, and infusion-related reactions. More serious risks include amyloid-related imaging abnormalities (ARIA), which can cause brain swelling, microhemorrhages, and, in rare cases, symptomatic hemorrhages. These risks necessitate careful patient selection and monitoring through regular MRI scans (Guo & Vaishnavi, 2023).

TREATING COGNITIVE SYMPTOMS

Five medications have US Food and Drug Administration (FDA) approval for the treatment of Alzheimer's disease (AD). They are:

- Cholinesterase inhibitors: donepezil (Aricept), rivastigmine (Exelon), and galantamine (Razadyne)
- Glutamate regulator: memantine (Namenda)

- Glutamate regulator/cholinesterase inhibitor: memantine/donepezil (Namzaric)

These medications are commonly prescribed to manage symptoms of Alzheimer's disease, particularly in the early to moderate stages. They have demonstrated statistically significant effects compared with placebos. However, these medications produce only a marginal improvement in cognition and functioning, and their benefits diminish after 1 to 2 years. Considering the potential side effects, which double in people older than 85 years, their use should be carefully weighed against the potential benefits.

Other medications are used to treat behavioral manifestations of major neurocognitive disorders, including AD. They will be discussed following the presentation of specific neurocognitive medications.

Cholinesterase Inhibitors

Because a deficiency of neural acetylcholine has been linked to AD, some medications aim to prevent its breakdown. These drugs function by inhibiting cholinesterase from breaking down acetylcholine into its components of acetate and choline. This allows for an increase in the availability and duration of action of acetylcholine, which leads to temporary improvement of some symptoms of AD.

The first FDA-approved cholinesterase inhibitor was tacrine (Cognex) in 1993 for the treatment of mild to moderate symptoms of AD. Tacrine was withdrawn from the market in 2012 due to a high frequency of side effects, including gastrointestinal effects, elevated liver transaminase levels, and liver toxicity.

Currently used cholinesterase inhibitors include donepezil (Aricept), rivastigmine (Exelon), and galantamine (Razadyne). The cholinesterase inhibitors are indicated for the mild to moderate stages of AD. Donepezil is FDA-approved for severe AD.

The most common side effects are gastrointestinal. These side effects are usually temporary, and a lower dose minimizes them. These medications are taken with food to reduce this side effect. Donepezil is available in tablet form and as an orally disintegrating tablet (ODT) that should not be crushed. Rivastigmine is provided in both a capsule form and an oral solution. Galantamine is available in a tablet, a capsule, and as an oral solution.

Cholinesterase inhibitors can also rarely cause bradycardia and incontinence due to their cholinergic-enhancing properties. They are used with caution when patients are taking nonsteroidal anti-inflammatory drugs (NSAIDs) due to the combined potential for gastrointestinal bleeding and ulceration.

The rivastigmine transdermal system (Exelon Patch) is applied once a day, making it useful for people who have trouble swallowing pills. The upper or lower back is recommended as the site of application because the patch is less likely to be removed by the individual. With this nonoral delivery method, there is no food requirement. It can cause skin irritation and should be discontinued if the irritation extends beyond the size of the patch.

Glutamate Regulator

Memantine (Namenda) is indicated for the treatment of moderate to severe dementia and is typically added after trying cholinesterase inhibitors. This medication works by regulating the activity of glutamate, a neurotransmitter that is present at higher levels in Alzheimer's disease (AD). Excessive glutamate can bind to receptors and allow too much calcium to enter neurons, causing damage. Memantine blocks these receptors, preventing excessive calcium influx and protecting brain cells.

Memantine tablets can be taken with or without food. After using memantine twice a day, patients may be switched to long-acting memantine XR for once-a-day dosing. These capsules can be swallowed intact or opened and sprinkled on food such as applesauce. They should not be divided, chewed, or crushed.

Common side effects of memantine include headache, constipation, and dizziness. Memantine XR may cause constipation. In clinical trials, the most common reason for drug discontinuation was dizziness.

Patients may be prescribed a combination of memantine and a cholinesterase inhibitor. Once tolerance to this combination has been confirmed, extended-release memantine (Namenda) and donepezil (Aricept) may be used together as Namzaric. Namzaric is FDA-approved for moderate to severe Alzheimer's disease symptoms. Namzaric is dosed once a day in the evening. The capsules can be taken with or without food, either whole, or sprinkled on food such as applesauce. They should not be divided, chewed, or crushed.

The most common side effects of Namzaric are those typically associated with its individual components, memantine and donepezil. These include dizziness, headaches, gastrointestinal issues (such as nausea, diarrhea, or loss of appetite), and sleep disturbances. While these side effects are common, they are not experienced by all patients, and the severity can vary.

MANAGING NON-COGNITIVE SYMPTOMS

Many individuals with dementia experience behavioral symptoms that significantly impact their quality of life, causing distress for both them and their caregivers. These behaviors may also contribute to the need for placement in a residential care facility. Common troubling symptoms are psychosis (hallucinations, paranoia), severe mood swings, wandering, anxiety, agitation, and verbal or physical aggression. In addition to being emotionally distressing, these behaviors can lead to physical harm, such as injuries from falls, infections, and incontinence.

Insomnia

Suvorexant (Belsomra) is an orexin receptor antagonist that is FDA-approved for the treatment of insomnia, including in individuals with dementia. It works by inhibiting the action of orexin, a neurotransmitter involved in regulating the sleep-wake cycle, thereby promoting sleep. Suvorexant is specifically indicated for patients experiencing insomnia, which is a non-cognitive symptom in dementia. Common side effects include daytime drowsiness, headache, and dizziness. More serious side effects, although rare, may include sleepwalking, complex sleep behaviors, and worsening depression or suicidal thoughts. Healthcare providers should closely monitor patients for any adverse effects, especially in the older adult population.

Agitation

Brexpiprazole (Rexulti), approved by the FDA in 2023, is an atypical antipsychotic for the treatment of agitation in dementia. It works by modulating neurotransmitters like serotonin and dopamine, which regulate mood and behavior. This medication is specifically indicated for managing agitation, which includes irritability, restlessness, and aggression.

As an atypical antipsychotic, brexpiprazole has a potentially lower risk of side effects seen with older antipsychotics, such as movement disorders. However, it should still be used with caution in older adults. Common side effects include dizziness, weight gain, and sedation. More serious side effects, such as an increased risk of stroke, heart problems, or neuroleptic malignant syndrome, must be closely monitored. The FDA stresses careful risk assessment and monitoring when using brexpiprazole, and it should be prescribed only when other treatments have not been effective.

While antipsychotic medications were once routinely used to manage behavioral symptoms of dementia, we now recognize that their use requires extreme caution due to the associated risks. Research has shown that these drugs can significantly increase the risk of stroke and death in this population, leading the FDA to issue a "black box" warning for these medications. The warning reminds healthcare providers that antipsychotics are not approved for treating dementia symptoms. Therefore, these drugs should only be prescribed in specific circumstances, such as when behavioral symptoms are due to mania or psychosis, when symptoms pose a danger to the individual or others, or when the person is experiencing significant distress, functional decline, or difficulty receiving care.

Antipsychotics should never be used to sedate or restrain people with dementia, and the lowest effective dosage should be prescribed for the shortest duration possible. Careful monitoring is required for potential adverse side effects. While antipsychotics remain the most commonly prescribed medications for agitation, some clinicians may opt for alternative treatments, such as mood stabilizers or seizure medications like carbamazepine (Tegretol®), depending on the individual's symptoms and needs.

CHAPTER 29

Psychotherapeutic Models

Registered nurses and nursing students prepared at the basic level are qualified to provide counseling, support, and education to their patients. They play an important role in promoting symptom stabilization and reinforcing healthy behaviors and interactions in the context of a therapeutic relationship.

Psychiatric-mental health advanced practice registered nurses are prepared to provide a more complex form of counseling known as psychotherapy. Often referred to as "talk therapy," psychotherapy includes a range of treatment techniques that help individuals identify and change self-defeating feelings, thoughts, and behavior.

Most of the therapies discussed in this chapter require advanced education for effective application and third-party reimbursement. However, it is important for nurses working and training in a psychiatric setting to be familiar with the types of therapies available. Becoming acquainted with these therapies offers several benefits, including the ability to:

1. Use basic concepts of various models as interventions, such as recognizing negative thought patterns as used in cognitive behavioral therapy or participating in reward systems when working with children and adolescents, as seen in behavioral therapy.

2. Understand the therapy being recommended to or being provided to a patient and be able to discuss the proposed therapy or the work with clarity.

This chapter provides snapshots of some of the most common and widely used psychotherapies. Most of these therapies can be applied to individuals, families, and groups. These therapies include the following:

- Cognitive behavioral therapy (CBT)
- Dialectical behavioral therapy (DBT)
- Mindfulness-based approaches
- Mindfulness-based stress reduction (MBSR)
- Mindfulness-based cognitive therapy (MBCT)
- Eye movement and desensitization and reprocessing (EMDR) therapy
- Exposure and response prevention (ERP) therapy
- Interpersonal therapy
- Behavioral therapy
- Modeling
- Operant conditioning
- Systematic desensitization
- Aversion
- Biofeedback
- Acceptance and commitment therapy
- Motivational interviewing
- Milieu therapy
- Group therapy

COGNITIVE BEHAVIORAL THERAPY

Cognitive behavioral therapy (CBT) is an active, time-limited, and structured approach. This evidence-based therapy is effective in treating a range of psychiatric disorders, including major depressive disorder, anxiety and phobias, along with chronic pain. The foundation of CBT is the principle that a person's feelings and behaviors are largely determined by the way people think about the world and their place in it (Beck, 1979). These cognitions, whether verbal or visual, are rooted in attitudes or assumptions developed from previous experiences. While some cognitions may be fairly accurate, others can be distorted, leading to emotional distress and maladaptive behaviors.

People develop schemas, or unique assumptions, about themselves, others, and the world in general. For instance, if a man holds the schema, "The only person I can trust is myself," he may expect that others have questionable motives, are dishonest, and will ultimately hurt him. Negative schemas can also include beliefs such as incompetence, abandonment, evilness, and vulnerability. These cognitive biases often operate unconsciously, meaning individuals are typically unaware of how these distorted perceptions influence their thoughts, emotions, and behaviors.

Rapid, unthinking responses based on schemas are known as automatic thoughts. These responses are particularly intense and common in psychiatric disorders such as depression and anxiety. Often, automatic thoughts, or cognitive distortions, are irrational and lead to false assumptions and misinterpretations. For example, if a woman views all experiences through the lens of her competency and adequacy, her thinking may be dominated by the cognitive distortion, "Unless I do everything perfectly, I'm a failure." As a result, she may react to situations in terms of personal adequacy, even when these situations are unrelated to her competence. Table 29.1 describes common cognitive distortions.

Table 29.1 Common Cognitive Distortions

Distortion	Definition	Example
All-or-nothing thinking	Thinking in black and white, reducing complex outcomes into absolutes	Although Valentina earned the second-highest score in the state's cheerleading competition, she consistently referred to herself as "a loser."
Over-generalization	Using a bad outcome (or a few bad outcomes) as evidence that nothing will ever go right again	Jackson had a minor traffic accident. He is reluctant to drive and says, "I shouldn't be allowed on the road."
Labeling	A form of generalization in which a characteristic or event becomes definitive and results in an overly harsh label for self or others	"Because I failed the advanced statistics examination, I am a failure. I might as well give up. I may as well quit and look for an easier major."
Mental filter	Focusing on a negative detail or bad event and allowing it to taint everything else	Ava's boss evaluated her work as exemplary and gave her a few suggestions for improvement. She obsessed over the suggestions and ignored the rest.

(Continued)

Table 29.1 **Common Cognitive Distortions—cont'd**

Distortion	Definition	Example
Disqualifying the positive	Maintaining a negative view by rejecting information that supports a positive view as being irrelevant, inaccurate, or accidental	"I've just been offered the job I thought I always wanted. There must have been no other applicants."
Jumping to conclusions	Making a negative interpretation despite there is little or no supporting evidence	"My fiancé, Juan, didn't call me for 3 hours, which just proves he doesn't love me anymore."
Mind-reading	Inferring negative thoughts, responses, and motives of others	Isabelle is giving a presentation and a man in the audience is sleeping. She panics—"I must be boring."
Fortune-telling error	Anticipating that things will turn out badly without sufficient evidence	"I'll ask her out, but I know she won't have a good time."
Magnification or minimization	Exaggerating the importance of something (such as a personal failure or the success of others) or reducing the importance of something (such as a personal success or the failure of others)	"I'm alone on a Saturday night because no one likes me. When other people are alone, it's because they want to be."
Catastrophizing	An extreme form of magnification in which the very worst is assumed to be a probable outcome	"If I don't make a good impression on the boss at the company picnic, she will fire me."

(Continued)

Table 29.1 **Common Cognitive Distortions—cont'd**

Distortion	Definition	Example
Emotional reasoning	Drawing a conclusion based on an emotional state	"I'm nervous about the examination. I must not be prepared. If I were, I wouldn't be afraid."
"Should" and "must" statements	Rigid self-directives that presume an unrealistic amount of control over external events	Natalie believes that a patient with diabetes has high blood sugar today because she is not a very good nurse and that her patients should always get better.
Personalization	Assuming responsibility for an external event or situation that was likely outside personal control	"I'm sorry your party wasn't more fun. It's probably because I was there."

Modified from Beck, A. T. (1979). *Cognitive therapy and the emotional disorders*. New York: International Universities Press.

Therapeutic techniques are designed to identify, reality-test, and correct distorted conceptualizations and the dysfunctional beliefs underlying them. Patients are taught to challenge their negative thinking and replace it with positive, rational thoughts. They learn to recognize when thinking is based on distortions and misconceptions.

Homework assignments play an important role in CBT. A useful technique is a four-column thought diary, where patients record the precipitating event or situation, the resulting automatic thought, and the accompanying feelings and behaviors. The final challenges the negative thoughts with rational evidence and thinking. Box 29.1 illustrates an entry in a thought diary.

DIALECTICAL BEHAVIOR THERAPY

Dialectical behavior therapy (DBT) is an evidence-based treatment developed to supper individuals with borderline personality disorder (Linehan, 1993). Research has also

Box 29.1 Thought Diary Entry

Event	Automatic Thought	Feeling 0 (low)–10 (high)	Alternate Thoughts
I went to my favorite restaurant. The server, Alyssa, who I know well, barely acknowledged me	Alyssa doesn't like me anymore. I must have said something stupid. I wonder who else doesn't like me here.	Hurt (6)	Alyssa doesn't feel well. She may be upset about something going on in her life. The restaurant was crowded and she may have felt overwhelmed

confirmed its effectiveness in individuals with comorbid personality disorders (such as obsessive–compulsive personality disorder) and other psychiatric disorders, including major depressive disorder, generalized anxiety disorder, substance abuse, and eating disorders.

DBT combines cognitive and behavioral techniques with mindfulness, which emphasizes being aware of thoughts and actively shaping them (see below). The goals of DBT are to help patients manage distress, improve interpersonal effectiveness skills, and enhance the therapist's ability to work with this population. Treatment begins by targeting suicidal behaviors, followed by interventions for destructive behaviors. Finally, DBT addresses quality-of-life behaviors across a hierarchy of care.

Mindfulness-Based Approaches

Mindfulness involves being fully present in the moment and focusing on the here and now, without judgment. In our culture, it is common to focus on or worry about the future, and many of us dwell on the past. However, what often gets missed is the present moment.

Mindfulness-Based Stress Reduction

Mindfulness-based stress reduction (MBSR) has roots in Buddhist and Hindu traditions. Jon Kabat-Zinn is credited with introducing mindfulness to Western culture through his MBSR program. Initially designed to treat chronic pain, the program has expanded to address other conditions, including major depressive disorders, anxiety disorders, and stress relief.

MBSR can be practiced during formal meditation sessions or informally throughout the day. For example, individuals can focus on an activity they may typically "zone out" during, such as brushing their teeth, doing the dishes, or taking a shower. The goal is to bring awareness to that activity in the present moment, concentrating on how all five senses engage with it rather than allowing the mind to wander.

Mindfulness-Based Cognitive Therapy

Mindfulness-based cognitive therapy (MBCT) is a focused approach that helps patients disengage from unhealthy cognitive patterns. The patterns that make individuals vulnerable to relapse of depression are those of rumination, where the mind repetitively focuses on specific negative thoughts. The main skill with MBCT is teaching patients how to shift mental gears.

Unlike conventional CBT, MBCT does not focus on changing core beliefs. Instead, it trains individuals to be more aware of physical sensations and of thoughts and feelings as mental events. Individuals come to see thoughts and feelings as aspects of experience that move through awareness but are not necessarily reality.

Eye Movement Desensitization and Reprocessing

Eye movement desensitization and reprocessing (EMDR) is an evidence-based approach to treating traumatized children and adults. EMDR therapy processes traumatic memories through a specific protocol. The clinician asks the patient to think about the traumatic event, while simultaneously engaging with other forms of stimulation, such as eye movements, audio tones, or tapping. The combination of cognitive focus and external stimuli promotes neurological and physiological changes that help individuals process and integrate traumatic memories.

Exposure and Response Prevention

Exposure and response prevention (ERP) is used to treat obsessive–compulsive disorder (OCD), eating disorders, phobias, panic disorder, generalized anxiety disorder, and social anxiety. This approach is similar to the behavioral approach of systematic desensitization but does involve relaxation techniques. ERP is a cognitively-based therapy that involves purposely exposing the individual to anxiety-provoking thoughts, images, and situations. The patient then makes a conscious choice to refrain from engaging in the ritual or compulsion. Over time, with continued exposure to the obsession and avoidance of the compulsion, the patient experiences a reduction in anxiety and obsessive thoughts.

A common metaphor used to explain this therapy is the idea of quitting "feeding the lion." In this analogy, the lion begging for food represents the obsessive thought, while feeding the lion is akin to the compulsion or ritual. When the individual chooses to stop "feeding the lion" (i.e., cease the compulsion/ritual), the lion might initially become agitated (i.e., anxiety may increase), but eventually, the lion goes away (i.e., anxiety decreases).

INTERPERSONAL THERAPY

Interpersonal therapy (IPT) is an effective short-term treatment, typically consisting of 12 to 16 sessions. This therapy is based on the assumption that psychiatric disorders are influenced by interpersonal interactions and the broader social context. The primary goal of IPT is to reduce or eliminate psychiatric symptoms by enhancing interpersonal functioning and increasing satisfaction with social relationships.

Interpersonal therapy has been shown to be effective in treating depression, particularly when it is linked to grief and loss, interpersonal conflict, role transitions, and deficits in interpersonal skills. The treatment is grounded in the idea that disturbances in key interpersonal relationships, or a difficulty forming such relationships, can contribute to the onset or maintenance of clinical depression. In interpersonal therapy, the therapist first identifies the core issue and then selects strategies tailored to address that specific problem area.

BEHAVIORAL THERAPY

Behavioral therapy is based on the assumption that maladaptive behaviors can change without the need for insight into their underlying causes. This approach is most effective when it targets specific problems with clearly-defined goals. Behavioral therapy has been demonstrated to be effective in treating conditions such as phobias, alcohol use disorder, and schizophrenia, among others. Five types of behavioral therapy include modeling, operant conditioning, systematic desensitization, aversion therapy, and biofeedback.

Modeling

In modeling, the therapist provides a role model for specific behaviors, and the patient learns through imitation. The therapist may model the behavior, provide another person to model it, or present a video for this purpose. For example, clinicians can help patients reduce their phobias about nonpoisonous snakes by having them first view filmed encounters between people and snakes in which the individuals remain calm and safe. Afterward, they view live encounters where people interact with the snakes in a similarly calm and safe manner.

Similarly, some behavior therapists demonstrate more effective patterns of behavior than those typically used, then have patients practice these new behaviors. For example, a student unsure of how to ask a professor for an extension on a term paper would first observe the therapist model an effective approach. The clinician would then help the student in practicing the new skill through a role-playing situation.

Operant Conditioning

Operant conditioning forms the foundation for behavior modification, utilizing positive reinforcement to encourage desired behaviors. For example, patients may receive tokens when they achieve specific goals or perform targeted behaviors. These tokens can then be exchanged for food, small luxuries, or privileges, forming a reward system known as a token economy.

Operant conditioning has proven effective in improving the verbal behaviors in children who are mute, autistic, and developmentally disabled. In patients with severe and persistent mental illness, behavior modification has helped enhance self-care, social behavior, and group participation. You may find this a useful technique useful as you progress through your clinical rotations.

A common example of positive reinforcement is a mother who takes her preschooler to the grocery store. When child begins to act out-demanding candy, nagging, crying, or yelling-various ways to reinforce or modify the child's behavior can be considered, as outlined in Box 29.2.

Systematic Desensitization

Systematic desensitization is a form of behavior modification therapy that involves creating behavioral tasks tailored to the patient's specific fears. It is similar to ERP, but also incorporates the practice of relaxation techniques. Patients follow four steps:

1. The patient's fear is broken down into its components by exploring the particular stimulus cues to which the patient reacts. For example, certain situations may precipitate a phobic reaction, whereas others do not. Crowds at parties may be problematic, whereas similar numbers of people in other settings do not cause the same distress.

2. The patient is exposed to the fear little by little. For example, a patient who has a fear of flying is introduced to short periods of visual presentations

---

Box 29.2 **Behavioral Reinforcement Approaches**

Action	Result
1. The mother gives the child the candy	The child continues to use this behavior. This is positive reinforcement of negative behavior
2. The mother scolds the child	Acting out may persist as the child receives attention, which positively rewards negative behavior
3. The mother ignores the acting out but gives attention to the child when he is acting appropriately	The child gets a positive reward for appropriate behavior

of flying—first with still pictures, then with videos, and finally in a busy airport. The situations are confronted while the patient is in a relaxed state. Gradually, exposure is increased until anxiety about or fear of the object or situation has ceased.
3. The patient is instructed on how to design a hierarchy of fears. For a fear of flying, a patient might develop a set of statements representing the stages of a flight, order the statements from the most fearful to the least fearful, and use relaxation techniques to reach a state of relaxation while progressing through the list.
4. The patient practices these techniques every day.

Aversion Therapy

Aversion therapy is used to treat behaviors such as alcohol use disorder, paraphilic disorders, shoplifting, violent and aggressive behavior, and self-mutilation. It involves pairing of a negative stimulus with a specific target behavior, thereby suppressing the behavior. This treatment is typically used when other, less drastic measures have failed to produce the desired effects.

Simple examples of extinguishing undesirable behavior through aversion therapy include painting bitter-tasting substances on the fingernails of nail biters or the thumbs of thumb suckers. Other examples of aversive stimuli are chemicals that induce nausea and vomiting, unpleasant odors, disturbing verbal stimuli (e.g., descriptions of unsettling scenes), costs or fines in a token economy, and denial of positive reinforcement (e.g., isolation).

Before initiating any aversive protocol, the therapist, treatment team, or society must answer the following questions:
• Is this therapy in the best interest of the patient?
• Does its use violate the patient's rights?
• Is it in the best interest of society?

If the therapist determines that aversion therapy is the most appropriate treatment, ongoing supervision, support, and evaluation of those administering it are essential.

Biofeedback

Through the use of sensitive instrumentation, biofeedback provides immediate and exact information regarding muscle activity, brain waves, skin temperature, heart rate, blood pressure, and other bodily functions. Indicators of the particular internal physiological process are detected and amplified by a sensitive recording device. An individual can achieve greater voluntary control over phenomena once considered to be exclusively involuntary if knowing instantaneously, through an auditory or visual signal, whether a somatic activity is increasing or decreasing.

The use of biofeedback was once reserved for clinicians with specialized training. However, with increasingly sophisticated technology, many people can now use some form of biofeedback themselves. Exercise trackers and smartwatches allow users to monitor sleep patterns and heart rates. One high-tech gadget is a clip-on device that tracks respiration changes indicative of tension, with a companion app suggesting relaxation techniques such as meditation. Additionally, a hand-held device measuring skin conductance (sweat) to indicates stress is paired comes with an app that teaches calming techniques.

Heart rate variability (HRV) testing has gained popularity for monitoring stress and recovery. Advanced wearables, such as fitness trackers and smartwatches, provide real-time HRV data through sensors that track heart rate variability using photoplethysmography (PPG) or electrocardiogram (ECG) technology. These devices typically pair with companion apps to analyze the subtle variations in time between heartbeats, offering insights into the user's stress levels and recovery state. HRV is often quantified on a scale, like 100 "points," for easier interpretation. A low HRV indicates stress, while a high HRV signifies relaxation. Users can track their baseline HRV and employ stress-relief techniques like mindfulness, relaxation, and physical activity to improve their HRV over time.

ACCEPTANCE AND COMMITMENT THERAPY

Acceptance and commitment therapy (ACT) evolved from behavior therapy, CBT, and mindfulness concepts. It is beneficial for patients who struggle with rumination over life's difficulties. During ACT, patients are guided to replace the internal struggle of emotions with acceptance of these feelings and work toward life goals. The six areas of focus in ACT are:

- Acceptance: allowing negative feelings and emotions to exist without trying to avoid or change them
- Cognitive defusion: noticing thoughts and feelings, without judgment, and learning techniques to deal with them in a non-threatening way
- Being present: bringing full awareness and attention to the present moment
- Self as context (observing Self): awareness of the "you" that experiences life, realization that one is more than an individual emotion or experience
- Values: positive qualities that the individual wants to work toward
- Committed action: setting goals and taking actions that align with personal values

MOTIVATIONAL INTERVIEWING

Motivational interviewing is an approach based on the transtheoretical or stages of change theory. It has gained popularity in its use as a brief, long-term, and supplementary intervention, particularly in the treatment of substance use disorders. It uses a person-centered approach to strengthen motivation for change. A key premise of motivational interviewing is that the individual must make the choice to engage in treatment.

Individuals may be at stage one, precontemplation, and need assistance in admitting there is a problem. If they have acknowledged the problem, contemplation, they may still not be ready to commit to addressing it. The goal of treatment is to assist in the development of awareness and a commitment. Preparation, or getting ready, and action, or changing, take place in early treatment phases. The maintenance stage is the ongoing commitment to a recovery program. Without continuing action, the individual will likely return to previous behavior, or relapse.

MILIEU THERAPY

Milieu (mil ẏ oo) is a word of French origin (mi "middle" + lieu "place") and refers to surroundings and physical environment. In a therapeutic context, it refers to the overall environment and interactions within that environment. It is an all-inclusive term that recognizes the people (patients and staff), the setting, the structure, and the emotional climate as important to healing. Regardless of whether the setting involves treatment of children, adult patients in a psychiatric hospital, substance users in a residential treatment center, or psychiatric patients in a day treatment program, a well-managed milieu offers patients a sense of security and promotes healing. Structured aspects of the milieu include activities, rules, reality orientation practices, and environment.

GROUP THERAPY

Group therapy is an evidence-based practice that allows multiple patients to be treated at the same time. Members benefit from the knowledge, insights, and life experience of both the leader and participants. A therapeutic group is a safe setting to learn new ways of relating to other people and to practice new communication skills. Groups can also promote feelings of belonging and a sense of cohesiveness (e.g., "We're in this together").

Group work is characterized by both content and process. Group content is the actual words that are used in the setting. Group process is the term used to describe everything else that goes on in a group. It refers to the way group members interact with one another such as being supportive, interruptive, or silent.

Registered nurses lead groups for education, tasks, and support. Advanced practice registered nurses are educated in the provision of theoretically based group therapy. Nurse leaders set the foundation for open communication and mutual respect. The degree to which the leader controls the direction of the group depends on the group's needs. Autocratic leaders do not encourage much interaction and exert control over the group. This leadership style works best for time-limited tasks such as community meetings. Democratic leaders promote group interaction while maintaining the role of leader. This style works well in most groups in the psychiatric setting. Laissez-faire leaders allow the group to control its direction. This works well in creative groups such as art or horticulture groups.

Yalom and Leszcz (2005) identify core principles that make a group therapeutic. These curative (healing) factors are powerful aspects of group work success.

CHAPTER 30

Neuromodulation Therapy

Although medication is the foundation of somatic (physical) treatments for psychiatric disorders and psychiatric symptoms, other options are available. Brain stimulation therapy began in 1938 when electroshock therapy was used to treat most psychiatric conditions. Since then brain stimulation therapies have become more sophisticated and are even considered high technology. These therapies all involve activating or inhibiting the brain directly with electricity. The following brain stimulation therapies are discussed in this chapter:

- Electroconvulsive therapy (ECT)
- Cranial electric stimulation (CES)
- Repetitive transcranial magnetic stimulation (rTMS)
- Magnetic seizure therapy (MST)
- Vagus nerve stimulation (VNS)
- Deep brain stimulation (DBS)

ELECTROCONVULSIVE THERAPY

Despite being a highly effective somatic treatment for psychiatric disorders, ECT has a long-standing negative reputation. This may be related, in part, to the outdated practice of restraining a conscious individual while inducing a full-blown seizure. Before the introduction of paralytic drugs, more than 30% of ECT patients experienced compression fractures of the spine (Welch, 2016). However, with modern anesthetic and paralytic agents, ECT is now a controlled, well-tolerated, and highly effective treatment.

Indications

ECT is FDA-approved for the treatment of depressive symptoms associated with major depressive disorder or bipolar disorder in individuals aged 13 years and older. Approximately 65% of ECT procedures are performed for depressive symptoms. However, since the FDA does not regulate medical practice, clinicians may also use ECT for other conditions, including as schizophrenia, schizoaffective disorder, and mania.

Risk Factors

The decision to use ECT requires careful consideration of its risks versus the risk of suicide and diminished quality of life due to untreated illness. Several medical conditions pose risks and require careful workup and management. Because the heart can be stressed at the onset of the seizure and for up to 10 minutes after, careful assessment and management of hypertension, congestive heart failure, cardiac arrhythmias, and other cardiac conditions are warranted (Welch, 2016). ECT also increases cerebral oxygen demand, blood flow, and intracranial pressure. Conditions such as brain tumors and subdural hematomas may increase the risk when using ECT.

Procedure

The ECT procedure is explained to the patient, and informed consent is obtained if the patient is being treated voluntarily. For a patient treated involuntarily, permission may be obtained from the next of kin, although in some states such treatment must be court-ordered.

Patients have a pre-ECT workup that includes a chest X-ray, an electrocardiogram (ECG), a urinalysis, a complete blood count, blood urea nitrogen, and an electrolyte panel. Benzodiazepines are discontinued before the procedure as they can interfere with the seizure process.

During the procedure, the patient is given a general anesthetic to induce sleep and a muscle-paralyzing agent to prevent muscle contractions and fractures. An electroencephalogram (EEG) monitors brain waves, and an ECG monitors cardiac responses. Brief seizures (30–60 seconds) are induced by an electrical current (as brief as 1 second) transmitted through electrodes attached to one or both sides of the head.

The usual course of ECT for an individual with major depressive disorder is two or three treatments per week to a total of 6 to 12 treatments. Continuation of ECT along with medication may help to decrease relapse rates.

Potential Adverse Reactions

Patients typically wake within 15 minutes of the procedure and are often confused and disoriented for several hours. The nurse and family may need to orient the patient frequently during the treatment course. Most people experience what is called *retrograde amnesia*, which involves memory loss of events leading up to and including the treatment itself.

CRANIAL ELECTROTHERAPY STIMULATION

Cranial electrotherapy stimulation (CES) is a noninvasive treatment using low-intensity electrical currents to stimulate the brain through electrodes placed on the scalp or earlobes. It is primarily used for individuals who have not responded to traditional therapies.

Indications

CES is FDA-approved for treating anxiety, depression, and insomnia, and is typically recommended for patients who have not found relief from other treatments. It is commonly used in outpatient settings and may appeal to those seeking a less invasive approach.

Risk Factors

CES is generally safe with minimal side effects, but precautions should be taken in certain cases. It is not recommended for individuals with a history of seizures or those with implanted devices like pacemakers. Pregnant women should avoid CES due to limited safety data.

Procedure

CES is performed in an outpatient setting, with electrodes placed on the scalp or earlobes. A low-intensity electrical current is passed through the skin for 20 to 60 minutes per session. Multiple sessions are required for optimal results, with a typical regimen involving daily treatments followed by tapering. CES can also be used at home under the guidance of a healthcare provider.

Potential Adverse Reactions

The procedure is generally well-tolerated with minimal side effects. Some patients may experience mild irritation at the electrode sites, dizziness, headaches, or a slight burning sensation. In rare cases, anxiety or restlessness may occur but usually subsides with continued use.

REPETITIVE TRANSCRANIAL MAGNETIC STIMULATION

Repetitive transcranial magnetic stimulation (rTMS) is a noninvasive modality used in the treatment of major depressive disorder. The rTMS system is an electromagnetic device that painlessly delivers a rapidly pulsed magnetic field to the cerebral cortex. These magnetic pulses activate neurons without inducing seizures.

Indications

The FDA has approved the use of rTMS for major depressive disorder. Specifically, this treatment is approved for adult patients who have failed to achieve satisfactory improvement from one prior antidepressant medication at or above the minimal effective dose and duration in the current episode. rTMS is also approved for the treatment of obsessive-compulsive disorder.

Risk Factors

Except- for braces and dental fillings, individuals with nonremovable metal in their heads should not receive rTMS. This procedure could result in the metal moving, heating up, or malfunctioning. Contraindicated metals include:
- Aneurysm clips or coils
- Stents in the neck or brain
- Deep brain stimulators
- Electrodes
- Metallic implants in ears and eyes
- Shrapnel or bullet fragments near the head
- Facial tattoos with metallic or magnetic-sensitive ink

Procedure

Outpatient treatment with rTMS takes about 30 minutes and is typically administered 5 days a week for 4 to 6 weeks. The patient remains awake and alert during the procedure. An electromagnet is placed on the patient's scalp, delivering short magnetic pulses pass into the prefrontal cortex. These pulses are similar to those used for magnetic resonance imaging (MRI) but are more focused. The pulses cause electrical charges to flow and induce neurons to fire or become active. Patients may experience a slight tapping sensation, scalp contractions, or jaw tightening during the procedure.

Potential Adverse Reactions

After the procedure, patients may experience scalp pain at the site of stimulation due to muscle contraction. Common side effects include headache, fatigue, and lightheadedness. No neurological deficits or memory problems have been observed. Seizures are a rare complication. Most side effects are mild and include scalp tingling and discomfort at the administration site. Post-procedure, patients may experience scalp pain at the site of stimulation due to muscle contraction.

MAGNETIC SEIZURE THERAPY

Magnetic seizure therapy (MST) combines certain elements from both ECT and rTMS. Like rTMS, MST uses magnetic pulses instead of electricity to stimulate a precise area of the brain (National Institute of Mental Health, 2024). Like ECT, MST induces a seizure. The seizure is accomplished by using higher-frequency pulses than the ones given in rTMS.

The goal of MST is to achieve the effectiveness of ECT while reducing its cognitive side effects. ECT leads to a much more widespread seizure induction. This widespread effect is probably responsible for cognitive problems after ECT. MST uses a more focal seizure expression with less involvement of hippocampal and deep brain structures.

Indications

Although MST is in the early stages of testing for psychiatric disorders, results are promising. Recent research indicates that MST has been effective in triggering remission in 30% to 40% of individuals treated for major depressive disorder and bipolar disorder. It is also being investigated as a treatment for schizophrenia and obsessive–compulsive disorder.

Procedure

The patient is anesthetized and given a muscle relaxant to prevent movement during the procedure. The motor activity of the right foot is monitored to track the duration of the seizure, and an EEG records brain seizure activity. Up to 600 pulses are delivered. Generally, two or three MST sessions are scheduled each week. Some studies have used up to 24 sessions or continued treatments until symptoms improve.

Potential Adverse Reactions

Common side effects following MST include headache, dizziness, nausea, vomiting, muscle aches, and fatigue. These side effects can be explained by anesthesia exposure and the induction of a seizure. Studies in both animals and humans have found that compared to ECT, MST produces:
- Fewer memory side effects
- Shorter seizures
- Shorter recovery times

VAGUS NERVE STIMULATION

Vagus nerve stimulation (VNS) was originally developed as a treatment for epilepsy. Clinicians later observed that, in addition to decreasing seizures, VNS appeared to improve mood in a population who normally experiences higher rates of depression. The mechanism behind VNS involves the vagus nerve, the longest cranial nerve, which extends from the brainstem to organs in the neck, chest, and abdomen. Electrical stimulation of the vagus nerve leads to increased neurotransmitters levels, enhancing mood and also improving the effectiveness of antidepressants.

Indications

The FDA has approved VNS as an adjunctive treatment for chronic or recurrent depression in adults aged 18 and older who have not responded to at least four antidepressant trials. This approval covers both unipolar and bipolar depression, provided there is a history of inadequate response to at least four antidepressant interventions. Patients are not required to have failed ECT to be eligible for VNS.

Procedure

The VNS implantation is typically performed on an outpatient basis. A pacemaker-like device is surgically implanted into the left chest wall, and a thin flexible wire is threaded up and wrapped around the vagus nerve on the left side of the neck. Following surgery, an infrared magnetic wand is held against the chest, while a personal computer or personal digital assistant is used to program the frequency of pulses. These pulses are usually delivered for 30 seconds every 5 minutes, 24 hours a day. Antidepressant effects typically develop in several weeks.

Potential Adverse Reactions

As a surgical procedure, VNS implantation carries the typical risks associated with surgery, such as pain, infection, and sensitivity to anesthesia. One common side effect is related to the placement of the lead near the vagus nerve, which is close to the laryngeal and pharyngeal branches. Voice alteration occurs in nearly 60% of patients. Other side effects include neck pain, cough, paresthesia, and dyspnea. These effects generally decrease over time. The device can be temporarily turned off by placing a special magnet over the implant, which may be particularly useful during public speaking or intense physical activity.

DEEP BRAIN STIMULATION

Deep brain stimulation (DBS) is a surgical procedure that uses electricity to directly stimulate specific sites in the brain. Electrical pulses are delivered continuously and are believed to reset the malfunctioning area of the brain.

Indications

DBS is an FDA-approved neurosurgical treatment primarily used for certain neurological disorders, including Parkinson's disease. Its application in psychiatric conditions has also been explored, with approval granted for obsessive-compulsive disorder (OCD). In 2022, DBS received Breakthrough Device Designation from the FDA to investigate its use for treatment-resistant depression. A systematic review and meta-analysis showed favorable effects of DBS in treating depression symptoms.

Procedure

Similar to VNS, a device is implanted in the chest wall to provide electrical stimulation. Unlike VNS, however, electrodes are implanted directly into the brain to modify brain activity. Before the procedure, the patient's head is shaved and attached to a frame to prevent movement. The patient remains awake during the procedure to provide feedback to the surgeon.

Two small holes are drilled into the skull under a local anesthetic, and a slender tube is threaded to specific areas of the brain where electrodes are inserted. In cases of major depressive disorder, several areas of the brain are targeted by DBS. For obsessive–compulsive disorder, electrodes are placed in the ventral capsule and ventral striatum, areas associated with obsessive thoughts and compulsive behavior.

After the placement of electrodes, the patient provides feedback and is then placed under general anesthesia. The electrodes are connected to wires inside the body that run from the head to the chest, where a pair of battery-operated generators are to continuously deliver electrical pulses and stimulate the brain.

Potential Adverse Reactions

DBS is a minimally invasive procedure but carries risks associated with any type of brain surgery, including:

- Bleeding in the brain or stroke
- Infection
- Disorientation or confusion
- Unwanted mood changes
- Movement disorders
- Lightheadedness
- Sleep disturbances

Because of its relatively recent introduction, not all side effects have been identified.

References

Alzheimer's Association. (2021). *2021 Alzheimer's disease facts and figures*. https://www.alz.org/alzheimers-dementia/facts-figures.

American Psychiatric-Mental Health Nurses Association, International Society of Psychiatric Mental Health Nurses, & American Nurses Association. (2022). *Psychiatric-mental health nursing: Scope and standards of practice*. (3rd ed.). Nursesbooks.org.

American Psychiatric Association. (2022). *Diagnostic and statistical manual of mental disorders, fifth edition, text revision (DSM-5-TR)*. American Psychiatric Association. https://doi.org/10.1176/qppi.books.9780890425787.

Beck, A. T. (1979). *Cognitive therapy and the emotional disorders*. International Universities Press.

Brennan, K., Sanchez, D., Hedges, S., Lynch, J., Hou, Y. C., Al Sayfe, M., Shunker, S., Bogdanoski, T., Hunt, L., Alexandrou, E., He, S., Mai, H., Rolls, K., & Frost, S. A. (2023). A nurse-led intervention to reduce the incidence and duration of delirium among adults admitted to intensive care: A stepped-wedge cluster randomised trial. *Australian Critical Care, 36*(4), 441–448. https://doi.org/10.1016/j.aucc.2022.08.005.

Brownell, K. D., & Walsh, B. T. (2018). *Eating disorders and obesity* (3rd ed.). Guilford.

Caplan, G. (1964). *Principles of preventive psychiatry*. Basic Books.

Centers for Disease Control and Prevention. (2018). *Data and statistics fatal injury report for 2017*. https://webappa.cdc.gov/cgi-bin/broker.exe. https://www.cdc.gov/mmwr/volumes/70/wr/mm7014e1.htm#:~:text=COVID%2D19%20death%20rates%20were%20highest%20among%20males%2C%20older%20adults,causes%20of%20death%20(6).

Centers for Disease Control and Prevention. (2023). *Data and statistics on children's mental health*. https://www.cdc.gov/childrensmentalhealth/data.html.

Centers for Disease Control and Prevention. (2024a). *Data and statistics on ADHD*. https://www.cdc.gov/adhd/data/index.html.

Centers for Disease Control and Prevention. (2024b). *Data and statistics on autism spectrum disorder*. https://www.cdc.gov/autism/data-research/index.html.

Centers for Disease Control and Prevention. (2024c). *Suicide data and statistics*. https://www.cdc.gov/suicide/facts/data.html#:~:text=Suicide%20deaths%2C%20plans%2C%20and%20attempts,1%20death%20every%2011%20minutes.

Donnelly, B., Touyz, S., Hay, P., Burton, A., Russell, J., & Caterson, I. (2018). Neuroimaging in bulimia nervosa and binge eating disorder: A systematic review. *Journal of Eating Disorders*, *6*(30). https://doi.org/10.1186/s40337-018-0187-1.

Ebert, C. H., Finn, C. T., & Smoller, J. W. (2016). Genetics and psychiatry. In T. A. Stern, M. Fava, & T. E. Wilens (Eds.), *Massachusetts General Hospital comprehensive clinical psychiatry*. Saunders.

Erikson, E. H. (1963). *Childhood and society*. Norton.

GoodRx. (2023). *Lofexidine*. https://www.goodrx.com/lofexidine.

Gordon, C., & Bereson, E. V. (2016). The doctor-patient relationship. In T. A. Stern, M. Fava, & T. E. Wilens (Eds.), *Massachusetts General Hospital comprehensive clinical psychiatry*. Saunders.

Gummin, D. D., Mowry, J. B., Spyker, D. A., Brooks, D. E., Osterthaler, K. M., & Banner, W. (2017). Annual report of the American Association of Poison Control Centers' National Poison Control Data System (NPDS): 35th Annual report. *Clinical Toxicology*, *56*(12), 1213–1415. https://doi.org/10.1080/15563650.2018.1533727.

International Council of Nurses. (2019). *The international classification for nursing practice catalog*. https://www.icn.ch/what-we-do/projects/ehealth-icnptm/icnp-browser.

Karakula-Juchnowicz, H., Banaszek, A., & Juchnowicz, D. (2023). Use of the opioid receptor antagonist naltrexone in the treatment of non-suicidal self-injury. *Psychiatria Polska*, *58*(4), 605–618. https://doi.org/10.12740/PP/OnlineFirst/161954.

Kerr, K. L., Moseman, S. E., Avery, J. A., Bodurka, J., Zucker, N. L., & Simmons, W. K. (2016). Altered insula activity during visceral interoception in weight-restored patients with anorexia nervosa. *Neuropsychopharmacology*, *41*(2), 521–528. https://doi.org/10.1038/npp.2015.174.

Kessler, R. C., Berglund, P., Demler, O., Jin, R., Merikangas, K. R., & Walters, E. E. (2005). Lifetime prevalence and age-of-onset distributions of DSV-IV disorders in the National Comorbidity Survey Replication. *Archives of General Psychiatry*, *62*(6), 593–602. https://doi.org/10.1001/archpsyc.62.6.593.

Kübler-Ross, E. (1973). *On death and dying*. Routledge.

Linehan, M. M. (1993). *Cognitive-behavioral treatment of borderline personality disorder*. Guilford.

Luo, Y. L. L., & Cai, H. (2018). The etiology of narcissism: A review of behavioral genetic studies. In A. Hermann, A. Brunell, & J. Foster (Eds.), *Handbook of trait narcissism*. Springer. https://doi.org/10.1007/978-3-319-92171-6.16.

Mahler, M. S., Pine, F., & Berman, A. (1975). *The psychological birth of the human infant*. Basic Books.

Memon, A., Rogers, I., Fitzsimmons, S. M. D. D., Carter, B., Strawbridge, R., Hidalgo-Mazzei, D., & Young, A. H. (2020). Association between naturally occurring lithium in drinking water and suicide rates: Systematic review and meta-analysis of ecological studies. *British Journal of Psychiatry*, *217*(6), 667–678. https://doi.org/10.1192/bjp.2020.128.

Mitchell, J. E., King, W. C., Courcoulas, A., Dakin, G., Elder, K., Engel, S., & Wolfe, B. (2015). Eating behavior and eating disorders in adults before bariatric surgery. *International Journal of Eating Disorders*, *48*(2), 215–222. https://doi.org/10.1002/eat.22275.

National Center for Complementary and Integrative Health. (2020). *Chamomile*. https://www.nccih.nih.gov/health/chamomile.

National Council for Mental Wellbeing. (2022). *How to manage trauma*. https://www.thenationalcouncil.org/wp-content/uploads/2022/08/Trauma-infographic.pdf.

National Council of State Boards of Nursing. (2018a). *A nurse's guide to professional behaviors*. https://www.ncsbn.org/brochures-and-posters/a-nurses-guide-to-professional-boundaries.

National Council of State Boards of Nursing. (2018b). *NCLEX-RN® examination: Test plan for the National Council Licensure Examination for Registered Nurses*. National Council of State Boards of Nursing. https://www.nclex.com/.

National Council of State Boards of Nursing. (2021). *NCSBN Clinical Judgment Measurement Model*. National

Council of State Boards of Nursing. https://www.nclex. com/clinical-judgment-measurement-model.page.

National Council of State Boards of Nursing. (2023). *Next generation NCLEX®: NCLEX-RN® test plan*. https:// www.nclex.com/files/2023_RN_Test%20Plan_English_ FINAL.pdf.

National Eating Disorder Association. (2018). *Glossary*. https:// www.nationaleatingdisorders.org/resource-center.

National Eating Disorder Association. (2023). *Types of psychotherapy*. https://www.nationaleatingdisorders.org/ types-psychotherapy/.

National Institute of Mental Health. (2012). *Older adults: Depression and suicide facts*. http://www.nimh.nih.gov/ health/publications/older-adults-and-depression/ older-adults-and-depression_141998.pdf.

National Institute of Mental Health. (2024a). *Statistics*. https://www.nimh.nih.gov/health/statistics.

National Institute of Mental Health. (2024b). *Bipolar disorder*. https://www.nimh.nih.gov/health/statistics/ bipolar-disorder.

National Institute of Mental Health. (2024c). *Brain stimulation therapies*. https://www.nimh.nih.gov/health/ topics/brain-stimulation-therapies/brain-stimulation-therapies.shtml.

National Institute on Alcohol Abuse and Alcoholism. (n.d.). *What is a standard drink?* https://www.niaaa.nih.gov/ alcohols-effects-health/overview-alcohol-consumption/ what-standard-drink#:~:text=In%20the%20United%20 States%2C%20one,which%20is%20about%2040%25%20 alcohol.

Peplau, H. E. (1952). *Interpersonal relations in nursing: Offering a conceptual frame of reference for psychodynamic nursing*. Putnam.

Peplau, H. E. (1968). A working definition of anxiety. In S. F. Burd & M. A. Marshall (Eds.), *Some clinical approaches to psychiatric nursing*. Macmillan.

Posner, K., Brent, D., Lucas, C., Gould, M., Stanley, B., Brown, G., Fisher, P., Zelazny, J. Burke, A., Oquendo, M. & Mann, J. (2009). *Columbia-suicide severity rating scale*. https://cssrs.columbia.edu/wp-content/uploads/ C-SSRS_Pediatric-SLC_11.14.16.pdf.

Prins, A., Bovin, M. J., Kimerling, R., Kaloupek, D. G., Marx, B. P., Pless Kaiser, A., & Schnurr, P. P. (2015). *The primary care PTSD screen for DSM-5 (PC-PTSD-5)*. https://www.ptsd. va.gov/professional/assessment/screens/pc-ptsd.asp.

Quality and Safety Education for Nurses (QSEN) Institute. (2012). *QSEN competencies*. https://www.qsen.org/competencies-pre-licensure-ksas.

Rahman, A., & Paul, M. (2023). *Delirium tremens*. StatPearls. https://www.ncbi.nlm.nih.gov/books/NBK482134/#:~:text=Delirium%20tremens%20was%20first%20recognized,to%2037%25%20without%20appropriate%20treatment.

Rogowska, M., Thornton, M., Creese, B., Velayudhan, L., Aarsland, D., Ballard, C., Tsamakis, K., Stewart, R., & Mueller, C. (2023). Implications of adverse outcomes associated with antipsychotics in older patients with dementia: A 2011-2022 update. *Drugs Aging, 40*(1), 21–32. https://doi.org/10.1007/s40266-022-00992-5.

Rosenvinge, J., & Petterson, G. (2015). Epidemiology of eating disorders part II: An update with special reference to the DSM-5. *Advances in Eating Disorders, 3*(2), 198–220. https://doi.org/10.1080/21662630.2014.940549.

Sadock, B. J., Sadock, V. A., & Ruiz, P. (2015). *Kaplan & Sadock's synopsis of psychiatry* (11th ed.). Wolters Kluwer.

Shear, K., Jin, R., Ruscio, A. M., Walters, E. E., & Kessler, R. C. (2006). Prevalence and correlates of estimated DSM-IV child and adult separation anxiety disorder in the national comorbidity survey replication. *American Journal of Psychiatry, 163*(6), 1074–1083. https://doi.org/10.1176/ajp.2006.163.6.1074.

Skodol, A. E., Bender, D. S., & Oldham, J. M. (2019). Personality pathology and personality disorders. In L. W. Roberts (Ed.), *Textbook of psychiatry*. American Psychiatric Association.

Spielman, A., & Glovinsky, P. (2004). A conceptual framework of insomnia for primary care providers: Predisposing, precipitating, and perpetuating factors. *Sleep Medicine Alert, 9*(1), 1–6.

Stone, D. M., Simon, T. R., Fowler, K. A., Kegler, S. C., Yuan, K., Holland, K. M., & Crosby, A. E. (2018). Vital signs: Trends in state suicide rates—United States, 1999–2016 and circumstances contributing to suicide—27 states, 2015. *Morbidity and Mortality Weekly Report, 67*(22), 617–624. https://www.cdc.gov/mmwr/volumes/67/wr/mm6722a1.htm.

Stroebe, M., & Schut, H. (1999). The dual process model of coping with bereavement: Rationale and description. *Death Studies, 23*(3), 197–224. https://doi.org/10.1080/074811899201046.

Substance Abuse and Mental Health Service Administration. (2022). *Screening, brief intervention, and referral to treatment (SBIRT)*. https://www.samhsa.gov/sbirt.

Substance Abuse and Mental Health Services Administration. (2023). *Key substance use and mental health indicators in the United States: Results from the 2022 National Survey on Drug Use and Health.* https://www.samhsa.gov/data/sites/default/files/reports/rpt42731/2022-nsduh-annual-national-web-110923/2022-nsduh-nnr.htm#:~:text=Major%20Depressive%20Episode%20among%20Adolescents,year%20MDE%20with%20severe%20impairment.

US Census Bureau. (2019). *Selected social characteristics in the United States.* https://data.census.gov/cedsci/table?tid=ACSDP5Y2019.DP02&hidePreview=true.

US Census Bureau. (2022). *Language use in the US: 2019.* https://www.census.gov/library/publications/2022/acs/acs-50.html.

US Department of Justice. (2013). *Crime in the United States 2013: Rape.* https://ucr.fbi.gov/crime-in-the-u.s/2013/crime-in-the-u.s.-2013/violent-crime/rape.

US Food and Drug Administration. (2021). *Online label repository.* https://labels.fda.gov/.

Vandeleur, C. L., Fassassi, S., Castelao, E., Glaus, J., Strippoli, M. F., Lasserre, A. M., Rudaz, D., Gebreab, S., Pistis, G., Aubry, J. M., Angst, J., & Preisig, M. (2017). Prevalence and correlates of DSM-5 major depressive and related disorders in the community. *Psychiatry Research, 250,* 50–58. https://doi.org/10.1016/j.psychres.2017.01.060.

Welch, C. A. (2019). Electroconvulsive therapy. In T. A. Stern, M. Fava, T. E. Wilens, & J. F. Rosenbaum (Eds.), *Comprehensive clinical psychiatry* (2nd ed.). Mosby.

Yalom, I. D., & Leszcz, M. (2005). *The theory and practice of group psychotherapy* (5th ed.). Basic Books.

Yonkers, K. A., Gilstad-Hayden, K., Forray, A., & Lipkind, H. S. (2017). Association of panic disorder, generalized anxiety disorder, and benzodiazepine treatment during pregnancy with risk of adverse birth outcomes. *JAMA Psychiatry, 74*(11), 1145–1152. https://doi.org/10.1001/jamapsychiatry.

Zipfel, S., Giel, K. E., Bulik, C. M., Hay, P., & Schmidt, U. (2015). Anorexia nervosa: Aetiology, assessment, and treatment. *The Lancet. Psychiatry, 2*(12), 1099–1111. https://doi.org/10.1016/S2215-0366(15)00356-9.

APPENDIX A

Patient-Centered Assessment

A patient-centered assessment such as this can be used to structure admission data. Key findings from an initial assessment provide direction for developing a nursing care plan. It is important to supplement most of the checkboxes included in this assessment tool with additional descriptions of abnormal findings. The assessment begins with general information, then covers essential information (e.g., substance use and sleep), and progresses to the more detailed mood and cognitive domains.

GENERAL INFORMATION

Name (or initials):
Age:
Gender identity: Sex assigned at birth:
Preferred pronoun: Sexual orientation:
Race:
☐ White ☐ Black or African American ☐ American
   Indian or Alaska Native
☐ Asian ☐ Native Hawaiian or Other Pacific Islander
Ethnicity:
☐ Non-Hispanic, Latino, or Spanish origin ☐ Hispanic,
   Latino, or Spanish origin
Language:
☐ English ☐ English as second language ☐ Need for
   interpreter/translator ☐ Other:
Height: Weight: Recent weight gain/loss (amount):
Marital status: ☐ Single ☐ Married ☐ Cohabitating
   ☐ Divorced ☐ Other:
Education: ☐ <High school ☐ High school
☐ Some associates/technical/trade ☐
   Associates/-technical/trade
☐ Some undergraduate ☐ Undergraduate

☐ Some graduate ☐ Graduate
Employment: ☐ Currently employed ☐ Full-time
    ☐ Part-time ☐ Unemployed
Occupation:
Residence: ☐ Rents ☐ Owns home ☐ Other:
Lives with:

PRESENTING PROBLEM

The presenting problem is the patient's own words as to the reason for being admitted or entering into treatment. Use a question such as "What is the reason you are being admitted (or treated) here?" Once a problem is identified you can use the patient's terms and phrases during the assessment.

RELEVANT HISTORY

1. Do you have any health problems?
2. Do you have allergies?
3. Do any family members have psychiatric problems?
4. Do you have a history of emotional, physical, or sexual abuse and/or neglect?
5. Have you ever experienced a traumatic event or traumatic events?

PSYCHIATRIC HISTORY

Treatment Dates	Therapist/Facility	Outcome

History of suicidality (ideation, attempt, method):
Current suicidality (ideation, plan, means):
History of violence/homicidality:
Current thoughts of violence/homicidality:
History of self-injury (e.g., cutting, head banging):
Current self-injury:

MEDICATION (INCLUDING OVER-THE-COUNTER)

Medication	Dose	Frequency	Dates of Use

ALCOHOL/SUBSTANCE USE

History of alcohol and/or substance use (when it started, how often, how much, legal problems associated with it):

Treatment for alcohol and/or substance use:

Current alcohol and/or substance use (how often, how much, last use):

RELIGIOUS, SPIRITUAL, SOCIAL, AND CULTURAL ASSESSMENT

1. What do you think are the causes of [insert chief complaint]?
2. Do you have a spiritual or religious affiliation?
3. What aspects of your spirituality or religious practices do you find most helpful?
4. Who are your main personal or social supports?
5. Are there practices within your culture that address [insert chief complaint]?
6. Are there restrictions on medical interventions or diet based on your spiritual, religious, or cultural beliefs and customs?

STRENGTHS, GOALS, AND COPING

Ask the patient to identify three strengths.

1. _____
2. _____
3. _____

Ask the patient to identify three goals for hospitalization/ treatment.

4. _____

5. _____

6. _____

Ask the patient to identify coping methods for stress, anxiety, and anger.

SLEEP PATTERN

Quantity: ☐ 0 to 2 hours ☐ 2 to 4 hours ☐ 4 to 6 hours
☐ 6 to 8 hours ☐ 9+ hours
Initiation: ☐ No problem falling asleep ☐ Difficulty falling asleep
Maintenance: ☐ Continuous sleep ☐ Wakes repeatedly
☐ Wakes and has difficulty returning to sleep
Quality: ☐ Refreshing ☐ Not refreshing

APPEARANCE

Eye contact: ☐ Direct ☐ Poor ☐ Intermittent ☐ Staring
☐ Intense
Pupils: ☐ Normal ☐ Constricted ☐ Dilated
Age: ☐ Appears stated age ☐ Appears older than stated age
Posture: ☐ Neutral ☐ Slouched ☐ Straight ☐ Tense
Gait: ☐ Normal ☐ Shuffling ☐ Staggering ☐ Spastic
Attire: ☐ Neat ☐ Unkempt ☐ Appropriate ☐ Inappropriate attire
Hygiene: ☐ Good ☐ Neglected
Skin: ☐ Healthy ☐ Impaired integrity

ATTITUDE

☐ Cooperative ☐ Engaged ☐ Disengaged ☐ Defensive
☐ Guarded ☐ Elusive ☐ Poor historian

BEHAVIOR

Psychomotor: ☐ Normal ☐ Hyperactive ☐ Restless
☐ Agitated ☐ Retarded
Movement: ☐ Akathisia ☐ Catatonia ☐ Echopraxia
☐ Waxy flexibility

☐ Verbal tics ☐ Motor tics ☐ Fine hand tremor ☐ Course hand tremor ☐ Dystonia
☐ Tardive dyskinesia (attach Abnormal Involuntary Movement Scale [AIMS] from Chapter 22)

MOOD

Mood is assessed by asking the patient, "How do you feel?" and then summarized by the nurse.
☐ Euthymic (normal) ☐ Depressed ☐ Sad ☐ Euphoric (elated) ☐ Angry
☐ Irritable ☐ Anxious ☐ Fearful ☐ Apathetic
☐ Anhedonic ☐ Alexithymic (unable to describe mood)

AFFECT

Affect is determined by observations of the nurse.
☐ Appropriate to situation ☐ Inappropriate to situation
☐ Congruent with mood ☐ Incongruent with mood
☐ Even ☐ Intense ☐ Blunt ☐ Flat ☐ Heightened
☐ Dramatic
☐ Constricted ☐ Fixed ☐ Immobile ☐ Labile

SPEECH

Presence: ☐ Present ☐ Absent/mute ☐ Aphasic
Rate: ☐ Slow ☐ Hesitant ☐ Normal ☐ Rapid
☐ Pressured
Volume: ☐ Soft ☐ Normal ☐ Loud
Articulation: ☐ Clear ☐ Mumbled ☐ Garbled
☐ Overemphasis ☐ Stuttered
Speech patterns: ☐ Echolalia (repeating others' words)
☐ Palilalia (repeating own words) ☐ Neologisms (creating new words)

THOUGHT PROCESSES

☐ Poverty of thought ☐ Normal quantity of thought
☐ Overabundance of thought
☐ Retarded ☐ Perseveration ☐ Circumstantiality
☐ Tangentiality ☐ Loose associations
☐ Flight of ideas ☐ Logical ☐ Disorganized ☐ Blocking
☐ Concrete thinking

THOUGHT CONTENT

Delusions: ☐ Paranoid ☐ Ideas of reference
☐ Persecutory ☐ Grandiose ☐ Erotomanic
☐ Somatic ☐ Jealousy ☐ Control ☐ Guilt ☐ Poverty
☐ Nihilistic ☐ Religious
Outside control: ☐ Thought broadcasting ☐ Thought
withdrawal ☐ Thought insertion
Intrusive thoughts: ☐ Obsessions ☐ Phobias
Preoccupation: ☐ Suicidality ☐ Aggression
☐ Homicidality ☐ Suspicions ☐ Fears

PERCEPTIONS

Hallucinations: ☐ Auditory ☐ Visual ☐ Tactile
☐ Olfactory ☐ Gustatory
Auditory hallucinations: ☐ Inside own head ☐ Outside
own head ☐ Pleasant/positive ☐ Negative ☐ Insulting
☐ Command ☐ Distractible
Frequency:
Other: ☐ Illusions ☐ Depersonalization ☐ Derealization
☐ Déjà vu

COGNITION

Alertness: ☐ Alert ☐ Clouded ☐ Drowsy ☐ Stuporous
Orientation: ☐ Person ☐ Time ☐ Date ☐ Place
☐ Situation
Attention and concentration:
Serial sevens (counting backward from 100 by 7 s)
☐ Able ☐ Makes mistakes ☐ Unable
Spelling a five-letter word (such as world) backward
☐ Able ☐ Makes mistakes ☐ Unable
Memory:
Immediate memory (repeating a set of words)
☐ Able ☐ Makes mistakes ☐ Unable
Short-term memory (repeating a set of words after an
interval)
☐ Able ☐ Makes mistakes ☐ Unable
Long-term memory (recalling a historical or geographical
fact)
☐ Able ☐ Makes mistakes ☐ Unable
Cognitive/visual functioning:
Complex task (draw the face of a clock)
☐ Able ☐ Makes mistakes ☐ Makes many mistakes
☐ Unable

INSIGHT

Recognition of psychiatric disorder
☐ Insight intact ☐ Some insight ☐ Insight absent
Participation in care decisions
☐ Actively participates ☐ Some participation
    ☐ No participation ☐ Resists participation
Understands that symptoms are part of a psychiatric
    disorder
☐ Insight intact ☐ Some insight ☐ Insight absent

JUDGMENT

☐ Judgment intact ☐ Judgment fair ☐ Judgment
    impaired ☐ Judgment critically impaired

APPENDIX B

Integrative Care

Disorder	Therapy	Description
Anxiety	Natural products/herbs	Supplements, vitamins, minerals, and herbs/botanicals are used to reduce anxiety. Examples: • Kava: rare cases of hepatotoxicity • L-Theanine: increases GABA and alpha activity • 5-HTTP: may be used for panic attacks
	Aromatherapy	Essential oils are used to enhance physical and mental well-being and for healing. Guidelines for safe use include dilution rates, caution with ingestion and use around eyes, and obtaining training for use in pregnancy, lactation, and with children. Examples: • Roman chamomile • Clary sage • Lavender • Mandarin • Neroli • Vetiver

Disorder	Therapy	Description
	Exercise	Exercise releases endorphins, provides distraction, and reduces tension. Exercise alters dopamine, serotonin, and norepinephrine; increases brain-derived neurotrophic factor; and reduces oxidative stress levels.
	Mind-body therapies: yoga, mindfulness-based stress reduction	Techniques such as yoga and mindfulness are used to enhance the mind's positive impact on the body. A specific yoga breathing technique may reduce obsessive-compulsive disorder symptoms.
	Expressive therapies	Music promotes relaxation and decreases autonomic arousal.
	Virtual reality–graded exposure therapy	Virtual images stimulate anxiety, which is paired with relaxation exercises.
	Electroencephalogram (EEG) or electromyography (EMG) biofeedback	Scalp sensors measure brain activity and patients learn how to regulate the body's responses to stress.
	Heart rate variability biofeedback	Heart rate changes are measured, and feedback promotes increased variability, lowers stress levels, and improves overall well-being.

(Continued)

Disorder	Therapy	Description
Attention-Deficit/Hyperactivity Disorder (ADHD)	Diet/nutrition	Food colorings, additives, sugar, and certain food allergens are avoided to decrease symptoms of ADHD.
	Natural products/herbs	Supplements, vitamins, minerals, and herbs/botanicals are used to decrease symptoms of ADHD. Examples: • Omega-3 fatty acids: high doses may decrease symptom severity • Zinc: may decrease hyperactivity • Acetyl-L-carnitine: may decrease symptoms of inattention
	EEG biofeedback	Scalp sensors measure brain activity, and patients learn how to regulate body responses. Symptoms of inattention, impulsivity, and hyperactivity are decreased.
	Mind-body therapies	Techniques such as yoga, mindfulness, and massage enhance the mind's positive impact on the body and decrease symptoms of ADHD.
	Exercise	Physical activity is used to reduce the symptoms of ADHD.

Disorder	Therapy	Description
Bipolar	Natural products/ herbs	Supplements, vitamins, minerals, and herbs/ botanicals are used to help stabilize mood. Example: • Omega-3 fatty acids: decrease mood swings when taken with a mood stabilizer
	Exercise	Physical activity is used to decrease symptoms of mania.
Depression	Natural products/ herbs	Supplements, vitamins, minerals, and herbs/ botanicals are used to improve mood. Examples: • St. John's wort: mild to moderate depression • Omega-3 fatty acids: in conjunction with antidepressants • SAMe: moderate to severe depression with or without antidepressants; risk of serotonin syndrome
	Exercise	Physical activity improves depressive symptoms.
	Bright light therapy	Light boxes decrease melatonin, reducing the symptoms of depression.
	Mind-body therapies: yoga	Yoga is an effective treatment for major depressive disorder.

(Continued)

Disorder	Therapy	Description
	Diet/nutrition	Regular meals consisting of fish, fruit, raw or cooked vegetables, and omega-3 fatty acids reduces depression. Vitamin D supplementation may reduce depressive symptoms.
	Massage therapy	A broad group of medically valid therapies involving rubbing or moving the skin are used to reduce depressive symptoms.
	Repetitive transcranial magnetic stimulation (rTMS)	Stimulation of the brain using a magnet on the scalp is used to help improve refractory depression.
	Intermittent theta-burst stimulation (iTBS)	A more intense form of rTMS reduces refractory depression.
Posttraumatic Stress Disorder (PTSD)	Virtual reality–graded exposure therapy	Virtual environments are used for progressive exposure therapy. Virtual environments may be even more effective than medication in PTSD and decrease symptoms by 30%.
	Acupuncture	May reduce symptoms of PTSD. Needles are inserted in the skin at key points (meridians) to modulate the flow of qi.

Disorder	Therapy	Description
	Eye movement desensitization and reprocessing (EMDR)	Patients explore disturbing memories while simultaneously focusing on external stimuli such as eye movements or hand tapping.
Schizophrenia	Natural products/herbs	Supplements, vitamins, minerals, and herbs/botanicals are used to alleviate symptoms of schizophrenia. Examples: • Omega-3 fatty acids • Folic acid: reduces positive and negative symptoms • Thiamine: used in conjunction with an antipsychotic • Glycine: improves functioning and decreases negative symptoms • Ginkgo biloba: used in conjunction with an antipsychotic.
	Mind-body therapies: yoga	Yoga enhances the positive interaction between the mind and body, which helps to decrease agitation and anxiety.
	Avatar therapy	Patients converse with an avatar that represents the hallucination. Avatar becomes less derogatory and more submissive over time, reducing the severity of the auditory hallucinations (Craig et al., 2018).

(Continued)

Disorder	Therapy	Description
Substance Use	Diet/nutrition	Relapse is reduced with diets low in sugar and caffeine and high in omega-3 fatty acids.
	Natural products	Supplements, vitamins, minerals, and herbs/botanicals are used to help reduce cravings, withdrawal, and the effect of substances on the body. Examples: • Amino acids such as taurine and L-tryptophan decrease cravings and help with withdrawal. • SAMe may decrease the risk of liver damage. • Kudzu decreases cravings and can help prevent relapse.
	EMG, thermal EMG, and EEG biofeedback	Patients are able to view the activity in the muscles and brain and learn how to self-regulate the body's response to stress. Biofeedback may decrease the relapse rate of alcohol use disorder.
	Exercise	Physical activity may decrease the relapse rate of alcohol use disorder.

Disorder	Therapy	Description
	Mind-body therapies: yoga	Yoga enhances the positive interaction between mind and body, which helps to decrease agitation and anxiety and reduces relapse.
	Cranioelectrotherapy stimulation (CES)	A weak electrical current in the head and neck reduces the severity of withdrawal for alcohol and opiates.

Index

Page numbers followed by *f* indicate figures, *t* indicate tables, and *b* indicate boxes.

NURSING DIAGNOSES BY CHAPTER

International Council of Nurses. (2019). *International Classification of Nursing Practice.* Retrieved from https://www.icn.ch/what-we-do/projects/ehealth-icnptm/icnp-browser